Ethical issues in
maternal–fetal medicine

This book brings together an unusually broad range of experts from reproductive medicine, medical ethics and law to address the important ethical problems in maternal–fetal medicine which impact directly on clinical practice. The book is divided into parts by the stages of pregnancy, within which the authors cover four main areas:

- the balance of power in the doctor–patient relationship and the justifiable limits of paternalism and autonomy;
- the impact of new technologies and new diseases;
- disability and enhancement (the 'designer baby'); and
- difference – to what extent the clinician should respect the tenets of other faiths in a multicultural society, even when the doctor believes requested interventions or non-interventions to be morally wrong. The aim throughout is to unite analytic philosophy and actual practice.

This is an important text not only for clinicians involved in human reproduction but also for philosophers and lawyers.

Donna Dickenson is the John Ferguson Professor of Global Ethics at the University of Birmingham. She is co-author of *The Cambridge Workbook in Medical Ethics*, and author of *Property, Women and Politics*.

Ethical issues in
maternal–fetal medicine

Edited by

Donna L. Dickenson

John Ferguson Professor of Global Ethics, University of Birmingham, UK

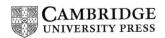

CAMBRIDGE
UNIVERSITY PRESS

PUBLISHED BY THE PRESS SYNDICATE OF THE UNIVERSITY OF CAMBRIDGE
The Pitt Building, Trumpington Street, Cambridge, United Kingdom

CAMBRIDGE UNIVERSITY PRESS
The Edinburgh Building, Cambridge CB2 2RU, UK
40 West 20th Street, New York, NY 10011-4211, USA
477 Williamstown Road, Port Melbourne, VIC 3207, Australia
Ruiz de Alarcón 13, 28014 Madrid, Spain
Dock House, The Waterfront, Cape Town 8001, South Africa

http://www.cambridge.org

First published 2002

Printed in the United Kingdom at the University Press, Cambridge

Typeface Minion 10/12pt   *System* Poltype® [v N]

A catalogue record for this book is available from the British Library

Library of Congress Cataloguing in Publication data

Ethical issues in maternal–fetal medicine / edited by Donna L. Dickenson.
        p.   cm.
Includes bibliographical references and index.
ISBN 0 521 66266 4 – ISBN 0 521 66474 8 (pb.)
1. Human reproductive technology – Moral and ethical aspects.   2. Perinatology – Moral and
ethical aspects.   3. Medical ethics.   I. Dickenson, Donna.

RG133.5. E8395 2001
176–dc21   2001025633

ISBN 0 521 66266 4 hardback
ISBN 0 521 66474 8 paperback

Contents

Contributors

Priscilla Alderson
Social Science Research Unit
Institute of Education
18 Woburn Square
London WC1H 0HS
UK

Rebecca Bennett
Centre for Social Ethics and Policy
Humanities Building
University of Manchester
Oxford Road
Manchester M13 9PL
UK

Françoise Baylis
Department of Philosophy
Dalhousie University
Halifax
Nova Scotia
Canada

Susan Bewley
Lead Clinician in Maternal–Fetal
Medicine
St Thomas's Hospital
Lambeth Palace Road
London SE1 7EH
UK

Cynthia R. Daniels
Political Science Department
Rutgers University
Hickman Hall
89 George St
New Brunswick
NJ 0891
USA

Donna L. Dickenson
Centre for the Study of Global Ethics
University of Birmingham
13 Pritchatts Road
Edgbaston
Birmingham B15 2TT
UK

John Harris
Centre for Social Ethics and Policy
Humanities Building
University of Manchester
Oxford Road
Manchester M13 9PL
UK

Sirkku Kristiina Hellsten
Department of Political Science/
Philosophy Unit
PO Box 35042
University of Dar es Salaam
Tanzania

Elina Hemminki
STAKES
Kiskontie 31
Helsinki 00280
Finland

Gillian M. Lockwood
Medical Director
Midland Fertility Services
3rd Floor
Centre House
Court Parade
Aldridge WS9 8RT
UK

Mary B. Mahowald
Department of Obstetrics and
Gynecology
University of Chicago School of
Medicine
Chicago
Illinois
USA

Eileen McDonagh
Department of Political Science
Meserre Hall 303
Northeastern University
Boston
MA 02115
USA

Jean McHale
Faculty of Law
University of Leicester
Leicester LE1 7RH
UK

Neil McIntosh
Department of Child Life and Health
University of Edinburgh
20 Sylvan Place
Edinburgh EH9 1UW
UK

Christine Overall
Department of Philosophy
Faculty of Arts and Science
Watson Hall
Queen's University
Kingston
Ontario
Canada K7L 3N6

Wendy Savage
Academic Department of Obstetrics
and Gynaecology
2nd Floor
St Bartholomew and Royal London
Hospital School of Medicine
51–53 Bartholomew Close
London EC1A 7BE
UK

Françoise Shenfield
Centre for Medical Ethics
UCL Medical School
The Rayne Institute
5 University Street
London WC1E 6JJ
UK

Susan Sherwin
Department of Philosophy
Dalhousie University
Halifax
Nova Scotia
Canada

Carson Strong
Department of Human Values and
Ethics
University of Tennessee Medical
College
Memphis
TN 38163
USA

Rosemarie Tong
Department of Philosophy
University of North Carolina at
Charlotte
9201 University City Boulevard
Charlotte
NC 28223
USA

Heather Widdows
Centre for the Study of Global Ethics
University of Birmingham
13 Pritchatts Road
Edgbaston
Birmingham B15 2TT
UK

Paquita de Zulueta
Department of Primary Healthcare and
General Practice
Imperial College School of Medicine
Charing Cross Campus
St Dunstan's Road
London W6 8RP
UK

Acknowledgements

Parts of the chapter by Carson Strong are adapted from his 1997 book, *Ethics in Reproductive and Perinatal Medicine: A New Framework*; the chapter is published with permission of Yale University Press. The chapter by Cynthia Daniels is adapted and enlarged from her article 'Between fathers and fetuses: the social construction of male reproduction and the politics of fetal harm' (1997), in *Signs: Journal of Women in Culture and Society*, vol. 22. Cynthia Daniels would like to thank Sam Frost, Robert Higgins, Suzanne Marilley and Linda Zerilli for their helpful comments and assistance on her chapter. Susan Bewley is greatly indebted to Dr Sophie Botros of the King's College Centre of Medical Law and Ethics, London, for comments and criticisms.

Introduction: recent debates in maternal–fetal medicine – what are the ethical questions?

Donna L. Dickenson

Centre for the Study of Global Ethics, University of Birmingham, UK

This book is arranged by the stages of pregnancy – in part because it is intended for a clinical audience, in part because the stages of pregnancy offer a narrative framework for understanding the recent debates in maternal–fetal medicine. This introduction, however, offers a different kind of descriptive framework – a conceptual one. In the second chapter, Carson Strong complements this introduction by suggesting a *normative* framework for use in debating issues in reproductive ethics generally, and maternal–fetal ethics in particular. (Reproductive ethics would also include other more 'high-tech' areas such as reproductive cloning, which are mostly omitted from this book because at present they are not immediately relevant to clinical practice, no matter how many column-inches of newsprint they occupy.)

Judging by the interests of the authors collected here, who come from a wide international and professional range of backgrounds, recent ethical debates in maternal–fetal medicine can be grouped into four principal areas:

(1) *Power in the obstetrician–patient relationship, and the justifiable limits of paternalism and autonomy.* Another less familiar way of phrasing this tension, as Jean McHale puts it in her chapter (6), is in terms of two dominant but conflicting rhetorics – 'choice' versus 'responsible parenting'.

(2) *The impact of new technologies and new diseases.* Here IVF (in vitro fertilization) and associated fertility technologies are twinned with HIV and AIDS because in both cases developments from outside ethical theory are driving ethical debate.

(3) *Disability and enhancement.* Although the concept of disability may appear purely clinical, a growing body of work views it as socially conditioned and value-laden. If there is no such thing as disability per se, in the extreme version of this view, then we must question the basis for interventions aimed at reducing disability in populations or preventing the birth of a 'handicapped' child to a particular couple. Similarly, at the other end of the scale, if 'normality' is not a clinical but a normative concept, what do we do about the desire to have children who are in some way 'better' than 'normal'? The possibility of genetic therapeutic manipulation accentuates problems about 'enhancement' – what is often

termed, perhaps with little justification, the 'designer baby' syndrome.

(4) *Difference*. Primarily an issue about culture, but also one about gender. To what extent must the clinician respect the tenets of other faiths in a multicultural society, even when patients or their families request interventions which the doctor believes to be morally wrong? The importance of gender enters in here not only when such interventions disadvantage women, but also because feminist theory, particularly in its psychoanalytical and postmodern versions, offers a way of understanding and foregrounding difference.

These issues are listed in 'descending order of popularity', so to speak. As we might expect, the largest number of contributions fall into the first category, the rather traditional but still problematic opposition of paternalism and autonomy in the obstetrical relationship. Into this grouping I have put the articles by Françoise Baylis and Susan Sherwin (18), Susan Bewley (8), Cynthia Daniels (7), Gillian Lockwood (10), Eileen McDonagh (14), Jean McHale (6) and Wendy Savage (17). Feminism informs both this first category and the fourth, although many fewer contributors have concentrated on difference – see Sirkku Hellsten (3) and Françoise Shenfield (9). Into the second category, the impact of new technologies and new diseases, fall the chapters by Donna Dickenson (15), Elina Hemminki (12), Mary Mahowald (16), Rosemarie Tong (5), Heather Widdows (11) and Paquita de Zulueta (4). The third set of issues, concerning disability and enhancement, is the focus of the chapters by Priscilla Alderson (13), Rebecca Bennett and John Harris (20), Neil McIntosh (21) and Christine Overall (19).

Power in the obstetrician–patient relationship

Referring to 'power in the obstetrician–patient relationship' will offend some physicians and strike others as inaccurate. In an age of audit and patient consumerism, they may argue, it is misleading to assume that it is doctors who have power over patients; the power dynamic is the other way around. In this section both sorts of power imbalance are explored; for example, Gillian Lockwood, a philosophically trained director of an English fertility services unit, discusses this issue from the point of view of the clinician who sometimes feels powerless to resist the patient's demands. Her chapter (10) concerns a would-be IVF patient with end-stage renal failure, who has had a kidney transplant, and who has a 10 per cent risk of dying within one to seven years of giving birth. The patient's initial kidney failure was due to severe recurrent pre-eclampsia in two earlier pregnancies, which both resulted in neonatal death after delivery at 26 weeks. Given that section 13 (5) of the Human Fertilisation and Embryology Act 1990 requires the clinician to consider the welfare of any child who may be born as a result of fertility treatment, should the clinician resist the woman's request in the name of the future child? In the best interests of the patient herself? It has been argued that this is the first time UK statute law has required doctors to make a value judgement about women's capacity to parent (Rennie, 1999); the test for abortion provision is less stringent and more medical. Does the existence of this legislation put the careful clinician at a power advantage or a disadvantage in dealing with doubtful requests by patients?

Nevertheless, the power of the doctor – the medical mystique is itself a force either to heal or to impede healing (Brody, 1992) – is still too widely ignored in conventional bioethics, which, very broadly speaking, generally conceives of the patient as autonomous and independent. To put it another way, conventional bioethics frequently lacks a political dimension (Dickenson, 2000). Although the principlist approach (Gillon, 1985; Beauchamp and Childress, 1989) includes justice as the fourth principle of medical ethics, the bioethical literature is far fuller on the first principle – that of autonomy. It has taken a feminist analysis to bring power relationships to the fore, and it is particularly appropriate therefore that power in the obstetrician–patient relationship should be the first category in this book, one of the aims of which is to bring together clinicians and feminist theorists.

The clinician who herself most embodies this synthesis is perhaps the English consultant obstetrician Dr Wendy Savage, who was the subject of a lengthy professional investigation in the mid-80s designed, many felt, to discredit her because she was dedicated to giving obstetric patients more power to choose. The investigation failed when it transpired that Dr Savage's record of safe and successful deliveries was actually better than that of her male colleagues, despite her opposition to medical paternalism. It is therefore very fitting that Wendy Savage should have contributed a chapter ('Caesarean section: who chooses – the woman or her doctor?') to this book.

Savage sets out the medical sequelae of Caesarean section in terms which make it clear that judicial interventions to enforce Caesareans on unwilling women put the patient at far greater risk. Emphasizing that the patient is the woman and not the fetus, Savage then details the history of enforced Caesarean judgments between 1992 and 1998. The initial judgment, *Re S* (1992), was based on an erroneous reading by the judge of the US Carder case (In *Re AC*, 1990) in which a terminally ill woman was forced to undergo a Caesarean section in an unsuccessful attempt to save the life of a fetus at the borderline of viability. The Carder case was overturned on appeal, but the High Court judgment missed that point. From then until 1998, English law, although based on this basic misunderstanding, moved closer and closer to overturning the traditional common law doctrine that the fetus is not a legal person (Scott, 2000). In the process, the Mental Health Act 1983 was also used to enforce Caesarean sections, although section 63 of that statute makes it clear that it must only be used to sanction forcible treatment for a mental disorder, never a physical one. The courts pulled back from the brink in 1998 with the *St George's Hospital* judgment (*St. George's Healthcare NHS Trust* v *S* [1998]), which reiterated that a competent woman has the right to refuse a Caesarean section, as she would any other procedure.

Savage also briefly considers the opposite situation, in which the woman requests a Caesarean section which the doctor opposes on the grounds that it is not clinically indicated and will increase the patient's level of risk. She argues that even a feminist clinician need not accede to any such request: 'So, whilst I as a doctor can support "a woman's right to choose" an abortion, and as a feminist I also support it, I do not think that CS on demand is every woman's right.' Here, as in Lockwood's case, the other aspect of power in the doctor–patient relationship comes to the fore – the case in which the clinician feels at a power disadvantage in resisting requests that are not in the patient's best medical interest.

The equivalent legal and political history for the US is set out by Cynthia Daniels (Chapter 7), but in terms which go beyond enforced Caesareans to include other forms of regulation of pregnant women – particularly those who abuse drugs. Women, Daniels argues, are seen as solely to blame for subsequent harm to fetuses, disregarding the documented connection between paternal exposures to toxins and fetal health. Male reproduction is construed in terms of virility, female in terms of vulnerability – with the exception of women of colour, who loom large in the American public debate about 'abusive' crack mothers. Yet sperm are also depicted as 'the littlest ones' at risk from environmental toxins. (We have seen much the same phenomenon in the UK, with publicity concerning the high levels of synthetic oestrogens in water and other sources, which are alleged to reduce male fertility.) Men are not to blame for the toxins to which they are exposed, however: 'Even in newspaper stories that address the connection between paternal exposures and fetal health, certain patterns of reporting emerge that function to reduce male culpability for fetal harm.' In terms of the doctor–patient relationship, then, Daniels's chapter should sensitize clinicians to the ease with which judgements can be made about female culpability for fetal harm – a cautionary note.

This same dilemma is tackled from a more explicitly clinical point of view by Susan Bewley (Chapter 8). Bewley, who is lead clinician in maternal–fetal medicine at St Thomas's Hospital, London, faces similar dilemmas to those which concern Savage – how far should a feminist obstetrician go in imposing treatment on women in the name of their own best interest, and/or that of the fetus? Bewley is willing to recognize the interests of the fetus to a greater, more pragmatic extent – or more correctly, to recognize the uniqueness of the maternal–fetal relationship, without necessarily assuming, in a naturalistic manner, that this uniqueness carries moral weight. Bewley maintains that the regulation of women who have chosen to maintain their pregnancy is also a different question from the abortion debate. The concepts which have evolved in the abortion literature are not really relevant to the clinician's dilemma in dealing with a drug-using pregnant patient.

In attempting to develop a conceptual framework which fits this particular clinical situation, Bewley draws on Frankfurt's distinction between first- and second-order desires (Frankfurt, 1971). It is a logical error to assume that a pregnant woman who continues to take drugs has a guilty intent to harm her fetus. 'Her first-order desire to take drugs overwhelms another first-order desire to do the best for her fetus, and possibly a second-order desire to be a drug-free woman. This is a double tragedy, as she harms her fetus, against her will, and her will is not free and autonomous.' Here Bewley and Daniels agree – the moral panic over 'crack mothers' is politically motivated but clinically unhelpful. Bewley's article is a model for what this book tries to achieve – the marriage of analytical and clinical arguments, put forward by a philosophically and legally aware clinician.

The British medical lawyer Jean McHale (Chapter 6) likewise considers the manner in which 'pregnancy over the last decade has become policed by those who advocate responsible motherhood'. As more widespread genetic information becomes available, she warns, 'it is likely to render us increasingly critical of those who make what we regard as being the "wrong" decision in relation to reproduction'. Can having a child at all be a 'wrong' decision? – particularly if it is known in advance that the child is likely to be so severely handicapped as to have little or no 'quality of life'. McHale is sceptical of this argument, suggesting that codes of practice stressing parental duties not to reproduce unless the offspring meet certain criteria are really just rationing tools. The argument that it is unfair for society to bear the 'costs' of the couple's penchant for reproduction, if their children are likely to be handicapped, meets with no friendlier reception from her. Pressing on beyond these politically motivated arguments, McHale asks whether there could conceivably be any remedy in law for enforcing a 'right not to be born'.

'Policing' motherhood is also a concern of the American political scientist Eileen McDonagh, who has contributed a groundbreaking chapter on 'Models of motherhood in the abortion debate'. In a previous book, *Breaking the Abortion Deadlock: From Choice to Consent* (1996), McDonagh sought to unite opponents and proponents of abortion behind an argument justifying abortion not in terms of the woman's right to choose, but of her consent to further continuation of the pregnancy. Conceding fetal personhood *in arguendo,* as most pro-choice activists do not, McDonagh argued that even if the fetus were a person, its claims would not necessarily 'trump' the mother's right to withhold consent to continuing the pregnancy and giving birth. (This is perhaps a more coherent argument in the US than in the UK, in that the *Roe* decision already turns on the woman's right to privacy rather than on the fetus's lack of legal personality.) In her chapter for this volume, McDonagh again breaks down the barriers between feminist and antifeminist arguments: 'The problem of abortion has been defined by pro-life activists (as we would expect), but also by pro-choice advocates (as we might not expect) on the basis of a very traditional model of motherhood, one invoking cultural and ethical depictions of women as maternal, self-sacrificing nurturers'. That is, by stressing the way in which unwanted pregnancy forces women into the stereotype of sacrificial victims, the model of motherhood used by pro-abortion campaigners is actually deeply conservative, and possibly counter-productive. In terms of the dynamic of autonomy and paternalism, it gives away too much hard-won ground.

McDonagh's chapter, like Daniels's, takes this section of the book out of the confines of the dyadic doctor–patient relationship and into the political arena. By contrast, Françoise Baylis and Susan Sherwin (Chapter 18) extend the political power dimension into a very familiar and 'ordinary' side of the obstetrician–patient encounter – 'non-compliance'. Baylis and Sherwin draw our attention to the way in which this apparently value-free term is used to reinforce the physician's power and to label the patient as an object of concern rather than a partner in the clinical relationship. 'In principle, professional advice is something that patients can choose to follow or not – this is the essence of informed choice... In some instances, however, failure to follow professional recommendations elicits pejorative judgements of non-compliance, and while these judgements are provoked by a failure to comply with specific advice, typically they are applied to the patient as a whole'. By alerting the conscientious practitioner to the ubiquitous presence of ethical issues, Baylis and Sherwin help to counteract the popular media assumption that the *only* serious questions in reproductive ethics are those about new technologies. That certain technology-related questions are also increasingly relevant to everyday practice, however, is the theme of the second section of the book.

The impact of new technologies and new diseases

The questions asked by McHale about limiting the rhetoric of responsible parenting recur in a more technology-driven form in the chapter by the American philosopher and feminist theorist Rosemarie Tong (Chapter 5). Pre-implantation genetic diagnosis (PIGD) extends the boundaries of what 'responsible' parents could and should do for their children, it might be argued. Likewise, the aims of medicine may conceivably be extended from doing no harm to this particular mother and fetus to producing the best babies possible. Perhaps this is a particular temptation in a largely privatized health care delivery system such as the US. As Tong remarks, physicians are unable to resist patient demands for genetic enhancement because there is no generally agreed set of aims of medicine with which to counter such demands – 'Medicine, it has been argued, is simply a set of techniques and tools that can be used to attain whatever ends people have; and physicians and other health care practitioners are simply technicians who exist to please their customers or clients, and to take from them whatever they can afford to pay'. Unless doctors are content to play this passive role, it is essential that they should think through the ethical issues surrounding new technologies and the increased demands to which they give rise. Should there be limits to genetic enhancement techniques? Should there even be limits to the obligation to seek to eliminate disease through the use of new technologies such as PIGD?

Advocates of PIGD present it as enhancing parental choice; Tong asks instead whether it might conceivably be a parental duty, either to future generations in general or to their own offspring. Although it seems plausible that there might be a duty to eliminate genetically transmitted diseases, to whom might we owe this duty? It is difficult to see how parents may owe a duty to children they will never have, which is the inevitable corollary of PIGD in that it enables the elimination of 'defective' fetuses. (Tong is sensitive to the value implications of 'defective', raising issues about disability and 'normality' which also recur in the chapters discussed next under 'Disability and enhancement'.) In her conclusion Tong finishes by arguing that there is a limited right to seek to perfect one's children genetically, and conceivably also a limited duty, but that society should seek to discourage parents from doing so.

The American medical ethicist Mary Mahowald (Chapter 16) raises similar issues about the duties of mothers faced with another set of 'choices' created by new reproductive technologies, particularly IVF. 'Although medical advances have considerably reduced the mortality and morbidity risks of childbearing for most women and their offspring, that same technology has introduced methods by which people who would not otherwise reproduce can have biologically related children. These methods are mixed blessings when the pregnancies they facilitate exacerbate the risks of gestation for women and their fetuses. They are also mixed blessings when, while providing a means to desired motherhood for some, they occasion pressures on others to undergo risks they would not otherwise encounter'. Higher-order pregnancies, as a form of iatrogenic harm occasioned by misapplication of fertility technologies, are the particular focus of Mahowald's attention.

The usual terminology for discussing such cases is 'fetal reduction', but Mahowald regards this concept as an oxymoron. No particular fetus is being 'reduced' – it is either being eliminated or preserved. Thus, Mahowald argues, the term 'fetal termination with pregnancy preservation' is preferable. This distinction is not merely semantic finickiness – 'fetal reduction' obscures the fact that some fetuses are being aborted, and yet even a 'pro-lifer' might agree that it is better to preserve some fetuses' lives if the alternative is the loss of all the fetuses. But which fetuses' lives? Can selective termination ever be justified, or is allowing 'targeting' of a particular fetus on grounds of sex, for example, simply wrong whether that sex is male or female? In a series of illuminating case examples, Mahowald teases out the ethical issues around selective termination, concluding that it may sometimes be justified but that practitioners need to be alert to possible abuses in justice which it may raise.

The still somewhat taboo question of what duties semen donors may have to their children is explored by Heather Widdows (Chapter 11). Widdows focuses on two main aspects of secrecy – donor anonymity and secrecy within the family, particularly non-disclosure to the child. Traditional arguments for secrecy are beginning to give way to counter-arguments for openness, but will donors still be forthcoming if their identities can be traced? Evidence from Sweden (the first country to introduce non-anonymous donation) indicates that after an initial dip in the number of donors, earlier levels of donation are regained, but with a different sort of donor, with more altruistic motivations.

In her section on secrecy in the family, Widdows covers issues such as accidental disclosure to the child, and the possible analogy between donor insemination (DI) and adoption. She explores what the best interests of the DI child are and discusses the importance of knowing one's genetic heritage in forming a stable identity. She also reflects on the effects of lying within the family, drawing on Kantian arguments. Finally, the validity of the arguments both for and against anonymity are considered, and the implications of changes in the practice of secrecy for donor insemination are outlined.

Elina Hemminki (Chapter 12), a Finnish epidemiologist and health technology assessment expert, approaches antenatal screening from an evidence-based medicine viewpoint. Her contribution is particularly valuable because, as an 'outsider' to medical ethics, she is able to pick up inconsistencies in how the reproductive ethics literature treats different interventions which actually raise many of the same questions. Whereas Tong and Mahowald primarily consider the individual woman or couple, Hemminki concentrates on populations, and on the ethical questions raised by mass screening. Is it right, for example, to impose on those undergoing screening an unavoidable risk of false positives and false negatives – which will never be altogether eliminated, no matter how precise the screening process? What about the impact of a positive test result on the wider family group – i.e. who also may be revealed to be at risk? How far does the duty to be screened extend, if there is such a duty?

'Fetal screening,' Hemminki writes, 'is based on certain values and beliefs, such as the importance of health, the feeling that a handicapped child is worse than none at all (particularly if there is an option of having a chance to try again) and the perception that handicaps cause suffering to the child itself, its

parents and/or to society. Through the organization of screening programmes and concomitant research, medicine and health care have been
given the authority to define which diseases and characteristics qualify for
these beliefs'. Directing our attention to the wider societal impact of screening, outside the dyadic doctor–patient relationship, Hemminki argues that
medicine has been given something of a poisoned chalice. What appeared at
first to be a straightforward part of the goals of medicine, the reduction of
disease in populations through genetic screening, is neither straightforward
nor necessarily part of the goals of medicine.

Similarly, the development of stem cell technologies may appear at first to
be an unmitigated blessing in terms of disease reduction, but the manner in
which stem cell lines are being established gives profound cause for fears
about abuse and exploitation. Donna Dickenson (Chapter 15) likewise
moves beyond the confines of the doctor–patient relationship, into wider
issues of justice. Most commentators have concentrated on the moral status
of the embryo, and those who have concluded in favour of developing stem
cell banks or lines have done so on the basis that the embryo used is not
harmed because it will in any case be destroyed (e.g. Nuffield Council on
Bioethics, 2000). In contrast, Dickenson concentrates on the risks of exploitation of pregnant women, and conversely on the arguments in favour of their
possessing a property right in stem cells derived from their embryos or
fetuses, in addition to the procedural right to give or withhold consent to the
further use of those tissues.

These rights can be viewed in a Lockean fashion, as derived from the
labour which women put into the processes of superovulation and egg
extraction (embryonic stem cells) or early pregnancy and abortion (embryonic germ cells). Alternatively, a marxist feminist interpretation would emphasize the added value which women put into the 'raw material' of gametes.
Uniting philosophical and jurisprudential argumentation, Dickenson argues
that it is legally fallacious and politically dangerous to assume that biotechnology companies should necessarily own the products derived from
women's labour in reproduction.

It is not only new technologies which pose ethical dilemmas; 'new' diseases
do so as well. The British general medical practitioner and lecturer Paquita de
Zulueta (Chapter 4) sets out a wide range of ethical issues that are not always
fully recognized in the care of HIV-positive pregnant women. Many of these
issues centre around responsibility for bringing infected children into the
world, or orphaning children, particularly in the Third World context. But
equally, in many cultures the notion of individual responsibility would be
alien to the question, as would the notion of conflict between the interests of
the HIV-positive individual and the wider community (for example, in civil
liberties questions).

De Zuleuta concentrates particularly on the ethics of anonymized testing, which sets utilitarian arguments in favour of reducing the incidence in the general population against the individual woman's 'right to know' – and perhaps to take prophylactic measures. She argues that arguments for anonymized testing are dominated by the 'old ethics' of medical paternalism, but that whereas paternalism is usually justified on the basis of the relationship of trust between the doctor and patient, that fiduciary relationship actually rules out anonymized testing. It is wrong, she argues, to use the newborn as a means to test maternal antibodies. In her conclusion, De Zulueta claims that (asymptomatic) pregnant women who undergo anonymized HIV testing are not patients, but rather healthy people who volunteer for testing in order to benefit the fetus. How can we balance the respect due to the pregnant woman's autonomy – particularly when she is not sick – with concern for the welfare of the woman and the fetus?

Disability and enhancement

Issues surrounding disability and enhancement are touched on by several of the authors already summarized, but they come to the fore in the chapters by Neil McIntosh, Priscilla Alderson, Christine Overall, and Rebecca Bennett and John Harris.

Neil McIntosh (Chapter 21), a consultant paediatrician in Scotland, offers a practising clinician's slant on disability, in the context of ethical issues in withdrawing life-sustaining treatment. He writes, 'Life-sustaining treatment implies that treatment is being given in order to maintain or create the best possible outcome for the child's future life. This future might be abnormal but it would be assumed to be compatible with the self-respect of the family and later of the infant and child. Such management should be in the best interests of the child concerned.' Yet what appears an unexceptionable position here is actually replete with difficult ethical judgements. It seems that McIntosh accepts a 'disability rights' perspective by acknowledging that 'this future might be abnormal'. However, the very notion of 'normality' is seen by some disabled people as itself a form of discrimination. At the end of his chapter, McIntosh offers a useful typology of uncertainty concerning the *probability* of severe disability and its effect on clinical decision-making, but what about the *utility* question? Is even severe disability necessarily a harm or loss?

This sceptical view emerges strongly among the people with disability interviewed by the English sociologist and children's rights advocate Priscilla Alderson (Chapter 13). Offering a qualitative research slant by interviewing adults who have conditions that are the object of antenatal testing, Alderson reviews contrasting positions on the advantages and disadvantages of prenatal counselling. The consensus among her interview subjects is that disability is not a biological construct, but a result of social restrictions.

There are disturbing implications of Alderson's results for both clinical practice and the abortion debate. Many of the conditions dealt with by McIntosh are more immediately life-threatening than those in the adults interviewed by Alderson; after all, these people *have* reached adulthood. Where does the ethically aware clinician draw the line between hopeless prolongation of an 'abnormal' life and sensitivity to the disability-rights view?

In terms of the abortion debate, Alderson appears to favour a movement away from antenatal testing for common disabilities and a return to unconditional acceptance of handicapped children as 'a gift of God'. If, as Dickenson argues, women's labour in pregnancy and childbirth gives them the Lockean right to control the circumstances in which they will perform that labour – and indeed whether they will perform that labour at all – there is no basis for imposing on pregnant women the duty to endure childbirth in the full knowledge that a severely handicapped child is likely to be the outcome. Alderson does, however, acknowledge the advantages of prenatal testing and termination when there is no other means of avoiding intolerable suffering on the part of the child and family. She was actually a member of the working party of the Royal College of Paediatrics on withdrawal and withholding of treatment from severely ill neonates and children, which handed down guidelines that accept the 'unbearable' situation, one in which repeated intervention is more than can be borne, as a legitimate reason for withholding treatment. (These guidelines are summarized in McIntosh's chapter.)

As Alderson asks whether the 'handicapped' fetus may be wronged by antenatal testing, the Canadian philosopher and feminist theorist Christine Overall (Chapter 19) questions, more broadly, whether born children can be harmed by the new reproductive technologies (NRTs). Three benefits of NRTs are often cited, Overall writes: existence itself; being born to parents who have actively sought parenthood; and the avoidance of disability. Where Alderson's and Overall's interests mesh is in this third 'benefit', although they come to opposite conclusions. Whilst Overall dismisses what she terms eugenicist claims that NRTs can and should produce 'better', 'enhanced' babies, she does conclude in favour of their use to minimize the incidence of disability.

Overall's scepticism about the philosophical validity of the first claim, that existence itself is a benefit, creates a productive tension with the work of Rebecca Bennett and John Harris. It is logically incoherent to claim that a being now in existence is 'better off' being born, Overall writes, because if that person had not been born, there would be no entity with which we can compare it. 'It's not as if children exist in a limbo, waiting to be given the opportunity to live via NRT's. Never having existed would not make some hypothetical child worse off; there is no child to harm . . . So, even if coming into existence is a type of benefit, failing to come into existence is not a harm.'

Bennett and Harris (Chapter 20) concede that this is a logical absurdity, but still maintain: 'It does seem reasonable to argue that as long as an individual does not have a life so blighted by suffering that it outweighs any pleasure gained by living, that individual has not been wronged by being brought to birth. It may well be that it does not make sense to talk of someone being made better or worse off by being brought into existence, but it does appear to make sense to talk about lives that are worth living and those that are so blighted by suffering that they may be considered "unworthwhile".'

Building on the example of deaf parents who prefer a deaf child, and would in a sense regard a 'normal' child as handicapped in the Deaf community, Bennett and Harris ask who is harmed if deaf parents elect to abort non-deaf fetuses and to deliberately bring a deaf child into the world. Here Bennett and Harris part company. Harris asserts that harm is done, on a utilitarian calculus, because more 'handicapped' children have been born, although no specific child has been harmed by being brought to existence, because it is impossible to compare existence with non-existence. (This argument rests, of course, on there being a lower utility in being born deaf, which is precisely what advocates for the deaf or disability activists would not accept.) Bennett, by contrast, does believe that a child who is deafened, or denied hearing by being denied a cure, is harmed by being unable to hear. However, a child born with congenital incurable deafness has not been harmed, and has not been denied anything she or he could ever possibly have had.

What is interesting about the example of the deaf community is how it turns 'disability' and 'enhancement' topsy-turvy. In the *Journal of Medical Ethics* article (Harris, 2000) from which Chapter 20 is drawn, Harris asks whether a deaf couple who choose to implant a deaf fetus over a hearing fetus are to be pitied if, by mistake, the 'normal' fetus is implanted instead. (If both states are really of equal value, which would be the expected position for a disability rights activist to take, presumably the couple should not be pitied, any more than a hearing couple would be if the woman gave birth to a deaf baby.) These sorts of questions lead naturally into the final topic analysed by authors in this collection, the nature of *difference*.

Difference: gender and culture

For the past 20 years feminist theory has been preoccupied with the notion of difference, dating perhaps from Carol Gilligan's *In a Different Voice* (1982, 1993 – 2nd edn.). Gilligan advanced the hypothesis that a different ethical 'voice' needed to be heard, one less concerned with the autonomy of the atomistic individual and more willing to recognize embeddedness in relationship. Although that voice was not only to be found in women, assessments of moral maturity in conventional psychological developmental testing tended to reward the autonomy model, and to find that model more frequently in boys and men. French psychoanalytic feminist theorists such as Hélène Cixous and Luce Irigaray provided an alternative emphasis on difference, grounded in Lacanian psychoanalysis and based on a revision of the 'mirror' stage to accommodate female experience. Postmodernism, also, contributed an accent on difference, to the extent that the very notion of 'woman' is undermined – differences within the category are as important as those between men and women to postmodernist feminists (Butler, 1987). Other feminists, however, doubt that without a unified notion of 'woman' there can properly be any such thing as feminism or feminist politics (Dickenson, 1997). Sceptics about the notion of 'difference' warn that 'an affirmation of the strengths of female "difference" which is unaware of [female suppression] may be doomed to repeat some of the sadder subplots in the history of Western thought' (Lloyd, 1993: p. 105).

The French clinician Françoise Shenfield (Chapter 9), a consultant in one of the few purely publicly funded IVF clinics in London, combines her clinical background with an interest in difference to suggest a new and thought-provoking analysis of human reproductive cloning. Drawing on the work of the French psychoanalytical feminist Julia Kristeva (e.g. Kristeva, 1984), Shenfield notes that 'Kristeva argues that we cannot respect and accept strangers if we have not accepted our own portion of strangeness, in other words, the stranger within ourselves. The implication for cloning is that the parent(s) seeking reproductive cloning cannot accept that strangeness, carried in the matrix of the gestating mother.' 'Because the identity of the subject is shaky, and subjectivity itself something to be constructed rather than a given, cloning poses a threat to our personal identity which we find difficult to tolerate. Another psychoanalytical question concerns the child thus conceived, rather than the parent: how will the child cope with building his or her sexual identity?' The 'newness' of Shenfield's argument itself seems a good argument for difference. The cloning debate has been treated very largely in conventional bioethical terms, as a matter of the domain of rightful choice of the rational consumer of medical care. Foregrounding difference and the construction of the subject, Shenfield suggests instead that rationality is less important than identity and subjectivity.

Writing from the viewpoint of public policy rather than psychoanalytical theory, the Finnish political scientist and development scholar Sirkku Hellsten asks the difficult question, 'Where does legitimate cultural difference in obstetric and gynaecological practice end, and discrimination against women begin?' Hellsten, who is currently working at the University of Dar es Salaam in Tanzania, is particularly concerned with female genital mutilation in sub-Saharan Africa, where it is viewed as an 'enhancement'. Are we morally obliged to accept that such a view deserves equal tolerance? Developing an argument from within the liberal, contractarian tradition, and adding a feminist concern with difference, Hellsten concludes that we are not so bound. She offers practical solutions to problems of multicultural working which allow clinicians to maintain their own moral view without affronting other cultures, drawing on her own experience.

'A framework for reproductive ethics'

Carson Strong (Chapter 2) provides a valuable overview in two senses, covering all four of the conceptual areas into which the other chapters fall, and also all the stages of pregnancy. Strong is primarily concerned to find a conceptual, normative and prescriptive 'ground zero' for making decisions in maternal–fetal ethics. Thus he takes our thinking back a step or two – rather than simply asserting, as many have done, that procreative freedom is valuable, he asks us to think about why it is valuable. 'Is procreative freedom valuable simply because freedom in general is valuable, or is there special significance to the fact that the freedom is procreative?' One might want to ask a further question – is women's procreative oppression the condition of men's procreative freedom? Does men's freedom rest on a prior 'sexual contract' in which women's freedom is consigned away? (Pateman, 1988). However, Strong is not necessarily unaware of this caveat. Indeed, his chapter can be seem as feminist insofar as it suggests that 'women's realm' – repro-duction – is essential to 'men's realm' – freedom.

Similarly, Strong encourages the reader to question whether all reasons for having genetic children are equally good. Must the liberal-minded clinician give equal worth to all reasons? Here the issues resemble those considered by Hellsten, and again, it is from philosophers and political theorists that the 'practical' professions of medicine and nursing can draw the most help. Strong considers three particular cases – one an enforced Caesarean, the second creation of preembryos in vitro, the third IVF in a postmenopausal woman – and applies his framework to shed some light on them. Essentially Strong argues for a consequentialist approach to what confers moral standing on infants, fetuses and pre-embryos, examining their degree of resemblance to the sorts of creatures whom it is socially beneficial to regard as persons.

Conclusion

I have not chosen to categorize these 21 chapters by the author's professional background, because it would be counter-productive in terms of the book's philosophy to do so. What is remarkable about the four issues that I have chosen is that they unite clinicians and non-clinicians, as indeed the book as a whole aims to do. The most striking example here is difference, where the two contributors are an IVF clinician (Shenfield) and a philosopher/political scientist (Hellsten). All of the categories, however, number at least one clinician among the contributors, in proximity to lawyers, medical ethicists, philosophers, political scientists and sociologists.

One thing which unites these disparate backgrounds is a concern with 'everyday ethics' – this is not a book about hypothetical situations, but about real clinical decisions. Sometimes the topics which the authors have chosen to cover, having been asked to bear 'everyday ethics' uppermost in mind, may seem surprising – for example, why should compliance in pregnancy raise ethical issues? After reading Baylis and Sherwin on compliance, together with the other articles in the book, I hope that the reader will be persuaded of two things: (1) that ethical debates in maternal–fetal medicine are unavoidable because the ambit of ethics is much more extended than might have been thought, but (2) that they are also neither insoluble nor entirely a matter of personal opinion.

References

Beauchamp, T.L. and Childress, J.F. (1989). *Principles of Biomedical Ethics*, 3rd edn. New York: Oxford University Press.
Brody, H. (1992). *The Healer's Power*. New Haven: Yale University Press.
Butler, J. (1987). *Subjects of Desire: Hegelian Reflections in Twentieth-Century France*. New York: Columbia University Press.
Dickenson, D.L. (1997). *Property, Women and Politics*. Cambridge: Polity Press.
Dickenson, D.L. (2000). Are medical ethicists out of touch? Practitioner attitudes in the US and UK towards decisions at the end of life. *Journal of Medical Ethics* **26**: 254–60.
Frankfurt, H.G. (1971). Freedom of the will and the concept of a person. *Journal of Philosophy* **67**: 5–20.
Gilligan, C. (1993). *In a Different Voice: Psychological Theory and Women's Development*, 2nd edn. Cambridge, MA: Harvard University Press.
Gillon, R. (1985). *Philosophical Medical Ethics*. Chichester: John Wiley and Sons.
Harris, J. (2000). Is there a coherent social conception of disability? *Journal of Medical Ethics* **26**: 95–100.
In Re AC [1990] 573 A 2d 1235 (D.C. App. 1990).
Kristeva, J. (1984). *Revolution in Poetic Language*. Tr. M. Walker. New York: Columbia University Press.
Lloyd, G. (1993). *The Man of Reason: 'Male' and 'Female' in Western Philosophy*, 2nd edn. London: Routledge.
McDonagh, E.L. (1996). *Breaking the Abortion Deadlock: From Choice to Consent*. Oxford: Oxford University Press.
Nuffield Council on Bioethics (2000). *Stem Cell Therapy: The Ethical Issues, A Discussion Paper*. London: Nuffield Council on Bioethics.

Pateman, C. (1988). *The Sexual Contract.* Cambridge: Polity Press.

Rennie, E. (1999). Access to donor insemination: Canadian ideals – UK law and practice. *Medical Law International* **4**: 23–38.

Re S (Adult refusal of treatment) [1992] 4 A11 ER 671.

Scott, R. (2000). Maternal duties toward the unborn? Soundings from the law of tort. *Medical Law Review* **8**: 1–68.

St George's Healthcare NHS Trust v *S* [1998] 3 W.L.R. 936 C.A.

2

Overview: a framework for reproductive ethics

Carson Strong

Department of Human Values and Ethics, University of Tennessee Medical College, Memphis, USA

Medical professionals now face a growing number of controversial issues involving human reproduction. To illustrate the variety of issues, consider the following three scenarios. In the first case, involving a pregnant woman at 36 weeks of gestation, the obstetrician believed there was placental insufficiency, a condition in which the fetus was not getting enough oxygen. The doctor recommended Caesarean delivery for the fetus's sake, but the woman refused the Caesarean, stating that she was putting her faith in God that everything would turn out well. At that point, the physician considered seeking a court order authorizing surgical delivery without the woman's consent (In *Re Baby Boy Doe*, 1994). This case raises important questions. What is the moral standing of the fetus, particularly the fetus that is relatively advanced in gestation? What reasons can be given in support of assigning priority to the woman's wishes? Are there cases in which refusal of treatment by pregnant women may be justifiably overridden?

In another case, a research team was attempting to learn how to mature ova in vitro. In normal reproduction, ova undergo a maturation process that prepares them for fertilization, but the process is not well understood. If ova could be matured in vitro, then new sources of ova for assisted reproduction would be available. For example, ova could be obtained from donors whose ovaries have been removed as part of therapeutic surgical procedures. In that event, donors would not have to receive hyperstimulation drugs, which can have adverse side effects. The research team wanted to find out whether its attempts to mature ova had been successful before offering this approach to patients. This would involve attempting to fertilize the ova in vitro, observing whether fertilized ova develop normally to the blastocyst stage, and then discarding them. However, some people object to any research that involves creating pre-embryos solely for research purposes.[1] Difficult questions are raised by this case. What moral standing, if any, do preembryos have? Is it ethical to create pre-embryos in the course of research and then discard them?

A third case involved a 63-year-old woman who lost her only child when he died in a motorcycle accident at the age of 18. Because she and her husband desired another child, she approached an infertility specialist and requested ovum donation. She wanted the donated ova to be fertilized with her husband's sperm and then transferred to her uterus, and her 65-year-old husband agreed with this plan (Carlson, 1994). This case also raises controversial issues. Is freedom to procreate important enough that we should permit postmenopausal women to become pregnant, if that is what they want?

One could give many more examples of new situations created by advances in reproductive and perinatal medicine. When we attempt to grapple with these many issues, we repeatedly come back to several central ethical questions. What is the moral standing of pre-embryos, embryos and fetuses? How much importance should be given to procreative freedom? Is procreative freedom valuable simply because freedom in general is valuable, or is there special significance to the fact that the freedom in question is *procreative*?

Need for an ethical framework

To resolve ethical issues in reproductive medicine, we need answers to these central questions. Although there is no way to *prove* what the correct answers are to these main questions, we can give arguments for and against different answers, and we can try to decide what answers are best supported by arguments. That is what ethics is all about – it involves looking at all sides of issues and trying to assess the relative merits of differing views. If we had reasonable answers to these central questions, then we would have what I am calling a *framework* for dealing with these issues. A framework is just a starting place. For any particular case or issue, it usually will be necessary to bring in additional considerations, facts and arguments in order to arrive at a conclusion. The framework is a way of articulating some of the basic principles from which one argues.

A framework can be based on religious beliefs, or it can be secular. This chapter focuses on a secular framework. Even though many of us have religious beliefs that influence our thinking about ethics, we still need a secular framework. This is because many of the cases in reproductive ethics raise policy issues – questions concerning what we as a society should permit or forbid. Should we allow ovum donation for 'older' women? Should we forbid the creating of pre-embryos solely for research purposes? It is not appropriate for the views of a particular religion to determine public policy, especially if it is a minority viewpoint. For example, it would be wrong to have a law stating that *no one* may use in vitro fertilization, simply because a particular religion holds that it violates God's commandments. By a 'secular' framework, I mean one whose defence does not depend on any particular religious viewpoint. The fact is, little attention has been given to articulating a secular ethical framework for reproductive and perinatal medicine. This is so, despite the fact that there has been much debate over individual issues.

I would like to suggest that an adequate framework should contain at least the following components. First, it should explore and assess the importance of reproductive freedom. What meaning and significance do we attach to having children? Why should procreative freedom be considered valuable? Secondly, a framework should put forward and defend a view concerning the moral status of offspring during the pre-embryonic, embryonic, fetal and postnatal stages of development. Thirdly, it should put forward an approach to the problem of assigning priorities when different ethical values or interests are in conflict. Its approach to prioritizing should be capable of taking into account all relevant ethical considerations, and it should provide practical guidance in resolving policy questions and individual cases. This chapter will put forward and attempt to defend such a framework.

Significance of freedom to procreate

Let us begin with reproductive freedom, which includes freedom to procreate and freedom *not* to procreate. It turns out that these two components of reproductive freedom are important for different reasons, so we shall consider them separately. To explore the significance of freedom to procreate, we need to ask why having genetic offspring is important to individuals. What reasons can be given for valuing the having of genetically related children? Are there good reasons to protect freedom to have genetic offspring?

To answer this question, I suggest that some insight can be gained by starting with what might be called 'ordinary procreation' – not involving in vitro fertilization, ovum donation or any type of assisted reproduction. I refer to the type of procreation in which a couple begets, by sexual intercourse, a child whom they rear. This is the more common type of procreation, in which parents raise children genetically their own. My strategy is to try to understand why having genetic offspring might be meaningful to people in this ordinary scenario, and then use this understanding to address the newer, more controversial situations.

Studies have identified a number of reasons people actually give for having genetic children, some of which seem selfish or confused (Pohlman, 1974; Arnold, 1975; Laucks, 1981). For example, some people desire genetic offspring as a way to demonstrate their virility or femininity. The views on which these reasons seem to be based – that virility is central to the worth of a man, and that women must have babies to prove their femininity – are unwarranted. They stereotype sex-roles and overlook ways self-esteem can be enhanced other than by having genetic offspring. By contrast, we want to consider whether reasons can be given that are capable of being defended. To be clear, what we are about to explore is not the descriptive question of what reasons people *actually* give, but the normative question of whether there are reasons that *could* be given to help *justify* the desire to have genetic children. There are several reasons that can be given, but for brevity only four will be mentioned here.[2]

First, having a genetic child might be valued because it involves *participation in the creation of a person*. When one has a child in ordinary procreation, a normal outcome is the creation of an individual with self-consciousness. The term 'self-conscious' implies not only being conscious, but also being able to reflect on the fact that one is conscious. Philosophers have regarded the phenomenon of self-consciousness with wonder, noting that it raises perplexing questions. What is the relationship between body and mind? How can the physical matter of the brain give rise to consciousness and self-consciousness? It is ironic that although we have difficulty giving satisfactory answers to these questions, we can create self-consciousness with relative ease. Each of us who begets or gestates a child who becomes self-conscious participates in the creation of a person. One might say that in having children we participate in the mystery of the creation of self-consciousness. For this reason, some might regard creating a person as an important event, perhaps one with spiritual overtones. Some might think of it as acting as an instrument of God's will. Others might consider it to be the fulfillment of religious duty. Thus, the idea of creating a person can have different types of special meaning. Perhaps not all who have children think about it in terms of creating a person, but this is a reason that can be given to help justify the desire for genetic offspring.

Second, having genetic children might be valued as an *affirmation of a couple's love and acceptance of each other*. It can be a deep expression of acceptance to say to another, in effect, 'I want your genes to contribute to the genetic makeup of my children.' Moreover, in such a context there might be an anticipation that the *bond* between the couple will grow stronger because of common children to whom each has a biological relationship. To seek intentionally the strengthening of their personal bond in this manner can be a further affirmation of mutual love and acceptance.

Third, procreation can provide a *link to future persons*. Some might value having such a genetic link, for various reasons. Some might think of it as a personal contribution to the future of the human community and its survival. For others, it might enter into a judgement about how one's life counts and how far its influence extends (Dyck, 1973).

A fourth reason is that having children can be meaningful in part because it involves experiences of pregnancy and childbirth. It should be acknowledged, of course, that some women do not find such experiences to be desirable. Discomforts can be significant, such as back pain, nausea and feeling tired. There can be other negative experiences, such as anxiety over the baby's health, fear of dying, insomnia, irritability and mood swings. And of course there is the pain of labour, or if Caesarean section is performed, the pain associated with abdominal surgery. Despite these negatives, some women find the experience on balance to be valuable. One of the satisfactions sometimes experienced by pregnant women is increased esteem or attention from others. Another is a feeling of joy sometimes experienced immediately after the birth of the child. Pregnancy is viewed by some as a learning experience that contributes to personal development and enrichment. Also, the satisfaction that derives from altruistic behaviour should not be overlooked, given that pregnancy can involve significant sacrifices for the sake of the fetus. These are some of the reasons a woman might give to explain why the experiences of pregnancy and childbirth are personally meaningful.

In stating these four reasons, I do not mean to imply that one *ought* to desire genetic offspring, but only that the desire can be defended. These are examples of reasons that are not silly or confused. Rather, they are reasons that deserve consideration. These reasons suggest that procreation can be valuable to an individual in part because it can contribute to self-identity, one's sense of who one is. For example, having participated in the creation of a person can be part of one's self-identity. Similarly, whether one has given birth or has obtained a certain kind of link to the future can be part of one's sense of who one is. These reasons also suggest that procreation can contribute to self-fulfillment, for it can result in marital love being enriched.

These reasons also help explain why *freedom* to procreate should be valued; namely, because procreation can be important to persons in the ways just discussed, including contributing to self-identity and self-fulfillment. Because of these considerations, interference with freedom to procreate can constitute a failure to give individuals the full respect they deserve as persons. This does not mean that freedom to procreate is never outweighed by other ethical concerns. Rather, it means that there are valid reasons to respect freedom to procreate, which implies that interferences with such freedom must be justified by appeal to overriding ethical considerations.

Importance of freedom not to procreate

Now let us consider why freedom *not* to procreate can be valuable. First, this freedom can be important for directing the course of one's life. Having children is a large undertaking that competes with other important goals and projects in one's life by placing demands on time, energy and resources. Thus, self-determination in making major life choices is promoted by freedom to decide whether to have children (or, for those who already have children, whether to have *additional* children).

Second, freedom not to procreate is important because it has a bearing on the freedom to make decisions concerning what happens to one's body. Bodily self-determination is relevant to decisions concerning sterilization, use of birth control pills and abortion, among other examples. Although bodily self-determination applies both to men and women, it has special significance for women because they bear the burdens of gestation.

The third reason focuses specifically on the interests of women. For women to gain political, social and economic equality, it is essential that they have freedom to control their reproductive lives. Equality for women requires, among other things, greater integration of women into positions of authority and influence in all fields of endeavour. Because childbirth and childrearing require much time and energy, the more heavily one's life is devoted to these activities, the more difficult it is to pursue education and careers leading to positions of authority. Society generally has put little pressure on men to participate in child-rearing, and women have shouldered most of the responsibilities in this area. For women as a group to be no longer held back, they must be free to make decisions about when and whether to try to have children.

This third reason has been articulated primarily by feminist writers, and it has received relatively little attention in mainstream medical ethics. Although there is considerable diversity of views among feminist writers, it is important to take note of common themes that run through the feminist literature on reproductive issues. Several authors have attempted to identify these main ideas (Overall, 1987: pp. 1–16; Andrews, 1989; Sherwin, 1989), and they include the following. First, a feminist perspective is founded upon an awareness that women have been and are the victims of unjustified limitations and barriers under a system of male dominance. Second, a feminist perspective seeks removal of this oppression of women and the bringing about of sexual equality. Third, with regard to reproduction, women should not be exploited. They should have control over their bodies, gametes and conceptuses. The medicalization of pregnancy and childbirth has resulted in a loss of control that should be reversed. Fourth, in formulating policies concerning reproductive issues, greater attention must be given to the input of women concerning their interests, needs and perspectives. It is important for mainstream medical ethics to give more attention to these concerns.

Moral standing of the fetus and embryo

Let us turn to the moral status of pre-embryos, embryos, fetuses and infants. It will be helpful to begin by discussing a number of secular views that have been put forward concerning when personhood begins. In this context, 'personhood' refers to a moral status that we might call 'full moral standing'. It involves having a substantial set of rights, including a strong right to life. All of the views that will be discussed have a feature in common; they all claim that personhood begins when some special characteristic is acquired. Each view, however, puts forward a different characteristic. We shall consider these views not only to identify their shortcomings, but also to point out the helpful insights they provide.

One view is that individuals become persons and acquire a right to life when they become *self-conscious* (Tooley, 1972). Because self-consciousness involves being able to reflect on the fact that one is conscious, it requires concepts and language – concepts such as *consciousness* and *self.* A paradigm example of a self-conscious individual would be a normal adult human being. By contrast, lower animals that lack concepts and language can be conscious but are not self-conscious.

However, there is a serious difficulty with the view that one must be self-conscious in order to be a person. The problem lies in its implications for infants. Infants are not self-conscious, given that they lack language and the concepts one must have in order to be self-conscious. Thus, according to the view in question, infants lack a right to life. However, this is at odds with our moral intuitions, according to which infants have moral interests that deserve protection, including a right to life. Therefore, the view in question should be rejected. Nevertheless, there is an important point to be gleaned from this view, namely, that everyone who *is* self-conscious has full moral standing precisely because they are self-conscious, even though one doesn't *have* to be self-conscious to have moral standing, as exemplified by infants.

A different view is that the *potential* to become self-conscious gives one personhood status (Devine, 1978). On this view, the embryo is a person because it has that potential. However, there is a problem with this view, which can be illustrated by the following scenario. Let us assume that it is possible to keep embryos alive in the laboratory, at least for a short period of time. Let us also assume that it is possible to transfer one of these laboratory embryos to a woman's uterus, which means that even when it is in the laboratory the embryo has the *potential* to develop into a self-conscious individual. Now, suppose that you walk into a laboratory and see that a fire has broken out. You see a child, approximately 10 years old, lying on the floor, suffering from heat and smoke. You also know that in this laboratory there is an embryo being kept alive by some equipment that is regulating its environment. You face a choice: either to carry out the child or to carry out the embryo with the life-support equipment to which it is attached. Assume that you are unable to carry out both of them. Which one should you rescue?[3]

Clearly, the morally correct choice is to rescue the 10-year-old child. This example shows that the embryo's potential to become self-conscious does not give it full moral standing. If it had full moral standing, then the decision concerning whom to rescue would be much more difficult. Nevertheless, this view suggests an important insight, namely, that the potential to become self-conscious has *some* moral significance. If an embryo's potential is actualized, then a person will come into existence, and that would be an event having moral import.

Some believe that the fetus becomes a person when it acquires *sentience* – that is, the capacity for feeling or perceiving (Sumner, 1981). However, the view that sentience by itself gives rise to personhood has broad implications that seem incorrect. Lower animals also are sentient. So, this view implies that animals have a right to life that is equal in strength to that of humans. This is a conclusion that will strike many of us as implausible. So, this view also should be rejected. But even so, sentience is a morally relevant characteristic. The reason is that one must be sentient in order to have moral interests. Plants, for example, are not sentient and therefore lack moral interests. Of course, you can nurture a plant and cause it to flourish, but the plant itself lacks any interest in whether you do this. By contrast, lower animals that are sentient have interests. For example they have an interest in avoiding pain and other unpleasant experiences. So, sentience is relevant to moral standing.

Another view is that the fetus becomes a person when it becomes *viable*. Those who hold this view often fail to realize that whether or not a given fetus is viable is relative to the state of our technology. The problem with the viability criterion can be seen by considering another version of the fire-in-the-lab example. This time, imagine that our technology has advanced to the point at which the embryo could be kept alive and developed in the laboratory until it grows into an infant. In other words, the embryo is viable in this scenario because so-called extra-corporeal gestation is possible. Again, you enter the lab, discover a fire, and have to choose between carrying out the 10-year-old child and carrying out the embryo and the equipment to which it is attached. The ethically preferable decision is still to rescue the 10-year-old, and this helps us to see that viability by itself does not give rise to personhood.

Others have argued that personhood begins with *birth* (Warren, 1989). The reason, they claim, is that when the infant is born it enters into a network of social relationships with other members of the human community. They claim that having this social role is what provides the basis for moral standing. The difficulty with this view is that the fetus can occupy a social role even before birth, involving relationships with various individuals. The pregnant woman, for example, can act in ways that promote or detract from the fetus's health. She can attend to the needs of her fetus by avoiding smoking and excessive alcohol use, eating nutritious meals and seeking treatment for medical problems of her own that can adversely affect the fetus, such as hypertension and diabetes. In addition, obstetricians can monitor the health status of the fetus and provide treatment or early delivery when necessary. For these reasons, a matrix of social relations between fetus and others is often present well before birth. Thus, it is difficult to argue that birth constitutes a sharp dividing line between those who are part of a network of social relationships and those who are not.

Nevertheless, the view in question helps explain why birth, as well as viability, are relevant to moral status. When a fetus becomes viable, its social role increases to some extent, particularly its role as a patient. This occurs because medical intervention for the sake of the fetus becomes feasible, in the form of early delivery followed by neonatal care. Having delivery as an option makes it important to identify health problems for which delivery would benefit the fetus, and thus obstetricians use available technologies to assess the viable fetus's medical status. Similarly, birth is morally relevant because typically it results in the infant becoming involved in a growing number and variety of social relationships.

In summary, none of the views discussed above provides an adequate account of moral standing. In looking for an alternative account, it will be helpful to make two distinctions. First, we need to distinguish between two senses of the term 'personhood'. The first sense is the one I mentioned above; it is normative and refers to a moral status that we might call 'full moral standing'. The second sense is descriptive and refers to the possession of self-consciousness, which typically is accompanied by other attributes including use of language, capacity for rational thought and action, ability to profess values and moral agency. Those who are self-conscious are persons in both senses of the term. Steinbock (1992: pp. 52–3) has suggested the terms *normative* and *descriptive* personhood, respectively, to refer to these two senses, and I shall use these terms.

The second distinction is between *intrinsic* and *conferred* moral standing. In the above discussion of the self-consciousness criterion, I pointed out that self-conscious individuals have full moral standing because of their inherent characteristics. In other words, self-conscious individuals have intrinsic moral standing because of the characteristics they possess. By contrast, it is conceivable that some individuals should be regarded as having moral status not because they have intrinsic moral standing, but because it is justifiable to confer moral status upon them. If embryos, fetuses, and infants have moral standing, it cannot be on the basis of their inherent characteristics alone, for they lack the characteristics needed for intrinsic moral standing; they are not persons in the descriptive sense. It is necessary, therefore, to consider whether it is justifiable to confer some degree of moral standing upon them. Should fetuses and infants be regarded as persons in the normative sense, even though they are not persons in the descriptive sense?

Let us consider how conferred moral standing for individuals who are not descriptive persons can be justified. Several authors have suggested that conferring moral standing on infants and at least some fetuses might be justified by the *consequences* of doing so (Benn, 1984; Feinberg, 1984a; Engelhardt, 1986; Warren, 1989). Treating infants with respect and tenderness can have good consequences for the persons they grow up to become. If they are treated abusively, then when they are adults others might suffer for it too, at their hands (Benn, 1984). Regarding infants as persons in the normative sense promotes important virtues such as sympathy and concern for others. Such concern offers a protection from the uncertainties as to when exactly humans become persons in the descriptive sense, and it helps protect persons who lose self-consciousness due to disease or injury (Engelhardt, 1986: p. 117). Treating infants well also promotes the desires of many people, since most of us care about infants and want them to be protected (Warren, 1989). Feinberg (1984a) has suggested that it is the infant's *similarity* to persons that makes the consequentialist arguments plausible.

This consequentialist approach to conferred moral standing seems promising. I suggest that what matters in the consequentialist argument is the degree of similarity an individual has to the paradigm of descriptive persons – to normal adult human beings. The reason is that the more similar individuals are to the paradigm, the more likely our ways of treating them will have the kinds of consequences identified by the authors discussed above. Not all possible similarities are morally relevant, however. For example, normal adult human beings have two eyes, as do most animals, but few would claim that this similarity supports conferring normative personhood status on all animals that have two eyes. It is necessary to identify *morally relevant* ways in which individuals can be similar to the paradigm. Advocates of the consequentialist approach to conferred moral standing have generally overlooked the relevance of the 'criteria' of personhood to their argument. Morally relevant characteristics discussed above include viability, sentience, the potential for self-consciousness and birth. Another similarity is physical resemblance to normal adult human beings. This similarity is relevant to the consequentialist argument because, psychologically, we are more likely mentally to associate paradigmatic persons with individuals who look like the paradigm than we are to associate them with individuals who do not look like the paradigm. Of course, similarity of physical appearance admits of degrees, and to some extent it is in the eye of the beholder. Nevertheless, it is clear that fetuses near term, for example, look more like paradigmatic persons than embryos do.

To consider the implications of this consequentialist approach based on degrees of similarity, let us begin with infants. The question is whether infants are similar enough to the paradigm to give plausibility to the consequentialist argument for conferred moral standing. Are they similar enough to make it reasonable to claim that a failure to confer a right to life upon them would result in adverse consequences of the sorts mentioned above? Normal infants possess a number of morally relevant similarities with the paradigm: they are viable; sentient; have the potential to become self-conscious; have been born; and are similar in appearance to the paradigm of normal adult human beings. Although some of these characteristics have been put forward as a sufficient condition for normative personhood of fetuses or infants, none of them alone constitutes plausible grounds for personhood. What often is over-looked is the significance of the aggregate possession of these characteristics. I suggest that the combination of these similarities is significant enough to justify conferring upon infants a right to life.

Let us apply these considerations to *fetuses* that are relatively advanced in development – fetuses that are viable and sentient. Such fetuses, assuming they are developmentally normal, possess a number of similarities to the paradigm: they are viable; sentient; possess the potential to become self-conscious; and to some extent have a physical appearance similar to the paradigm. However, the similarities are slightly less for these advanced fetuses than for infants because infants have been born and typically are more involved in social roles. These considerations support the view that advanced fetuses should have a conferred moral status that is close to, but not quite as high as, that of infants.

What about pre-embryos and embryos? Here we obtain very different results. Here the argument for conferred moral standing is weak because pre-embryos and embryos lack viability, sentience, a social role and any physical resemblance to descriptive persons. They have very little similarity to the paradigm. However, conferring a minor degree of moral status upon the pre-embryo and embryo is justifiable because they have at least one morally relevant characteristic, namely, their potentiality.

Finally, presentient fetuses occupy an intermediate position. They have the potential to become self-conscious, and to some extent they can occupy a social role. However, the degree of dissimilarity with the paradigm, together with the fact that as nonsentient creatures they lack moral interests, suggests that a conferred right to life would not be warranted. Nevertheless, some degree of moral consideration would seem justifiable, based on their limited similarity to the paradigm of self-conscious human beings.

As the reader can see, this view holds that moral standing increases as the fetus develops. However, it is not what one might call a 'gradualist' view – it does not claim that moral standing is continuously increasing with each day's development. A gradualist view makes distinctions that seem too fine. For example, it implies that an eight-cell pre-embryo has greater moral standing than a four-cell pre-embryo – perhaps only slightly greater but nevertheless greater. It implies that with each small increase in development of fetal organs there is a corresponding increase in fetal moral status. However, it is not at all clear that such small differences should count morally. By contrast, the view proposed here holds that moral standing increases with the acquisition of an increasing number of morally relevant similarities to the paradigm, as out-lined above.[4]

Assigning priorities

Ethical issues in reproductive medicine can be characterized as conflicts between ethical values. The term 'ethical values' covers all the ethical rules, principles and concerns relevant to reproductive ethics. These concerns include role-related duties, virtues, rights, respect for persons and consideration of the consequences of actions. Examples of more specific values that often are relevant to ethical issues in reproductive medicine include the following: reproductive freedom; the well-being of procreators and potential procreators; the well-being of offspring; the well-being of society; the well-being and autonomy of women individually and as a group, respect for life; and scientific freedom, among others.

In resolving value conflicts, one must choose from among several approaches to assigning priorities. To identify these approaches, we need to consider the following question: at what level of generality should the assigning of priorities to conflicting ethical values be made? When we attempt to answer this question, we see that there are four main possibilities:

(1) The prioritization is considered to hold *whenever* the values in question conflict.
(2) The prioritization is made in the context of a certain issue, or type of case. The prioritization is considered to hold for all cases of that type. The same prioritization would not necessarily hold in other types of cases in which the values in question conflict.
(3) The prioritization is made in the context of individual cases and might differ in different cases of a given type.
(4) For some issues or types of cases, the prioritization takes place in the context of individual cases, as in approach (3), and for other issues or types of cases the prioritization is considered to hold for all cases of that type, as in approach (2).

The first approach involves assigning a hierarchical ranking to values or groups of values. Once the ranking is made, it is fixed, and it is applied to all cases and issues without exception. An example of this approach is an ordering put forward by Robert Veatch (1981), in which a group of nonconsequentialist principles always takes priority over the principle of beneficence. The difficulty with this approach is that it fails to deal adequately with the complexity of morality. For any given value or set of values that supposedly is ranked first, we can always think of a situation in which that value or set of values is overridden by other values. With regard to Veatch's ordering, for example, there are situations in which the principle of beneficence – and more specifically, the principle that we should prevent harm to others – takes priority over the nonconsequentialist principle of autonomy. I have in mind situations in which it is justifiable to prevent individuals from harming third parties.

In the second approach, a ranking of values is made that stays fixed for all cases in which a given issue arises. To illustrate, consider the issue of whether to carry out requests by single women for artificial insemination, in which a central conflict is between the reproductive freedom of the woman requesting artificial insemination and, arguably, prevention of harm to the child who would be brought into being. The view that this issue should be resolved by always giving priority to prevention of supposed harms to the child – and that requests for artificial insemination by single women should never be honoured – is an example of the type of prioritization in question. Moreover, for *every* issue, the approach in question identifies a preferable value (or set of values) and assigns priority to the chosen value(s) in every case in which the issue arises. Although its inflexibility would seem to be a drawback, this approach seems to be assumed by many authors in reproductive ethics. The difficulty with this approach is similar to that of the first approach. Even when we focus on a particular issue, the view that a certain ethical value, or set of values, should *always* have priority often reflects an oversimplification of the moral situation. For a given value or set of values that supposedly is given priority for a certain issue, often we can think of a case of the type in question in which that value or set of values is overridden by other moral considerations.

According to the third approach, for each issue values are ranked in the context of each specific case. This approach seeks a balancing or compromise of the main conflicting ethical values involved in a given issue. This involves giving priority to one value (or group of values) in some cases but assigning priority to a different value (or group of values) in other cases of the type in question. This approach is referred to as case-based, or 'casuistic', reasoning (Jonsen and Toulmin, 1988; Strong, 1988). Casuistry, as it is called, avoids much of the oversimplification of the first two approaches. Also, it reflects well how decision-making in bioethics usually does and should take place. It does this by taking seriously a common characteristic of ethical issues in the clinical setting – variation among cases. For a given type of ethical conflict, there usually are a number of morally relevant ways in which it can vary from one case to the next, and these variations can make a difference in the decisions that ought to be made. On the other hand, although this approach is more flexible than the first two, it falls short of the degree of flexibility that is needed to deal adequately with the complexities of bioethics. Although in general, cases should be decided individually, for some issues there might be compelling reasons to prioritize similarly in all cases. For example, based on broad concerns about positive eugenics, it might be argued that physicians should refuse *all* requests for prenatal genetic testing for nondisease characteristics, such as intelligence, height or body build, rather than deciding on a case-by-case basis. The third approach is not amenable to this type of broad critical assessment of an issue (Arras, 1991).

The fourth approach is preferable to the third because, although it recognizes the validity of case-by-case decision-making generally, it also acknowledges that for some issues there can be broad social considerations that provide reasons for adopting a uniform policy across all cases. Thus, it allows such broad considerations to be taken into account. Moreover, the fourth approach does not require that some prioritizations be made at the level of issues – it simply leaves open that possibility. It holds that there is a presumption in favour of ranking values in the context of individual cases, but that this presumption might sometimes be overridden. Thus, the fourth approach allows us to grapple with the 'big picture' – to ask where we are going and where we should be going in regard to human reproduction – and to formulate policies that take into account the big picture. Because the fourth approach includes the type of reasoning involved in the third approach, it too is casuistic. It is helpful to have terms to distinguish these two versions of casuistry. Thus, I refer to the third approach as *strict* casuistry and the preferred fourth approach as *modified* casuistry.

Application of the framework

The main components of an ethical framework have been presented. It should be noted that an important test of an ethical framework is its usefulness in resolving issues. The length of this chapter limits my ability to elaborate on the implications of the framework and to give examples illustrating its usefulness. However, a few brief examples will perhaps be suggestive. Let us consider the cases mentioned at the beginning of the chapter.

One of the issues mentioned was maternal refusal of treatment needed for the fetus. One of the reasons these cases cause consternation for the health professionals involved in them is that doctors perceive the fetus as having a relatively high moral status. Often these conflicts arise relatively late in gestation, during a period when, based on our framework, the fetus has a substantial moral standing. Nevertheless, according to the framework the moral standing of the late gestation fetus is not quite as high as that of infants. It is not quite equivalent to the status of full personhood. On the other hand, the pregnant woman does have full personhood status. For this reason, it is not easy to justify imposing an invasive treatment upon a mentally competent pregnant woman against her wishes. Her having a moral standing greater than that of the fetus does not logically entail that forced treatment could never be justifiable. However, it does support the idea that there should be a very strong presumption in favour of respecting the woman's wishes. In other words, it would take very compelling reasons to justify overriding her wishes. In practically all cases in which forced maternal treatment is contemplated, the reasons are not sufficiently compelling.[5]

Another issue concerned whether it is ethical to create pre-embryos solely for research purposes. Objections to such research are based on the view that pre-embryos have substantial moral standing and that such use is disrespectful toward them. On this view, creating pre-embryos for research and then destroying them is a failure to treat them as ends in themselves. In reply, the framework provides a reasonable defence of the view that pre-embryos have a relatively small degree of moral standing. They are dissimilar to the paradigm in so many morally relevant ways that it is implausible to maintain that they ought to be treated as ends in themselves.

Because of their potentiality, pre-embryos can reasonably be claimed to have some degree of moral standing. To say that they have *some* moral standing implies that they should be treated with some degree of respect, although the amount of respect called for is far less than that owed to descriptive persons. But what is involved in giving 'respect' to pre-embryos? Even though they have only a small degree of moral standing, it might be asked whether respect for them requires that they not be created solely for research purposes. This raises the question of how to decide what actions we must perform to show adequate respect for pre-embryos. Our ethical framework suggests an approach to answering this question. It holds that the pre-embryo's moral standing is based on consequentialist considerations. In deciding whether certain actions should be carried out (or not carried out) in order to be adequately respectful toward pre-embryos, we therefore should consider the consequences of performing and not performing those actions.

When we apply this approach to the question of creating pre-embryos solely for research purposes, our examination of consequences includes consideration of the advancement of scientific knowledge. A main point is that prohibiting the creation of pre-embryos solely for research purposes prevents some types of important research. For example, research into maturation of oocytes is desirable for the reasons discussed at the beginning of the chapter. Another area of research involves cryopreservation of oocytes. The ability to freeze mature oocytes would be useful for several reasons. First, oocyte freezing could replace pre-embryo freezing when couples use in vitro fertilization (Dawson, 1990). Some couples would consider this desirable because it would avoid the ethical issues associated with disposing of extra pre-embryos. Second, some women diagnosed with cancer might want to store their oocytes before chemotherapy or radiation treatment. Third, freezing would facilitate ovum donation because it would no longer be necessary to synchronize the cycles of donor and recipient. Given these potential uses, questions about safety would need to be explored. For example, would freezing oocytes damage their chromosomes? Research on this question would require fertilizing thawed oocytes in vitro, allowing them to develop, and testing the pre-embryos genetically (Trounsen, 1990). However, this would involve creating, testing and then discarding pre-embryos.

In these and other areas of research, there are potential medical benefits that appear to outweigh any adverse consequences that might reasonably be expected to result from creating pre-embryos solely for research purposes. Thus, it can be argued that respect for pre-embryos does not require that we refrain from creating them for research purposes, provided the research has sound scientific design, is conducted with the informed consent of those donating the gametes and promises to give valuable information.

A third issue concerned ovum donation for postmenopausal women. Several arguments have been put forward against ovum donation in these cases. First, it has been argued that there is an increased probability that one or both parents would die before the child is raised, and thus there is a risk that ovum donation to an older woman will be *harmful* to the child. In reply, this objection overlooks the fact that the actions that supposedly harm the child are the very actions that bring the child into being. Because the objection overlooks this, it misuses the concept of 'harm'. To see this, we must consider what it means to be harmed. A key point is that individuals are harmed only if they are caused to be worse off than they otherwise would have been (Feinberg, 1984b: pp. 31–64). Therefore, the claim that ovum donation to postmenopausal women risks harming the child amounts to saying that the children whose parents die are *worse off than they would have been if they had not been conceived*. However, it is unreasonable to make this claim. Some will say that the claim fails to make sense because it tries to compare nonexistence with something that exists. Others will claim that it makes sense but is false. The latter claim is based on the view that sometimes it can make sense to say that a child is worse off than she/he would have been if she/he had not been created, namely, when the life is filled with suffering to such a degree as to overshadow any pleasurable or other positive experiences the child might have. This claim might be made, for example, if an infant were born with a debilitating, painful and fatal genetic disease. The view in question goes on to point out that having a parent die is not equivalent to having a life so terrible that one would have been better off never having been born. Although there would be psychological trauma associated with parental death, one would expect the children's lives also to contain positive experiences, so that they would regard their lives as worth living. Thus, whether incoherent or false, the claim that the children in question are *harmed* by being brought into being should be rejected.

Second, it can be objected that such ovum donation should not be permitted because pregnancy and childbirth involve increased risks to the older woman. This objection draws from a body of literature dealing with the effects of advanced maternal age on pregnancy. In most of this literature, it is worth noting, advanced maternal age is defined as 35 or older. Although there are conflicting reports within this literature, overall it supports the view that advanced maternal age (≥ 35) is associated with an increased incidence of complications of pregnancy, including diabetes, hypertension, *abruptio placenta, placenta previa* and Caesarean section (Berkowitz et al., 1990; Cunningham et al., 1997: pp. 572–7). In this literature, little data is available concerning pregnancy complications for patients over the age of 45. Thus, the degree of risk for women over 45 is unknown.

In response to this objection, several points can be made. First, maternal risks can be reduced by screening potential ovum recipients for health problems, including diabetes and cardiovascular problems, and by closely monitoring the mother's health status during pregnancy (Sauer et al., 1993). Second, patients should be permitted to assume at least *some* degree of risk, if that is their choice, provided they are mentally competent and adequately informed of the risks. In this context, being adequately informed would include being told that the degree of risk is unknown for older women who are free of prenatal health problems.

In addition, positive arguments can be given supporting ovum donation for older women, based on the reasons for valuing freedom to procreate discussed in the framework. To begin, it is worth noting that some of those reasons can be considered important to 'older' persons. A relatively older couple might value procreation because it involves participation in the creation of a person, because it can affirm mutual love, or because it provides a link to future persons.

These are reasons why having genetic offspring can be important to persons. Let us consider the extent to which these reasons have implications for ovum donation, where the recipient will be the gestational but not the genetic mother. First, the recipient's male partner would be the genetic father of any children who are created by the oocyte donation, and the reasons identified could be important to him. He would participate in the creation of a person and have a genetic link to future persons. Also, although his partner is not the genetic mother, he might regard their mutual desire for her to gestate his genetic offspring to be an affirmation of each other's love. Second, several of the identified reasons would be relevant to the oocyte recipient. Through her gestational role, she would participate in the creation of a person. She, too, might regard her procreative contribution as an affirmation of mutual love. Although she would not have a genetic link, she would have a familial link to future persons, based on her role as gestational and social mother. All things considered, ovum donation for older women can satisfy reasonable desires, the fulfillment of which can promote the self-identity and self-fulfillment of the individuals involved. These considerations support the view that, at least in some cases, it is ethically justifiable for physicians to provide ovum donation to older women.

These examples point out several main ways the framework can be helpful in resolving cases and issues. A defensible view concerning the moral status of pre-embryos, embryos, fetuses and infants is helpful in addressing many issues in reproductive ethics, including enforced treatment during pregnancy and research using pre-embryos. The framework's exploration of reasons for valuing freedom to procreate is useful whenever new issues arise in which freedom to procreate is implicated, including ovum donation for older women. The exploration of reasons for valuing freedom not to procreate and the framework's approach to assigning priorities to conflicting values are also useful in dealing with the variety of issues that arise.

Endnotes

1 The term 'pre-embryo' refers to the product of gametic union from fertilization until the appearance of the embryonic axis (the primitive streak) at approximately 14 days after fertilization (Ethics Committee, 1990). 'Embryo' refers to the product of gametic union from the beginning of the third week after fertilization until the end of the seventh week after fertilization.
2 For a discussion of additional reasons that can help justify the desire for genetic offspring, see Strong (1997: pp. 18–22).
3 This scenario is similar to one suggested by Leonard Glantz and stated in Annas (1989).
4 This view of moral standing based on morally relevant similarities was put forward in Strong (1991a).
5 A more thorough defence of this view can be found in Strong (1991b; 1997: pp. 177–93).

References

Andrews, L.B. (1989). Alternative modes of reproduction. In *Reproductive Laws for the 1990s*, ed. S. Cohen and N. Taub, pp. 361–403. Clifton, N.J.: Humana.

Annas, G. (1989). A French homunculus in a Tennessee court. *Hastings Center Report* **19**: 20–2.

Arnold, F. (1975). *The Value of Children: A Cross-National Study*. Honolulu: East–West Population Institute.

Arras, J.D. (1991). Getting down to cases: the revival of casuistry in bioethics. *Journal of Medicine and Philosophy* **16**: 29–51.

Benn, S.I. (1984). Abortion, infanticide, and respect for persons. In *The Problem of Abortion*, ed. J. Feinberg, pp. 135–44. Belmont, CA: Wadsworth.

Berkowitz, G.S., Skovron, M.L., Lapinski, R.H. and Berkowitz, R.L. (1990). Delayed childbearing and the outcome of pregnancy. *New England Journal of Medicine* **322**: 659–64.

Carlson, M. (1994). Old enough to be your mother. *Time* **143** (January 10): 41.

Cunningham, F.G., MacDonald, P.C., Gant, N.F., Leveno, K.J., Gilstrap, L.C., Hankins, F.D.V. and Clark, S.L. (1997). *Williams' Obstetrics*, 20th edn. Stamford, CT: Appleton & Lange.

Dawson, K. (1990). Introduction: an outline of scientific aspects of human embryo research. In *Embryo Experimentation*, ed. P. Singer, H. Kuhse, S. Buckle, K. Dawson and P. Kasimba, pp. 3–13. Cambridge: Cambridge University Press.

Devine, P.E. (1978). *The Ethics of Homicide*. Ithaca: Cornell University Press.

Dyck, A.J. (1973). Procreative rights and population policy. *Hastings Center Studies* **1**: 74–82.

Engelhardt, H.T., Jr. (1986). *The Foundations of Bioethics*. New York: Oxford University Press.

Ethics Committee of the American Fertility Society (1990). Ethical considerations of the New Reproductive Technologies. *Fertility and Sterility* **53**(Suppl. 2): i–vii, 1S–104S.

Feinberg, J. (1984a). Potentiality, development, and rights. In *The Problem of Abortion*, 2nd edn., ed. J. Feinberg, pp. 145–50. Belmont, CA.: Wadsworth.

Feinberg, J. (1984b). *Harm to Others*. New York: Oxford University Press.

In *Re Baby Boy Doe, a fetus* (1994). 632 N.E. 2nd 326 (Ill. App. 1994).

Jonsen, A.R. and Toulmin, S. (1988). *The Abuse of Casuistry*. Berkeley: University of California Press.

Laucks, E.C. (1981). *The Meaning of Children: Attitudes and Opinions of a Selected Group of U.S. University Graduates*. Boulder, CO: Westview.

Overall, C. (1987). *Ethics and Human Reproduction: A Feminist Analysis*. Boston: Allen and Unwin.

Pohlman, E. (1974). Motivations in wanting conceptions. In *Pronatalism: The Myth of Mom and Apple Pie*, ed. E. Peck and J. Senderowitz, pp. 159–90. New York: Crowell.

Sauer, M.V., Paulson, R.J. and Lobo, R.A. (1993). Pregnancy after age fifty: application of oocyte donation to women after natural menopause. *Lancet* **341**: 321–3.

Sherwin, S. (1989). Feminist and medical ethics: two different approaches to contextual ethics. *Hypatia* **4**: 57–72.

Steinbock, B. (1992). *Life Before Birth: The Moral and Legal Status of Embryos and Fetuses*. New York: Oxford University Press.

Strong, C. (1988). Justification in ethics. In *Moral Theory and Moral Judgments in Medical Ethics*, ed. B.A. Brody, pp. 193–211. Dordrecht: Kluwer.

Strong, C. (1991a) Delivering hydrocephalic fetuses. *Bioethics* **5**: 1–22.

Strong, C. (1991b) Court-ordered treatment in obstetrics: the ethical views and legal framework. *Obstetrics and Gynecology* **78**: 861–8.

Strong, C. (1997). *Ethics in Reproductive and Perinatal Medicine: A New Framework*. New Haven: Yale University Press.

Sumner, L.W. (1981). *Abortion and Moral Theory*. Princeton: Princeton University Press.

Tooley, M. (1972). Abortion and infanticide. *Philosophy and Public Affairs* **2**: 37–65.

Trounsen, A. (1990). Why do research on human pre-embryos? In *Embryo Experimentation*, ed. P. Singer, H. Kuhse, S. Buckle, K. Dawson and P. Kasimba, pp. 14–25. Cambridge: Cambridge University Press.

Veatch, R.M. (1981). *A Theory of Medical Ethics*. New York: Basic Books.

Warren, M.A. (1989). The moral significance of birth. *Hypatia* **4**: 46–65.

Generic issues in pregnancy

Multicultural issues in maternal–fetal medicine

Sirkku Kristiina Hellsten

Department of Political Science/Philosophy Unit, University of Dar es Salaam, Tanzania

Introduction

This chapter sets the debate between universalization of ethical norms and relativist demand for cultural autonomy in the matters of morals within the practical context of maternal–fetal medicine and reproductive health care. The debate between universalism and relativism is particularly central in the field of maternal–fetal medicine, because the universal protection of individual's rights and such values as equality and personal autonomy are usually the very basis for the improvement of women's and children's health around the world. Nevertheless, in many cultures, particularly in many traditional (sometimes also called communitarian) communities, these values are rejected and individual rights are systematically denied to women and children – often in the name of cultural integrity, customary values and the defence of collective rights, all within the same human rights discourse. This chapter attempts to give a theoretical background that can help health care professionals make difficult ethical choices in multicultural environments. Most of the practical examples mentioned in this article are from Tanzania, for the simple reason that during my visiting lectureship at the University of Dar es Salaam these local customs, the problems involved in them and attempts to solve these problems are the ones that have become most familiar to me.

The thorny ethical dilemma for the health care professionals working in an international or widely multicultural environment is the following. On the one hand, it is evident that the promotion of women's and children's health and well-being not only means finding the best possible medical cure available, but also indicates commitment to the promotion of the individual's social status in families, communities and in social order in general. On the other hand, sometimes promoting individuals' rights and autonomy, particularly women's and children's rights and autonomy, can lead into culturally based ethical disagreement and value clashes which, for their part, may turn the patients as well as their whole communities away from the help and cure they need the most.

To deal with these multicultural issues and their relation to human rights in medical care, we need agreement on ethical norms that can be applied across national and cultural borders. Finding such norms is, however, not an easy task. After all, a global set of ethical norms not only needs to be applicable everywhere, it also has to be sensitive to differences in cultural traditions as well as differences in needs between individuals (and between groups of individuals) in their social contexts. In other words, global bio-ethics needs to try to get away from the misguided polarization between universalism and relativism, on the one hand, and between individualism and collectivism, on the other hand. Sometimes this same debate is discussed within the framework of liberalism and communitarianism, that is, between the protection of individual rights and the promotion of the common good (Kuczewski, 1998; Etzioni, 1999).

If we are to find any globally acceptable set of norms, we need to take recent feminist bioethical challenges seriously and try to find a way to promote universal values in a manner that takes the particularity of cultures as well as the special needs of individuals in different situations seriously. This presupposes that we, on the one hand, acknowledge that it is not only collectivist cultures that fall into the trap of cultural relativism. Even liberal pluralism based on the universal respect for individual rights can easily turn into relativist subjectivism, which exaggerates an individual's autonomy, giving the illusion of free choice in a situation in which social pressure directly affects one's decisions and actions. On the other hand, we need to understand that universalism and individualism are not logically tied to-gether. Instead, the demand for the respect of collectivist values is usually set within international human rights standards and thus, must gain its plausi-bility by universalization of collective rights. In other words, the culturally relativist demand that we treat the ethical views of different cultures as equals is based on contradictory arguments – the relativity of cultural values and ethical norms is defended by appealing to universal respect for tolerance, equality and *collective* rights.

Finally, in order to find a way to agree on the values that can be universally promoted, we need to make a distinction between the prescriptive and descriptive uses of terms that we use to denote particular cultural features. In other words, when we talk about 'collectivist' culture we have to differentiate between its universally acceptable, positive elements and its negative features and practices. Thus, we cannot automatically presume a collective culture to be 'oppressive' towards its individual members; it can as well be democrati-cally supportive of them. Alternatively, when we talk about 'individualist' culture, we cannot presume support for individuals' self-development and realization of their moral autonomy. Instead we might face 'egoism', 'social alienation', 'moral indifference' or even 'moral incapacity' within such a culture.

All in all, I claim that the main problem in finding global bioethical norms is not incompatibility between universalist and relativist reasoning or be-tween individualist and collective ethical positions per se. First, within individualist societies, human rights lack universal protection; in particular, women's rights are easily ignored. Second, even if we can find a set of values and norms based on these values that can be globally accepted, we do not pay enough attention to their promotion in practice – what are the most acceptable means to promote the shared values and norms in particular cultural contexts?

Liberalism and conflicting interests in medical decision-making

When we talk about multicultural issues in maternal–fetal medicine, we often start by setting up a polarization between two quite different bioethical frameworks. These approaches are, on the one hand, universalism, which focuses on universal human rights, and on the other hand, relativism, which emphasizes the relativity of cultural belief and value systems. As long as these polarizations remain, there is a tendency to create two opposite bioethical positions – that is, universalist liberal individualism and relativist communitarian collectivism. Since these positions are also seen as incompatible, a productive dialogue and ethical concurrence between them appears to be logically impossible. In relation to human rights protection, however, it often appears that both positions appeal to the universal request for rights protection. Individualists demand respect for the rights of individuals and relativists for the rights of social collectives and cultural entities. Thus, despite their apparent incompatibility, they both claim to make plausible demands from international law and universal human rights. What is the philosophical justification for these demands?

Bioethical thinking in Western pluralist and multicultural democracies is typically based on liberal concepts of justice, demanding the universalization of such individualist values as respect for individual autonomy, protection of individual rights and the promotion of equality and tolerance. Liberal individualism demands that we treat everybody equally, no matter what their gender, race, lifestyle or cultural background is. It also presumes that we consider individuals to be autonomous moral agents capable of choosing their own values and ways of life. On the other hand, this means that we need to let individuals decide on the way they want to live their lives and what kind of cultural identity to maintain. In other words, neither the state nor another individual is allowed to tell somebody what kind of life is 'the good life' (Rawls, 1971, 1993; Hellsten, 1999: pp. 69–83).

In a modern pluralist society, we are asked to tolerate different lifestyles and respect diversity in cultural backgrounds within the liberal universalist ethical framework. In maternal–fetal medicine and reproductive health issues this means that we are expected to respect a patient's autonomy and rights, including the right to maintain one's cultural values and beliefs. Even within a liberal framework there are limits to tolerance – differences in beliefs and lifestyles can be accepted only if they do not harm someone else or violate someone else's rights. Sometimes, however, the actual harm is difficult to detect or prove (Kukathas, 1992: pp. 105–39) .

In modern pluralist society, the most difficult ethical and multicultural issues are usually those involving conflicting rights and interests of different individuals. There is also the question of the status of one's autonomy. In maternal–fetal medicine, for example, we may sometimes disagree about whose rights have the priority – a mother's rights or her future child's rights. For instance, whilst the proponent of abortion defends women's autonomous choice as a moral agent and their right to control their own body, the opponent may believe (on religious or other grounds) that the fetus is already a moral person and thus has rights that have to be taken into consideration.

The choice medical professionals have to make is usually between conflicting rights and interests of individuals in question. In most cases of maternal–fetal medicine this would often be the choice between respecting a pregnant woman's right to decide what happens to her own body and protecting an innocent child from avoidable harm and damage. Besides abortion issues, rights and interest may also conflict when the woman's actions and lifestyle (drugs, tobacco smoking, alcohol, sexually risky behaviour or unprotected sex) may directly or indirectly jeopardize the health of the fetus (Matthieu, 1996: p. 9). (See also chapters 7 and 17 for further discussion.)

In a pluralist society the diversity of our value and belief systems may make it difficult to find an agreement on whose rights and interests should be protected in any given case. Sometimes it may seem that a woman's rights and interests (in remaining free from outside interference and control) should have priority. At other times the child's rights and interests in having a decent quality of life may seem to override the respect for a mother's autonomy. However, in general these disagreements can usually be debated – if not always conclusively resolved – within a shared ethical framework that in itself accepts that all individuals have some universal and equal rights.

From the universal protection of human rights to 'laissez-faire ethics'

When medical decisions are made within a Western liberal bioethical framework, the first ethical guideline is that individual rights should always be protected, which takes priority over promotion of the common good. This guideline is also at the core of international protection of universal human rights. The universalist position also promotes equality. The core guideline in the promotion of equality is that individuals are treated as equals despite their differences – whether we talk about random and natural differences (differences that individuals cannot themselves choose but are born with) such as gender, race and ethnicity, or we focus on the differences in people's choices concerning their values, ways of living or cultural identities. This also means that scarce resources should be allocated justly and evenly.

In medical practice, the liberal concept of justice protects patients' autonomy by means of informed consent in decision-making. Sometimes this abstract demand for the equal protection of autonomy may turn into a fear of paternalism. Any type of interference in someone else's choices is in itself seen as a violation of autonomy. The result, oddly enough, is a form of relativist reasoning called subjectivism.

Particularly in this time and age, when tolerance is in general promoted and the plurality of belief systems, value choices and cultural identities appears to have some intrinsic moral value, there is plenty of room for uncertainty about how best to respect autonomy within different social settings and cultural contexts. The problem is that the liberal concept of justice, in its universal request for respect for individual autonomy, tends to ignore social influences and community pressures. Subjectivist thinking exaggerates individual autonomy and may regard even socially coerced decisions as independent choices. Thus, while those of us who have been socialized with the Western individualist ethical outlook are ready to reject cultural relativism because of its tendency to give a community priority over individual rights, we may still get trapped into relativist reasoning on the individualist level, in the form of subjectivism. Subjectivism can be described as a degenerate form of individualism which turns the universal demand for tolerance and individual rights into a laissez-faire ethics and moral indifference, leading in the end to incapacity to make moral judgements (Hellsten, 1999: pp. 69–83).

Let us take an example of how subjectivism works within a multicultural environment – female circumcision, now more properly called female genital mutilation (FGM). Despite its harmful physical effects, this tradition is still practised in various communities around the world; sometimes it still exists even within modern, multicultural society, practised by members of traditional cultures who claim they are merely using their right to maintain their particular cultural identity. The reasons given to defend this practice vary from one culture to other. In some places it is believed that a girl who does not go through it, will not be able to get married and have children. These beliefs turn into reality in communities in which the tradition still lives strongly. Some other cultures see FGM as a precondition for women's fidelity and social harmony of the community. Elsewhere it might be protected by religious beliefs (Hellsten, 1999: pp. 69–83).

From the point of view of maternal–fetal medicine and reproductive health care, FGM is, however, a harmful practice, which has no medical justification.

Quite the contrary, it is an extremely painful and traumatic experience, which causes serious health damage to women. Mothers and their unborn children have to endure the consequences of this practice. For instance, while giving birth the mother can suffer from rupture and excessive bleeding. Female genital mutilation in its various forms (circumcision proper/sunna, excision, infibulation) has such immediate dangers to a woman's health as haemorrhage and shock from acute pain, infection of the wounds, urine retention and damage to the urethra or anus. Gynaecological and genitourinary effects include haematocolpos, keloid formation, implantation dermoid cysts, chronic pelvic infection, calculus formation, dyspareunia, infertility, urinary tract infection and difficulty of micturition. Obstetric effects are perineal lacerations, consequences of anterior episiotomy, for example blood loss, injury to bladder, uretha or rectum, late urine prolapse, puerperal sepsis, delay in labour and its consequences, for example vesicovaginal and rectovaginal fistulae or fetal loss. The baby, for its part, may suffer birth defects and brain damage because of a difficult labour (UNICEF, 1995: pp. 54–6; Hellsten, 1999: pp. 69–83).

However, what has made the interference in the practice of FGM so controversial from the liberal, individualist point of view is that social coercion disguises itself as individuals' autonomous choice. In many cases it is not only the community and/or parents who insist on maintaining the practice; the young women and girls themselves may appear to accept it willingly, even ask for it. In some rare cases, even when their parents have understood the medical dangers of the practice and have decided not to put their daughters through it, the girls themselves may still insist on having the operation (UNICEF, 1995, pp. 54–6).

This apparent submission to FGM and the acceptance of other harmful traditions has made it sometimes difficult to decide which limits an individual's autonomy more: her social context or the paternalism practiced by health care professionals. In general, however, it is globally recognized that this practice is maintained by social coercion and pressure – mothers are afraid of social ridicule and rejection by their communities. Because of the direct physical harm caused by FGM, this tradition is now considered a violation of individual rights (particularly as a violation of women's and children's rights) and hence taken to be a human rights issue. In other words, it is considered justified to try to stop or change the practice of this cruel, culturally tied tradition.

Traditional societies and cultural relativism

Subjectivist reasoning was a result of apparently conflicting demands within the liberal concept of justice, which, on the one hand, demanded that we give the rights of individuals priority over any cultural claims, and on the other hand, allowed individuals the freedom to choose their cultural identities. After all, sometimes it is difficult to know exactly when some lifestyles or cultural identities are autonomously chosen, and when they are the result of strict socialization and indoctrination. At least in a pluralist society, we can plausibly argue that immigrants who choose to leave their country for whatever reason and live within a liberal society, also have to be ready to adopt the norms of their new home country. Particularly if they have left their own country because of its political intolerance or disrespect for individuals' lives and rights, they should be more than ready to do away with the traditions which themselves violate individuals' integrity.

Finding a framework for ethical agreements becomes more complicated, however, when health care professionals themselves cross borders and work in a country with different value and belief systems from their own. In such a situation relativism lurks behind every corner – in a curious way, the degeneration of liberal individualism into subjectivism gets support from collectivist relativism. First, as discussed above, the fear of paternalism easily leads into subjectivist reasoning and disregard of the special needs and particular social context of an individual. While universalization of values may sound justified in theory, in practice Westerners have often been accused of too easily disregarding the rationality of 'primitive people', their traditions and their choices of values and norms. The fear of paternalism still makes many liberals wonder whether interfering in an alien culture's practices is in itself a violation against the universal demand for tolerance and moral autonomy. Second, since some communities protect traditional practices by appealing to the relativity of the cultural norms and to the human rights principles of freedom and non-interference, liberal individualism appears to be merely one ethical outlook among many other ones. It then has no special position within other cultural beliefs and no right to try to assimilate other cultures to its values. Third, since the attempts to change particular practices might actually end up harming rather than helping individual members of the given community, some health care professionals may feel that it is better not to get involved at all. It becomes tempting to let other cultures find their own way to deal with their social and health problems. If the offered health care is not welcomed on the given conditions, why even bother?

Women's health in a patriarchal society

When working in an international environment, health care professionals may notice that the liberal framework of universalist individualism does not appear to suffice in solving the ethical problems they face in their daily work.

Particularly when Western medical knowledge and technology is applied in developing countries with more collectivist cultural practices, there can often be clashes between different value and belief systems. This is especially evident in maternal–fetal medicine and reproductive health care, which must first take into account the special needs of women, and secondly find a way to satisfy these needs appropriately in diverse circumstances.

Due to social inequality, discrimination and direct violence against women in many parts of the world, mere medical care is not enough to advance maternal–fetal care and reproductive health. In order to improve the overall situation, health care professionals have to identify the symptomatic social causes of the physical problems, such as women's low position within their society. Particularly in patriarchal societies the questions of individual rights and gender equality become central, because in these societies the protection of women's health is not a high priority. In order to explicate the relation between the issues of culture, the issues of human rights and the issues of women's health, I want to take a look at some concrete patriarchal cultural traditions which effectively hinder the advancement of women's health care in many traditional communities.

The main problem is that a patriarchal social system in general gives women very low social status. The principal duty of a woman in such a society has historically been to bear her husband's children (particularly sons) and to serve as the foundation of the family. The cost to women's health of discharging this duty is often unrecognized, and women's and children's ill health is still often explained through fate, destiny and divine will, rather than through the neglect of reproductive health services and social injustice (Cook, 1995: p. 263; Howard, 1995: pp. 301–13).

In many patriarchal societies there is strict control of women's sexual and reproductive behaviour and denial of their special needs and rights. This control results in unjust allocation of health care resources, as well as in violent and harmful practices such as FGM. In addition to genital mutilation there are many other traditions that are seen as necessary in order to suppress and guide women's sexual behaviour. Some of these traditions may be less violent than FGM, but in the long run they may often be as harmful. For instance, in the Tanzanian coastal region one such tradition is the 'teaching of life skills', which requires that girls stay indoors (usually in small and dark mud huts) for between three months and three years. These girls miss education as well as proper health care during this time.

Such direct violence as wife-battering and rape directly risks the health of a pregnant mother, as well as the development of a fetus, in every part of the world. In many patriarchal communities, more generally, treatment of women and girls as inferior to men and boys affect women's and children's health and development (e.g. Howard, 1995: p. 307). In some traditional African communities, for instance, women get less food or food of lower nutritional value than men, despite the fact that their energy consumption is as high or even higher than that of men due to the hard domestic and agricultural work they do. This workload is seldom relieved even during pregnancy. During their pregnancy women are also deprived of special types of food because of traditional beliefs. In Tanzania, among the Maasai tribe, pregnant women continue their normal workload, but are denied foods high in fat and are made to vomit every morning. In some other African tribes pregnant and/or lactating mothers are not allowed to eat eggs and chicken. The purpose of these diets is to keep the mother's weight low, as well as the child's birth weight, to avoid a difficult labour that can lead to the death of either mother or child. The solution itself, however, often contributes to the problems, because the result of these nutritional practices is that in many cases children are stillborn, or are born with a very low birth weight (UNI-CEF, 1995: pp. 4–6).

All these traditions and attitudes are still strongly supported not only by the men in these societies, but at least in public apparently also by the women themselves. In many places mothers choose the best food for their husbands and usually also for their sons. Mothers themselves and the daughters eat what is left over. Many attempts to change these traditions have failed, because it is seen as insensitivity to cultural preferences. Thence, because many of the practices and forms of behaviour are so tightly interwoven in the cultural structure of the society, women themselves may turn out to be also their strongest proponents (UNICEF, 1995: pp. 4–54). For example, during a conference on women's rights and domestic violence, held in Dar es Salaam, many Kenyan women agreed publicly that they needed to be periodically beaten by their husbands to become better and more obedient wives (*Daily News* (Tanzania), 19 April, 1999).

In such a situation, a health care professional with a different cultural background has a difficult task in trying to improve women's health and position within her community while simultaneously remaining sensitive to cultural difference. If medical and other interventions are seen as disrespecting the tradition of a particular community, the result may be that the old customs are even more strongly defended and the care needed is rejected as 'foreign' influence. In the end, again it is women and children who suffer most.

In addition to the cruel practices and direct violence which are used to prevent or punish suspected female sexual impropriety, women and children are often the undeserving victims of the effects of many sexually transmitted diseases, particularly AIDS. Men's infidelity, and women's inability to refuse sexual contact with men because of their weak social position, contribute alarmingly to the spread of AIDS. In Western health care practice, AIDS is often excessively medicalized. While this medicalization may help avoid stigmatization of patients in the West, seeing AIDS merely as a medical issue ignores the wider social–cultural aspects involved in its spread and treatment in the developing world. First, focusing on AIDS merely from the medical point of view may disregard the social structures that contribute to the spread of AIDS. Culturally accepted rape, socially or physically pressured prostitution and widely practiced polygamy all deny women a fighting chance against AIDS. Ironically, seeing AIDS as merely a medical problem may actually stigmatize women as victims of the disease, in a situation in which they often could not have done anything to avoid getting the HIV virus. Since talking about sex is still taboo in many communities, the information on the virus is not passed on properly and the real causes of the disease are misunderstood or merely disregarded (McFadden, 1992: pp. 157–69; Heise, 1995: pp. 238–55; Jones, 1999: pp. 223–37). Medical practitioners coming from outside with 'liberal' ideas are easily shunned and their views rejected.

Other types of maternal–fetal problems include early and unwanted pregnancies as well as unsafe abortions. While it is often understood that too early, too late and, in general, too frequent pregnancies can cause serious health problems to mothers, many of whom often are children themselves (under 18 years), old habits die hard. Family planning is often not accepted, and may even be taboo. Medical professionals who have to work with these issues may face a dilemma about how to approach the matter and how to educate not only women but also their husbands and/or male partners. In Musoma Rural District in Tanzania, for instance, 25 per cent of the young girls admitted having been forced or raped in their first sexual intercourse. Globally, between 20 to 30 per cent of all women report having been physically assaulted by an intimate partner at least once in their life, according to the Washington-based Health and Development Policy Project. In 1993 the World Development Report of the World Bank estimated that gender violence causes more deaths and disability among women aged 15 to 44 than cancer, malaria, heart disease, traffic accidents or even war. Many abused women suffer in silence because of poverty, shame, ignorance or lack of confidentiality and appropriate health care.

In many traditional communities with very scarce health care resources, better family planning is essential. However, in these same communities, marriage and motherhood often define one's womanhood. Women may take unusual risks to become pregnant and to carry a child to term even if they are infected by the HIV virus, and even if they know what serious medical complications it may have for their children. These women may want to have children and/or carry their pregnancies to term, regardless how short or painful their own or their children's lives might be. On the other hand, in these same societies pregnant women who are not married are often stigmatized, shamed and shunned by their community. Thus having an abortion may be the only way for these girls and women to protect their future. Since in many cases they do not want others to know about their pregnancy, unsafe abortions and self-abortions are typical. This results in serious health problems (Cook, 1995: pp. 256–71; Heise, 1995: 238–55; Jones, 1999: 223–37; also Yamin and Maine, 1999: pp. 563–607). A study conducted at the Muhimbili Medical Center in Dar es Salaam, for instance, has shown that 50 per cent of women between 15 and 24 years of age have been hospitalized because of abortion related complications.

A further challenge for maternal–fetal medicine is the vicious circle that follows when young girls with unplanned pregnancies drop out of school, and thus miss out on the information they would need in order to improve their own and their children's health and to plan the size of their family. They also miss the chance to get an education that would help them to take more general control over their own lives. After all, those who have the least access to information, to health services, to the right to make critical decisions and choices, are the easiest victims of any serious disease. In order to advance women's and children's health and well-being, it is necessary to try to educate women and advance their social status. At the same time, however, we need to acknowledge that the advice given or the methods of care suggested can sometimes lead the patient and her family to reject essential medical help, turning instead to self-help or the less professional and sometimes straightforwardly harmful advice and treatment of traditional healers. In Mara Region in Tanzania, for instance, a high number of women seek help from traditional healers rather than professionals with modern (often Western) medical training. The result has been that many of them die annually from complications, such as prolonged labour pains, excessive bleeding and bursting of the womb when giving birth, because of the use of untested traditional medicine during labour (Howard, 1995: pp. 301–13). Sometimes this rejection of modern medicine occurs because the patient and/or her family and community feel offended by the physician's interference in their value or belief systems. Sometimes the cause lies in the particular treatment (family planning, abortion, Caesarean delivery, prenatal testing or blood transfusion) which in itself offends against particular cultural norms.

Feminist bioethics and respect for difference

From a universalist point of view in maternal–fetal medicine and reproductive health care, the immensity of women's health problems in many societies, particularly in the developing world, is related to the social constraints on women's lives. In order to improve women's health we not only need more health care and medical resources, we also need to improve women's social position and promote women's rights within their communities. However, controversial as it may sound, attempts to respect an individual's rights and autonomy within some traditional and mainly patriarchal cultures may very easily provide further justification for the suppression of women and children within these cultures.

Let us take an example of how liberal promotion of the same standards everywhere and insensitivity to social influence can reinforce existing structural discrimination and injustice. One attempt to promote maternal health and women's position in a society has been to establish a system of maternal benefits. The idea of maternal benefit and child allowance is to secure women an economically more independent position. However, in order for this proposal to succeed, the society has to have already adopted the liberal concept of justice and to be committed to enhancing women's rights. While the idea in itself promises more equality to women, importing it and applying it directly to a male-dominated culture may create serious problems in practice. In a society in which patriarchal attitudes remain, providing maternity benefits can sometimes weaken rather than improve women's position. In order to get the benefits, men pressure women to have more children; the money is controlled by the men, making women even more dependent. The practical conclusion might easily be that it is better not to promote women's rights in these societies, but to take an alternative approach in order to improve women's health. This conclusion, however, is a set-back to international human rights protection as well as for the quest for a global bioethics.

In order to avoid this misguided logic, recent feminist bioethical approaches offer some guidance. First of all, feminists point out that universalism in prevalent Western bioethics is based on blindness to difference. Feminists believe that difference-blindness may in practice disregard the special needs of individuals and particularly women. Feminists point out that 'womanhood' in general is seen as a form of abnormality, deviance from the ideal norm of *a man*. So-called universalism often fails to take into account how much influence our personal differences as well as social circumstances have on our health, health care and medical practices. In its attempt to treat everybody equally, universalism may in reality disregard the differences between people (whether we talk about race, ethnicity or gender) that should be taken into account when we have to decide on medical advice or treatment for a particular person (Wolf, 1999: pp. 65–81). Since our concept of equality is based on an illusionary, idealistic standard of normality, we may discriminate against those who do not fit this norm.

In medicine, the idea of equality may then easily turn into an ideal of similarity. Treating everybody exactly the same may mean failing to understand the special problems which particular groups of people, for instance African women, may encounter in their social circumstances and in their medical care. In many cases individual patients benefit more from medical treatments in which the particularities in their personal situation are taken into consideration.

Second, the feminist criticism of the Western abstract form of liberalism shows that the same is true when it comes to the promotion of universal human rights standards. Despite the demand for universality, these standards themselves are historically based on the experience of men. Thus they either inadvertently or deliberately ignore many human rights violations particularly relevant to women (such as domestic violence, rape and other forms of sexual and reproductive violence and coercion). In fact, such violations of women's rights have become to be considered to be in many parts of the world as natural 'privileges' of men.

Since human rights standards were originally set by men and justified by the idea of social contract which, even in the West, historically excluded women from equal participation as less rational and less human, there still appear to be problems in including women within the scope of human rights. As Catharine MacKinnon (1998) has pointed out, there is always a way to find jurisdictional, evidentiary, substantive, customary or habitual reasons to overlook these violations and to disregard women's special needs. Thus, those human rights violations that are done to women are actually sometimes defended by the very human rights standards that should be there to prevent these violations. Appeals to cultural identities, autonomy and tolerance can be used to justify women's global subordination by men, not only by traditional communities but also in apparently democratic societies which claim to promote equality (MacKinnon, 1998: pp. 105–15).

Many human rights violations escape the human rights net, because women in general as a group (and particularly not as individuals) are still not seen as naturally meeting the standard of the ideal of humanity. Their special needs make them more vulnerable, but the demand for equal treatment justifies overlooking this vulnerability. In other worlds, the demand that everyone should be treated the same may effectively ignore the special needs of women and disregard sexually based violence towards women. When and if women's special needs are taken into account, the ideal of individual rights turns into a discourse of women's collective rights as women. Talking about collective rights makes 'women's rights issues' appear to be some kind of deviation from 'universal human rights issues', as any minority or cultural rights demand is. Womanhood then remains a deviation from the ideal of our 'common humanity', and women cannot meet the traditional standards for human rights (MacKinnon, 1998: pp. 101–15).

If we want to promote equality in practice and not merely as an abstract ideal, particularly in maternal–fetal medicine, we need to pay attention not only to diagnostic differences, but also to differences in socio-politico-cultural circumstance. Equality may sometimes require that we do not try to provide all the same services to everybody everywhere, but rather that we try to find the most appropriate way to promote health in particular situations. This means that we must take seriously the feminist criticism of Western abstract universalism. Particularly, we need to pay attention to how the ideal of equality is to be realized in everyday life. It cannot merely mean some abstract ideal of common humanity, because such a concept of humanity is often interpreted in social and medical practice as the fundamental similarity of all human beings, without paying attention to the differences in their needs and special circumstances.

It should be noted here also that while feminist bioethics provides important criticism of abstract universalism, its own focus on difference is often questionable, again because of the danger of falling into relativist reasoning. Particularly if it is mainly gender difference that is emphasized, there is an evident danger that we may construct a distinct moral outlook, which cannot provide the normative basis for globally acceptable ethical guidelines. Thus, feminist bioethics should not give up on the ideals of common humanity for fear of losing the notion of universal human rights altogether – leaving instead only women's rights, children's rights, minority rights, disability rights and so on *ad infinitum*. If that happens, the demand to protect women's rights may plausibly be seen to conflict with a 'competing' demand to protect patriarchal cultural practices, instead of being properly taken to be a demand for protection of individual rights within not only a particular community, but in all communities.

The contradiction of relativism

Relativism is usually considered to be an opposite view to the universalist ethical outlook. Its normative emphasis is on the incompatibility of different value and belief systems – it claims that there are no universal principles of justice that would apply to all cultures. In the form of relativism known as subjectivism, this means that individuals may not interfere with each other's value choices. In cultural relativism it suggests that members of one society cannot legitimately interfere with the social practices and traditions of other societies (Hellsten, 1999: pp. 69–83). Conservative traditionalists who resist cultural change and progress tend to appeal to cultural relativism; but ironically, so do health care professionals from individualist and traditionally liberal cultures, who may be tempted to justify inequality in the name of tolerance for the individual's autonomy and choice. Ethical relativism appears to be a strong and devious opponent in our quest for a global bioethics. However, I argue next that it can be beaten by its own internal logical contradictions.

The main logical problem of relativist reasoning is that if it is to be considered as a plausible normative ethical stand, as first pointed out by Bernard Williams in his *Morality* (1972), it cannot altogether reject the ideal of universal values. In a form of cultural relativism, social collectives have moral priority, but behind this priority there is a presumption of universal respect for difference and choice. The whole idea of cultural or collective rights is based on the very same universal and rather liberal ideals of tolerance and autonomy in choices. In other words, while individualists demand universal respect for individual rights, cultural relativists demand universal respect for collective rights (Williams, 1972). Since, according to the relativist argument, one set of values should not be considered superior to any other one, relativism in itself cannot provide justification for either the collectivist or the individualist ethical order. In the end, relativism merely argues that neither the individualist nor the collectivist ethical outlook can claim universal status, however simultaneously it defends the absolutist idea that there are some type of moral rights that should be universally protected. Therefore, the self-contradiction of relativism actually provides a productive starting point for the quest for a global bioethics.

Individuals and social collectives

In international human rights declarations there is now wide agreement that there exist universal rights. The dispute is about whether these rights are individual rights or collective rights. The defence of cultural rights, however, has proven to be problematic. First, they tend to conflict with individual rights. Second, there is an evident problem in identifying the relevant social unit whose rights are to be respected. However, cultures are social collectives, and social collectives are always composed of individuals; they can only claim their rights through their individual members. Thus, the whole concept of collective rights is built on false premises, because the development of cultures is also attained by the work, interaction and ideas of the individual members of the culture, and in the end by cultures' demands for the rights of their members (or at least for some of them, if not always for all equally) (Kukathas, 1992: 105–39; Hellsten, 1999: 69–83).

If individual rights truly were globally equally promoted and respected, there would not be a need for special protection of minorities and other disadvantaged social entities. Promotion of collective rights does not mend the existing social injustices. Instead it opens the door to further suppression of individual rights in the name of the common good and/or cultural identity.

The logical and practical impossibility of collective rights, however, does not mean that we have to reject all collectivist values. Nor does it mean that all features of individualism are in themselves desirable. After all, while the logical incoherence of relativism opens a door towards global bioethics, it does not directly provide us with an indisputable set of norms. Instead, it guides us towards shared values by showing that even supporters of relativism have to agree that there are some autonomy-based rights, whether individual or collective, that we must see as universal – including the right to tolerance for the differing views to which relativism calls our attention. Now that we have dissolved the ethical polarization between relativism and universalism, the next step is to undermine the polarization between individualism and collectivism.

If there is some agreement on the universality of rights, tolerance and equality, we have a basis for evaluating practices within a particular culture against those ethical standards we already share. In other words, while we have no basis by which to condemn an entire culture for particular practices which in themselves violate the shared ethical principles, we have the basis to evaluate these practices themselves. All cultures have different practices and norms, some of which may be more compatible with the universal values of tolerance, equality and rights than others. These practices do not necessarily correspond to the distinction between individualism and collectivism. In order to find a way to global ethical agreement on what practices are to be abandoned and which encouraged, we have first to understand the fundamental differences as well as the similarities in ethical norms between individualist and collectivist cultures. When we are comparing, for instance, Western individualist conceptions of health and health care against those of the more collectivist cultures of the East or South, we may appear to start from profoundly different ethical outlooks in medical practice.

In collectivist cultures, the starting point for health care choices and medical treatment is not usually an individual, the patient herself, but rather her close social environment and in particular her family. For instance, in many Eastern countries such as Japan, China, Philippines and Indonesia, as well as in many African communities, people do not usually practice self-determination in the explicit fashion required in the individualist, Western part of the world. The medical decision-making is rather based on family-determination. A family member's health problem is an issue and responsibility for the whole family. Thus, special fiduciary obligations have to be recognized – the family must take care of the sick. A family's duty to help the patient is not only to provide material and economic aid, but also to help her to make decisions, and sometimes even to make the decisions for her. Thus, social responsibility includes the burden of listening to medical information from physicians, making difficult choices or signing treatment authorizations. When the chosen representative of the family talks with the physician, his or her duty is to make everything work smoothly in the best interest of the patient. In this type of medical culture, the relationship between a mother and her unborn child is seldom a matter to be discussed and dealt with merely by the physician and the potential mother. Instead it concerns the whole family, often including not only both parents, but also the extended families of both parents (Fan, 1999: p. 557; Nakata et al., 1998: pp. 601–15).

When a community is based on respect for the common good and respect for collectivist values, it is important that we try to make a distinction between the positive and negative sides of collectivism. For instance, it should be acknowledged that the promotion of social ties can serve either authoritarian or liberal ends – to suppress certain members of a community or to protect an individual within her community. In fact, without a commitment to families, communities and the well-being of social collectives as a whole, it is in the end impossible to guarantee individual rights. Instead, the result would be the Hobbesian state of nature, the war of all against all. After all, without any social context and social protection, individual rights lose their meaning. Thus, while it is true that a collective society may suppress individual autonomy and disrespect equality, it can also promote democracy in decision-making. The most important and the most difficult task is to find the balance between individuals' rights and social duties.

We need to distinguish between 'collective' and 'oppressive', as well as between 'individualist' and 'individual-respecting' – much as either individualist liberals or collectivist traditionalists may distrust that contrast. If we talk about collectivism within a patriarchal community which oppresses women, the family-centred mode of health care smothers mothers' chances to make decisions for themselves and for their children. However, in a culture in which families are democratic and caring units of social cooperation, sharing responsibility in time of trouble may contribute to improvement in the patient's medical condition and provide great relief to the patient. Although family-centred decision-making is oppressive in patriarchal societies, in societies that already respect equality, it may have positive effects on both public and individual health. By comparison, in an extremely individualist society, lack of social support may add to the health problems of women (Cheng et al., 1998: pp. 616–27; Nakata et al., 1998: pp. 601–15) .

This collectivist, family-centred decision-making model is sometimes also called 'familism' (Fan, 1999: pp. 549–62) or 'communalism' in Africa (Wiredu, 1996: pp. 71–3, 114–9). Behind this family-centred decision-making model can be found very different cultural understandings of what constitutes one's moral personhood. In the individualist ethical framework, the individual is seen as a moral agent who is at the centre of the decision-making process, but in collective cultures an individual's moral status depends on her relation to others, her role (as a mother, wife, daughter, sister or in-law of someone) in a larger community and her place in the universe. For instance, in Chinese ethical thinking, based on a Buddhist world view, medical decisions can take a different turn because people have to follow what is seen as the natural cause of things in the cosmos. In the Buddhist thinking, nature means something like the power of spontaneous self-development and what results from that power. Interfering in the cause of nature is thought to have bad consequences. From the point of view of reproductive health care and maternal–fetal medicine, this belief might result in the family's unwillingness to allow physicians to conduct any testing or other prenatal treatments which can affect the development of the fetus and thus change the fate of the child (Fan, 1999: pp. 555–9; for Japan, Nakata et al., 1998: pp. 608–9).

In maternal–fetal medical practice, the positive side of collectivism would mean, first, that family involvement in decision-making is justified only when the subject of the treatment welcomes it and is informed about the decisions concerning her and her future child. Her duty to her family, community or society as a whole cannot violate her rights in a way that would risk or harm her health or the health of her child. Second, since social ties have such an influence on our choices, physicians and nurses have to try to find out what are the choices which are truly desired by the patient herself and what is socially pressured.

Cultural identity vs. moral identity

In the quest for a global bioethics and universal protection of human rights, the main challenge is to avoid the relativist trap and to introduce modern medicine and health care in a culturally sensitive manner which promotes individuals' rights without striving for cultural assimilation. Introducing new treatments, attitudes or ideas may at first be considered offensive, but it does not in itself show disrespect towards a particular tradition or way of life. Cultures themselves are not stable entities, rather they develop (whether this development is progress or decay) with the actions and choices of their individual members. Absorbing new ideas and methods of care does not mean that a community is giving up its cultural identity, rather, the new means can empower and strengthen the community through the well-being of its members.

When members of different cultures and social collectives demand their rights, their demands themselves need to be based on choice rather than social coercion. In addition to such clearly collectivist values as solidarity, caring, mutual cooperation and social responsibility, these values must also include the universal acceptance of the demand for tolerance and equal respect. If the members of these cultures cannot within their communities live in accordance with these values they want to promote, the true nature of saving cultural identity can be questioned. In other words, if a particular community is not itself ready 'to practice what it preaches', its preaching loses its authority.

When the universal demand for tolerance and equal respect for cultural identity is taken seriously, cultural choices are seen as an essential part of the development of one's moral identity. This moral identity, however, can be fully realized only when an individual has a chance to make independent ethical choices against her own cultural beliefs, and when she can judge her cultural practices against those of other cultures. Evaluating one's values does not mean that one must choose between two entirely different value systems of dissimilar cultures. Instead, it should be a choice between particular values within diverse systems.

A person's moral identity cannot be equated with cultural identity, rather, moral identity is a precondition in our choices of lifestyles, traditions and cultural allegiances. In other words, when cultural diversity and respect is emphasized, it needs to be recognized that a person's moral identity is always influenced by her cultural background. However, it should not be wholly equated with her culture. The stronger our moral identity is, the better we can change and develop our cultural practices without losing our cultural identities. In fact the more moral character we have developed, the more we learn to appreciate the good in our cultural background.

In a global context this means that sometimes we need to interfere with practices that we see as unjust, and to help both the victims of this oppression and the oppressors to recognize the injustice practiced. Once the injustice is brought out in the open, it is more difficult to defend in public. This is the case above all when these practices cause serious health risks to individuals. After all, these individuals as members of particular communities (as is particularly the case with women and children) themselves guarantee the further existence and flourishing of these communities and cultures (Benhabib, 1995: p. 238).

Towards a global bioethics

From the point of view of global bioethics, we have to find the proper ways to make a distinction between positive and negative cultural features. In order to do this, we need to recognize the following points. First, we need to see which ethically disturbing practices are genuinely due to cultural beliefs, and which to ignorance or lack of education. Second, we need to acknowledge which ethical issues are the result of fundamental cultural differences (e.g. between respect for individual autonomy and collectivist decision-making processes). Finally, we have to differentiate those ethical issues which *appear* to be culturally bound but in fact are a consequence of invalid logic and/or misinterpretations of the values that we may already share.

After we have identified the foundational cause for ethical disagreements, we need to find the right way to educate people with different cultural and social backgrounds. We need not only to understand the traditional roles of different groups in this society, but also to use these groups as our messengers. We need to be sensitive to the differences in cultural attitudes and to give more emphasis to the role of the family and community in health care and in social development in general. This can help to plan the education and medical care accordingly. In many cultures, individuals and particularly individual women, are powerless without the support of the rest of the community. When communities as a whole understand that common good can be achieved only through the well-being of their individual members, they can develop grass-root level progressive forces. This means that in addition to access to basic maternal health care and family planning services, medical professionals have to make connections with the traditional leadership (chiefs, religious leaders and elders) within a particular community. Partnership between health services, formal political systems and traditional social systems will be necessary in order to find an inter-culturally acceptable strategy for delivering the proper health services. Consultations with communities and community-based service provision are needed to identify community concerns and to design mutually satisfactory ways to promote better health. In Ghana, for instance, a pioneering rural project on basic health care (funded by USAID, the Rockefeller Foundation, and the Ministry of Health of Ghana) has focused on community-based health care, resulting in increased immunization coverage and greater use of family planning methods. The community members themselves are involved in choosing the health care methods as well as with the results (*Guardian* (Tanzania), July 9, 1999).

Conclusion

Many reproductive health problems are caused by women's unequal access to medical and other resources, as well as by oppressive sexual, health and birth practices. Particularly in patriarchal cultures, the real reasons for women's chronic reproductive disabilities or premature death in labour/childbirth are often heavy burdens of work, poor nutrition of women and girls, too early and continual pregnancies and generally excessive childbearing, often accompanied by direct physical violence. But a patriarchal culture is not necessarily collective. Even within individualist cultures there remain attitudes and practices that treat women as less valuable than men. Women's special needs are often ignored, whether deliberately or inadvertently, either in the name of universal respect for overestimated autonomy or in the name of cultural rights. All in all, human rights standards themselves tend to ignore the complexity of women's social position and are used to justify practices and behaviour which, if done to men, would be automatically considered as human rights violation.

If we take seriously the feminist challenge to modern bioethics when we deal with patients from different cultural backgrounds, we can find a proper way to promote the health and well-being of women and children without ignoring difference, social ties and local cultures. In Tanzania, the Ministry for Community, Development, Women's Affairs and Children (led by a woman minister) is itself, at least in principle, an example of an attempt to pay more attention to the role that communal values, social ties and gender play in development. In order to promote health as well as justice, we need to take into account the local context and the particular physical, social and cultural circumstances of the particular patient. This means that the delivery of health services to individuals has to start by focusing on their characteristics and powers of their communities, instead of promoting standardized benchmarks.

Sensitivity to differences between individuals and social collectives, and a focus on the positive features of particular cultural systems, help us to turn communities into progressive rather than regressive forces in the improvement of maternal and fetal health. Strong communal and family values, different cultural beliefs and social practices should not be condemned, rather they should be objectively considered as an integral part of development. No culture is inherently unreasonably resistant to development and change towards better living conditions as long as enough sensitivity and respect is shown towards its particular, local characteristics.

To summarize, this chapter aims to show that it is not impossible to find a shared set of values that can be universally promoted in different types of cultures, without requiring cultural assimilation. Individuals' rights can and should be promoted even within collectivist cultures. While this means abandoning repressive social structures, it does not have to mean turning away from close social ties and solidarity. In the same way, collectivist values such as social responsibility and caring can and should be promoted in individualist cultures. This does not have to mean that we are returning to traditionalism. While social collectives can oppress their individual members, there is no reason why they could not also empower their members. While individuals may disregard their communities, there is no logically valid or morally legitimate reason why they should not work for the good of these communities – as long as we treat the individual members as equally valuable.

References

Benhabib, S. (1995). Cultural complexity, moral interdependence, and the global dialogical community. In *Women, Culture and Development*, ed. M. Nussbaum, pp. 235–55. Oxford: Clarendon Press.

Cheng, M., Wong, K.K. and Yan, W.W. (1998). Critical care ethics in Hong Kong: cross-cultural conflicts as East meets West. *Journal of Medicine and Philosophy* 23: 616–27.

Cook, R. (1995). International human rights and women's reproductive health. In *Women's Rights, Human Rights: International Feminist Perspectives*, ed. J. Peters and A. Wolper, pp. 256–75. New York: Routledge.

Etzioni, A. (1999). *The Limits of Privacy*. New York: Basic Books.

Fan, R. (1999). Critical care ethics in Asia: global or local? *Journal of Medicine and Philosophy* **23**: 549–62.

Heise, L. (1995). Freedom close to home: the impact of violence against women on reproductive health. In *Women's Rights, Human Rights: International Feminist Perspectives*, ed. J. Peters and A. Wolper, pp. 238–55. New York: Routledge.

Hellsten, S.K. (1999). Pluralism in multicultural liberal democracy and the justification of female circumcision. *Journal of Applied Philosophy* **16**: 69–83.

Howard, R. (1995). Women's rights and right to development. In *Women's Rights, Human Rights: International Feminist Perspectives*, ed. J. Peters and A.Wolper, pp. 301–13. New York: Routledge.

Jones, N. (1999). Culture and reproductive health: challenges for feminist philanthropy. In *Embodying Bioethics, Recent Feminist Advances*, ed. A. Donchin and L.M. Purdy, pp. 223–237. Lanham, MD: Rowman and Littlefield.

Kukathas, C. (1992). Are there any cultural rights? *Political Theory* **20**: 105–39.

Kuczewski, M. (1998). Medical decision-making: a role for the family. *The Responsive Community* **8**: 11–12.

MacKinnon, C. (1998). Crimes of war, crimes of peace. In *Outlook: A Selection of Readings for the 50th Anniversary of the Universal Declaration of Human Rights*. Washington, DC: US State Department.

Matthieu, D. (1996). *Preventing Prenatal Harm, Should the State Intervene?*, 2nd edn. Washington, DC: Georgetown University Press.

McFadden, P. (1992). Sex, sexuality and the problems of AIDS in Africa. In *Gender in Southern Africa: Conceptual and Theoretical Issues*, ed. R. Meena, pp. 157–95. Harare: Sapes Books.

Nakata, Y., Goto, T. and Morita, S. (1998). Serving the emperor without asking: critical care ethics in Japan. *Journal of Medicine and Philosophy* **23**: 601–15.

Rawls, J. (1971). *A Theory of Justice*. Cambridge, MA: Harvard University Press.

Rawls, J. (1993). *Political Liberalism*. New York: Columbia University Press.

UNICEF (1995). *The Girl Child in Tanzania: A Research Report*. Dar es Salaam: UNICEF.

Williams, B. (1972). *Morality*. Cambridge: Cambridge University Press.

Wiredu, K. (1996). *Cultural Universals and Particulars: An African Perspective*. Bloomington: Indiana University Press.

Wolf, S. (1999). Erasing difference: race, ethnicity and gender in bioethics. In *Embodying Bioethics: Recent Feminist Advances*, ed. A. Donchin and L.M. Purdy, pp. 65–81. Lanham, MD: Rowman and Littlefield.

Yamin, A. and Maine, D. (1999). Maternal mortality as a human rights issue: measuring compliance with international treaty obligations. *Human Rights Quarterly* **21**: 563–607.

4

HIV in pregnancy: ethical issues in screening and therapeutic research

Paquita de Zulueta

Department of Primary Healthcare and General Practice, Imperial College School of Medicine, London, UK

Introduction

Human immunodeficiency virus (HIV) infection in pregnancy creates complex and challenging moral dilemmas, both for pregnant women and for those involved in their care. A recent breakthrough in research has shown that mother-to-child transmission (vertical transmission) can be reduced with the use of anti-viral drugs (Connor et al., 1994), with obstetric interventions – Caesarean section in particular (European Mode of Delivery Collaboration, 1999) – and with avoidance of breast-feeding. These findings have made pregnant women the focus for preventative and therapeutic strategies, and for public health policies. They have provided the impetus for further research into cheaper and simpler ways to reduce vertical transmission in resource-poor countries. They have also generated ethical challenges and dilemmas at both the individual and the global level.

Setting the scene

HIV-related disease, AIDS, now kills more people worldwide than any other disease. In 1998, two and a half million people died from AIDS. A report in 1999 from the United Nations AIDS program (UNAIDS, 1999) cited the prevalence in 1998 as being 33.4 million, a rise of 10 per cent (nearly six million new cases), from the year before. This shows a disturbing lack of progress in prevention nearly 20 years into the epidemic. People living in sub-Saharan Africa account for two-thirds of those infected with the virus. The majority of these infections are acquired from heterosexual or vertical transmission.

Females in sub-Saharan Africa are particularly vulnerable to HIV infection. Rates in girls are three to four times that of boys (Malloch Brown, 2000). This is owing to a variety of socio-cultural factors, such as sexual behaviour, poverty, migrant labour and gender inequality. Women account for 43 per cent of all HIV-infected people over 15 years of age (UNAIDS, 1999). It was predicted that by the year 2000, six million pregnant women would be infected with HIV (Scarlatti, 1996). HIV infection is transmitted to 15–25 per cent of babies born to HIV-infected women in Europe and America, and to 25–35 per cent of those born in Africa, India and Thailand (Peckham and Gibb, 1995; Newell et al., 1997).

The majority of children acquire HIV infection from their mothers, such that the number of infected children parallels the number of infected women. The United Nations reported that in 1997 there were approximately 600 000 babies infected annually with HIV-1 through vertical transmission – about 1600 daily – and that 90 per cent of these were born in Africa (UNAIDS, 1998a). In fact, according to Peter Piot, executive director of the UNAIDS agency, half of all newborn babies in Africa carry the HIV virus (Anonymous, 1999a).

This exceedingly bleak outlook is relieved in part by the discovery that the following measures can reduce vertical transmission:

- Avoidance of breast-feeding decreases transmission after birth by about 14 per cent (Dunn et al., 1992).
- More importantly, the large randomized controlled trial conducted by the Paediatric AIDS Clinical Trial Group (PACTG) in 1994 showed unequivocally that perinatal treatment with an anti-viral drug, zidovudine (AZT), significantly reduced vertical transmission of the HIV virus by about two-thirds in more developed countries – from around 25 per cent to 8 per cent (Connor et al., 1994).
- Furthermore, refining anti-viral therapy and selectively performing planned Caesarean section has given even better results (European Mode of Delivery Collaboration, 1999).
- Vitamin supplements have not been clearly shown to reduce transmission, but have improved the adverse pregnancy outcomes associated with HIV infection in resource-poor countries (Fawzi et al., 1998).

In fact, provided that the resources are available, vertical transmission rates can now be reduced to less than two per cent (Tudor-Williams and Lyall, 1999). In other words, vertically acquired HIV is a near-preventable condition.

In the affluent, developed countries, up to 1994, HIV-positive women were faced with the grim choice of either continuing with a pregnancy that carried a 1:5–6 risk of their offspring being infected (if bottle-fed), or of having a termination. In addition, until the advent of highly active retroviral treatment (HAART) in the mid-1990s, the prognosis for an HIV-infected individual was bleak. Women found to be HIV- positive faced the prospect of a fatal progressive illness. (The time taken for AIDS to develop can vary greatly – the average is around nine years.) But now HIV-infected individuals in these countries can hope for an increased longevity, with the maintenance of an independent, reasonable quality of life for several years (Cohn, 1997). Nevertheless, they need to take complex regimes of three or more anti-viral drugs (de Cock, 1997), with many adverse effects. Some people have difficulty tolerating the treatment physically or psychologically. The disease, albeit more controllable, remains incurable. This has important ethical implications – sometimes overlooked in the discussion of perinatal HIV. Nevertheless, pregnant women in these countries can at least be confident that their offspring can escape infection, and, that if they accept treatment, they themselves may benefit from earlier diagnosis (de Cock and Johnson, 1998).

It is a tragic irony, however, that the countries with the highest prevalence tend to be those with the fewest resources to combat the disease – 19 out of 20 people infected with HIV cannot benefit from HAART. The majority of pregnant women cannot benefit from these modern, evidence-based treatments and interventions.

For those living in developing countries, the new treatments are virtually unobtainable owing to prohibitive costs (Anonymous, 1998; UNAIDS, 1998a; Bayley, 2000; Cochrane, 2000). For example, the 076 regime costs $1000 in the United States. Many countries in sub-Saharan Africa spend as little as $6 a year for health care per person per year (Bayley, 2000; Cochrane, 2000).

In resource-poor countries, antenatal care itself may be minimal or non-existent (Graham and Newell, 1999; Marseille et al., 1999; Mofenson, 1999). The cost and complexity of AZT treatment, according to the PACTG 076 protocol, makes it unobtainable for countries that may only be able to spend a very small percentage of their gross national product (GNP) on health care. It is only those who participate in trials (or the very privileged) who stand a chance of receiving prophylactic therapy.

Hence the majority of HIV- positive women living in poor countries face the prospect of bringing into the world children who may be infected, or orphaned at an early age.

Even reproductive choices may be limited. In some countries, women are expected to bear children, and fecundity is associated with high status. Partners do not often collaborate in reducing risks and conceptions (Schott and Henley, 1996).

Studies in the early 1990s in Kenya and other African countries have shown that the epidemic has had little impact on attitudes and subsequent childbearing (Ryder et al., 1991; Temmerman et al., 1995). Political-will to confront the problem has also been slow to manifest itself in many African countries. But there are signs of change (Altman, 1999). It is disappointing that at the time of writing, President Mbeki of South Africa appears to be reversing this positive trend. Rather than endorsing a programme of national funding for perinatal zidovudine (prevalence in pregnant women is around one in five), he is exploring the evidence for AIDS not being caused by HIV – a very unorthodox view (Anonymous, 2000a).

In conclusion, the gross inequity in resources, particularly in health care provision, that exist today between the affluent and the poor countries is brought into sharp focus by the contrasting fates of those with HIV. There are, however, some hopeful signs of progress. The UN Security Council, chaired by the vice-president of the USA, convened in January 2000 to discuss actions to tackle the problem of AIDS – the first time that a health-related issue has ever been discussed. Pharmaceutical countries have agreed to reduce the costs of their drugs for distribution in some poorer countries (Anonymous, 1999b). The World Bank has pledged its support (Anonymous, 1999c; Cochrane, 2000). In addition, some countries, such as Uganda and Senegal, have managed to reduce transmission by vigorous public health education programmes (Anonymous, 2000b).

HIV testing and screening in pregnancy

The discovery that vertical transmission can be reduced has had a major impact on named-testing policies in countries where resources are available to implement preventative measures. Before 1994, anonymized antenatal unlinked HIV screening, or surveillance, had already been widely adopted by public health and political institutions in several countries, in order to monitor the prevalence of HIV in the antenatal community (Heath, Grint and Hardiman, 1988; Peckham et al., 1990; Hudson et al., 1999). For example, in the UK, it began in 1990, as part of the Department of Health's Unlinked Anonymous HIV Prevalence Monitoring Programme, and continues until the present day. Pregnant women are considered an 'epidemiological useful' group because they represent a stable sub-group of the heterosexually active population at 'normal risk'. They are usually in regular contact with health professionals, and have blood tests taken routinely.

I shall now consider the potential implications of a positive result, the nature of the relationship between the health professional and the pregnant woman, and the process of consent, as these are all relevant to a discussion about the ethics of anonymized and named testing.

The implications of a positive result

A pregnant woman is likely to experience considerable distress on discovery of her positive status (Manuel, 1999), particularly as she may feel more vulnerable and dependent on others, and she has the added responsibility of motherhood ahead of her. She may contemplate real risks of rejection from her partner, family and friends.

For those working, employment may be put into jeopardy. Life or medical insurance may be difficult to obtain.

In a resource-rich country, if a pregnant woman does agree to HIV testing, the assumption is that if she proves to be HIV-positive, she will comply with the treatments to prevent vertical transmission. This assumption has been borne out by empirical research (Gibb et al., 1997; Lyall et al., 1998). A woman, however, may not be aware of the chain of events that will proceed from the discovery of a positive status in pregnancy. In addition to taking anti-viral treatment, she may be advised to have a planned Caesarean section. Some women may object. In English law, the competent woman's right to refuse treatment is absolute, even if her fetus is put at risk from her decision. Once born, however, the interests of the child are paramount, and parental views may be overridden if they are seen to conflict with the child's welfare. Babies can still gain protection from infection if given antiviral treatment within 48 hours of birth, even if the mother has refused to take medication or have a Caesarean section (Wade et al., 1998).

If a woman is known to be HIV-positive, health professionals may recommend that her recently born child is tested for HIV, arguing that it is in the best interests of the child. Diagnosis can now be made as early as one to three months of age (Corbitt, 1999), and early diagnosis leads to improved prognosis (Evans et al., 1995; Richardson and Sharland, 1998). The infected child, without treatment, usually survives only five years or less in developing countries. With treatment, survival may be until the age of 15, or beyond. Parents might not wish for their child to be tested. Knowledge of their child's positive status could have a profoundly negative impact on their relationship with him or her. It is beyond the scope of this discussion to consider the poignant dilemma for parents of whether or not to disclose to their child his or her incurable infection and uncertain life expectancy, or to explore the burden of imposing life-long unpleasant treatment on a child, and of protecting him or her from stigma.

A British legal case in September 1999 highlighted the difficulties (Anonymous, 1999d; Verkaik, 1999). A woman, known to be HIV- positive, gave birth. She had not taken anti-retroviral treatment in pregnancy and had breast-fed from birth. There was therefore a significant risk (20–25 per cent) that the child would be infected. Health professionals were alarmed. The couple refused to have their child tested for HIV. They did not believe that HIV was an infection that responded to antiviral treatment. Social Services made an application under the 1989 Children Act. The child (now four months old) was made a ward of court, and the court overruled parental refusal and ordered the test. If the child tested positive, treatment was to be instituted. The woman, however, was not ordered to stop breast-feeding. The couple fled the country with their child. Had the child been found to be HIV-positive, one can speculate on the difficulties in implementing a complex anti-viral regime with non-compliant parents.

HIV-positive mothers in developed countries are advised to abstain from breast-feeding, but guidelines for women respect their right to make a choice

(Department of Health, 1999). It is evident from the case above, however, that women may find that breast-feeding causes disapprobation, and may even result in their infants being considered 'at risk'. Decisions regarding their child's welfare may then be taken out of their hands. Abstention from breast-feeding creates particular difficulties in countries and cultures where breast-feeding is the norm, and bottle-feeding stigmatizes a woman (Graham and Newell, 1999). In addition, bottle-feeding may be risky in areas where hygiene is low and may be prohibitively expensive (UNAIDS, 1998b).

Voluntary named testing poses particular ethical problems in poorer countries (Temmerman et al., 1995; Karim et al., 1998). HIV prevalence may be considerably higher in some of these countries, such that in theory the cost-effectiveness of screening is correspondingly much greater than in the affluent countries (Marseille et al., 1999; Postma et al., 1999; Soderlund et al., 1999). But without the resources for treatment, as is often the case, the benefits to women are less clear. Knowledge of HIV status may be particularly burdensome to those living in some countries, creating not only stigma and social isolation, but also abandonment or violence from partners and/or family (Temmerman et al., 1995; Duke, 1999; McGreal, 1999; Wiktor et al., 1999). HIV testing in this context should not be undertaken without providing counselling and support. The women can be given strategies to help cope with the disease, prepare for the future, reduce risk behaviour and make reproductive choices. But as one researcher expressed it: 'There is not much that we can offer African women once we have told them the bad news' (Temmerman et al., 1995: p. 970).

Even if women accept testing, they do not necessarily wish to receive the result. Presumably this is owing to the risk of stigma and social discrimination. Temmerman et al. (1995) found that most of the women participating in a research trial in Kenya did not actively request their test result. One-quarter dropped out of a research study once they learnt they were test-positive. This has been a common finding in research studies in Africa (Dabis et al., 1999; Guay et al., 1999; Wiktor et al., 1999).

The relationship between the health professional and the patient

As I have discussed elsewhere (de Zulueta, 2000a), the relationship between a health professional and a patient can be characterized as a fiduciary one. Respect for a patient's autonomy cannot be divorced from acting in her best interests, as it is usually the patient who knows what is best for her. Others share this view. For example, Pellegrino and Thomasma (1988: p. 55), both professors of medical humanities, say: 'Respecting wishes of patients is an essential feature of acting in their best interests'. Margaret Brazier, a professor of law, and Dr Mary Lobjoit (Brazier and Lobjoit, 1999) also endorse the notion of the fiduciary relationship between the health professional and the patient, and describe it as a therapeutic alliance or partnership.

The health professional is therefore entrusted to put the patient's interests first, and to hold certain things (such as confidential information) 'in trust'. As Brazier succinctly expresses this: 'It is trite to describe the health professional's relationship with his or her patient as a relationship of trust, yet the description encapsulates the very heart of the relationship' (Brazier and Lobjoit, 1999: p. 187). The health professional has a duty to promote the well-being of both the mother and the unborn child, but should only provide care that the mother agrees to. The woman, as an autonomous agent, confers on the fetus the status of being a patient (McCullough and Chervenak, 1994).

If we believe that respect for autonomy is a fundamental principle in health care, then we should give pregnant women the opportunity to know their HIV status. 'The information is material to making informed choices about her own and her baby's future' (Boyd, 1990: p. 176). Pregnant women are not typical patients. They are not ill, but are undergoing a normal physiological process. They voluntarily seek help from health professionals to maximize their own and their baby's welfare. Arguably it is even more of an imperative to respect their autonomy.

Consent

The importance accorded to patient consent reflects the respect with which health professionals regard their patients. Consent can be defined as both a legal and an ethical requirement. Failure to seek the patient's consent is not only a moral failure, but, in English law, also leaves the doctor liable to the tort or crime of battery or to the tort of negligence. For consent to be legally valid, it must be competent, informed and voluntary. The information required is such that the patient understands in broad terms the nature and purpose of the procedure, and the principal risks, benefits and alternatives (*Chatterton v Gerson*, 1981). Voluntariness implies freedom from coercion.

Consent is a *process*, not an event, and involves a continuing dialogue between the health care professional and the patient, such that there is genuine shared decision-making. Patients should control the amount and timing of information. I submit that in the case of anonymized testing, and in the case of 'routine' voluntary named testing, consent is often vitiated by a lack of understanding and information, and sometimes by coercion.

The ethics of anonymised unlinked screening for HIV in pregnancy

With anonymized testing, there is a tension between the perceived interests of society (the public good) and those of the individual. The conclusion taken by the working party of the UK Institute of Medical Ethics (IME), that the benefit to the public from anonymized testing outweighs any individual harm (Boyd, 1990), is no longer tenable.

Despite the fundamental therapeutic change for pregnant women (at least in resource-rich countries) since 1994, anonymous antenatal testing inexorably continues in the UK and in several other developed countries (Nicoll et al., 1998). This may be justified in countries where the resources are not available to offer counselling or treatment, and where the data may be used to galvanize the developed world into providing aid. It seems harder to justify in wealthy countries. In fact, anonymized testing has been abandoned in some places, as it is considered unethical (Richards, 1999). So what are the current justifications?

Anonymized testing provides accurate prevalence figures relatively cheaply and easily. These figures, it is argued, can then be used to provide the justification for allocating more resources to the treatment and prevention of the disease, particularly in areas of high prevalence. They can also provide information as to the cost-effectiveness, or desirability, of offering voluntary named testing. They provide valuable information for health educators and health professionals. Public health physicians and HIV specialists argue that there is a continuing need to monitor prevalence and trends, as these may change (Pinching, 2000; Nicoll and Peckham, 1999), and that the data can be used to audit the success of a voluntary named testing programme. These arguments are persuasive, but they fail to take into account the professional's duty of care.

Another justification that appears in the literature is the proposal that consent to having a blood test implies consent to having it tested for HIV, and that the patient has given her blood away and has no property rights over it. This is dismissed by Brazier as a red herring. She points out that the when the blood is taken, the *intention* is always to test it for HIV, and that the patient should be informed of this. It could be argued that it is up to women to decide whether they wish to have an HIV test done anonymously. But I would counter-argue that it is unprofessional and unethical to encourage individuals to relinquish benefits that may affect third parties (human fetuses), even if these are not 'legal persons'. Grubb and Pearl (1990) take the view that public policy should deny women this opportunity.

Finally, it could be argued that if an informed mother agrees to anonymized testing, she does not *intend* to deprive the fetus of benefit, as she does not know if she harbours the virus. This argument is also used to justify the health professional's behaviour – no harm is intended, and there is no responsibility to act upon the result since it is unobtainable. But a professional cannot abrogate his or her duty to inform the mother of the benefits of diagnostic testing. If we consider other instances of screening, such as cervical screening, or, more appropriately, genetic screening for susceptibility to a treatable cancer, it would seem bizarre and immoral if professionals sugges-ted to patients that they should not receive the results of such tests.

Anonymized testing may represent an abuse of trust in the health profes-sional. A woman attending an antenatal clinic carries the reasonable expecta-tion that all tests and procedures are done either directly to benefit her or her unborn child (de Zulueta, 2000a). This assumption is reinforced if the test is done by a health professional, precisely because the relationship is one of trust. As one mother poignantly expressed it: 'But surely if they found something wrong they'd tell you, wouldn't they?' (Kahtan, 1993). Policy-makers exploit this trust in obtaining blood for anonymized testing.

All babies in the UK and several other countries have blood taken for the Guthrie test at around six days after birth (the heel prick test). Some of this blood is used for anonymized testing of maternal antibodies to HIV. The baby is used as a vehicle for testing the mother. It is *accepted* practice not to seek parental consent. The case for abuse of trust is even stronger than with anonymized testing of pregnant women, as the mothers are even more likely to assume that all tests are for the baby's benefit. Since the baby relies entirely on others to protect his interests, it is arguably even more unethical to use the baby 'merely as a means, rather than as an end in himself', to paraphrase Kant.

In order to make an informed choice, the woman needs to understand the nature of the test itself, as well as the advantages and disadvantages of not receiving the *result* should it be positive. Kennedy and Grubb (1994) take the view that the doctor's duty to inform may extend to informing a patient of the risks of non-treatment. They cite a case when a doctor was found in breach of duty for failing to inform a woman of the potential consequences of not agreeing to a cervical smear.

Are antenatal women adequately informed to give valid consent to anony-mized testing? The IME took the view that the widespread distribution of a leaflet published by the Department of Health and Central Office of Informa-tion (1989) 'largely satisfied' their recommendations that it gave patients adequate information and allowed them the option to refuse (Boyd, 1990: p. 176). But this assumes that women read the leaflets, and that they are in a language which they can understand. In addition, the leaflet issued by the Department of Health, in circulation after 1994, does not refer to treatments available for reducing vertical transmission. Nor does it refer to the risks of breast-feeding. In any case, the notion of passive consent, that is to say that consent is implied unless there is a verbal refusal, is ethically unsound and 'a concept quite alien in English law' (Brazier and Lobjoit, 1999: p. 183).

Some statements make it clear that policy-makers actually *do not wish* for informed consent (Department of Health, 1997: p. 73). In clinics that pro-vide universal testing (see later), the women should have received the relevant information from a pre-test discussion with the midwife, and the opportunity to have a named test. But the contradiction in undertaking both named and anonymized tests is striking. 'On the one hand she is receiving the strong message that she should accept testing "for the good of her baby". Yet on the other hand she is being asked to accept testing whereby she and her baby cannot benefit!' (de Zulueta, 2000b: p. 25).

Do women understand the nature and purpose of antenatal testing? Anecdotal and empirical evidence (Kahtan, 1993; Chrystie et al., 1995) shows that the majority of women do not understand anonymized testing. In addition, it is doubtful that all women know that their blood is being tested anonymously for HIV. In one study only five per cent fully understood the nature of the testing, and a significant proportion believed that they would be informed should the result be positive (Chrystie et al., 1995).

The standards committee of the General Medical Council in 1988 took the view that unlinked anonymous HIV testing breached no fundamental ethical principle (Anonymous, 1988). In the light of my arguments, this statement can no longer be upheld. The principle of autonomy is frequently infringed by the process of anonymized testing, and, as Brazier says, 'Consent truly is a myth' (Brazier and Lobjoit, 1999: p. 179). The moral justifications for violating autonomy are considerably weakened by the knowledge that there are methods to prevent vertical transmission. Women must be made aware that by relinquishing the opportunity to receive the result of the HIV test, they are depriving themselves and their future children of potential benefit.

The ethics of named testing

The Department of Health's Unlinked Anonymous Surveys Steering Group in 1989 rejected mass voluntary testing as an alternative to anonymized testing. The harms of voluntary named testing – social discrimination, stigma and the lack of a curative treatment if found to be HIV-positive – were considered to outweigh the benefits. Gill, a consultant epidemiologist, and colleagues, summarized the position against voluntary testing in 1989: 'If the necessary HIV surveys use the universal named case finding method they will be complex, expensive, and subject to participation bias. They may cause considerable and avoidable distress in populations with very low prevalence'(Gill et al., 1989: p. 1296). This statement appears to be borne out by empirical evidence. The uptake for anonymized testing in the UK in 1996 was 99.9 per cent, but below 25 per cent for voluntary named testing (Gibb et al., 1998). This paternalistic practice of withholding the truth is now viewed as an infringement of patient autonomy. Furthermore, empirical evidence shows it to be contrary to the wishes of most patients (Novack et al., 1979; Buckman, 1996). As argued above, the benefits of named testing, and the arguments in favour of truth-telling are further strengthened, particularly as third parties are placed at risk by non-disclosure.

The different methods of implementing named testing are as follows. 'Opting out' is the practice whereby the HIV test is offered as one of the normal routine antenatal tests, and the woman is given the option to refuse after pre-test briefing or discussion (which I shall describe below). This is also referred to as universal or routine testing. 'Opting in', by contrast, makes the test available to all, but places the burden on the woman to request it. The latter system was rejected by the IME on the grounds that women who were unaware of being at risk would not benefit, and that those who did consider themselves at risk could expose themselves to discrimination and stigmatization. In addition, this 'request policy' has been shown to be inefficient in identifying those at risk (Gill et al., 1989). The IME, even in 1990, recommended 'opting out' testing. Targeting women who are considered to be at risk, a 'selective policy', has been perceived as discriminatory (Mercey, 1998; Sherr et al., 1998/9) and inefficient (Hawken et al., 1995; Noone and Goldberg, 1997).

Following 1994, there was a shift in policy, and antenatal women in resource-rich countries were targeted by policy makers and public health institutions for strategies to reduce the transmission of HIV to infants. The majority of industrialized countries adopted a universal testing policy (whereby all women were offered the test), and developed their own guidelines. The European Collaborative study collected and collated data on antenatal testing from 15 members of the European community (Thorne et al., 1996). Policies ranged from mandatory or near-mandatory testing, to no policy at all (Hudson et al., 1999).

Governments decide, according to resources and priorities, at what level of prevalence a universal policy will be introduced. This will vary greatly between poor and rich countries. Women at high risk in 'low-prevalence areas' may well miss out; this resource allocation dilemma is one well known to all screening programmes, and difficult to resolve. This merits further discussion, but suffice to say that if resources are available, there is a strong argument for recommending a universal policy for all pregnant women (Hudson et al., 1999). In 1994, the UK Department of Health endorsed a policy of universal voluntary testing in 'areas of high prevalence' (defined as HIV prevalence of one in five hundred or less), and issued guidelines (Department of Health, 1994). The Centres for Disease Control and Prevention (CDC) recommended this testing policy in the US for *all* pregnant women, and published inter-professional guidelines (CDC, 1995). In the US, doctors are advised to offer the test to women and to obtain written consent or refusal in order to avoid litigation. The reasons for refusal must be carefully documented, and the woman advised to have the test on each subsequent visit (Grimes et al., 1999). Some countries, such as France and the Netherlands, have made it mandatory for health professionals to offer the HIV test. Unsurprisingly, uptake in these countries is high (as well as in Sweden and the US). In the UK it is much lower but rising (de Cock and

Johnson, 1998; Nicoll et al., 1998). High uptakes have been followed by a decline in paediatric AIDS (Nicoll et al., 1998; Nicoll and Peckham, 1999).

The latter observation has fuelled the impetus for increasing uptake. In fact, in some places, mandatory testing is favoured in order to guarantee a maximum uptake, and therefore to ensure benefit to the greatest number of babies born from women with HIV. The American Medical Association recently voted in favour of mandatory testing of pregnant women, although mandatory testing is a legal requirement in only a few states such as Texas and New York (Phillips et al., 1997; Sherr, 1999). Phillips et al. (1997) found that in San Francisco the majority of health professionals favoured mandatory antenatal testing. Testing without consent is common (Sherr, 1999). Even some pregnant women favour routine testing without consent, as found, for example in Kenya (Marjan and Ruminjo, 1996). It would appear that these women may prefer not to have the burden of choice.

The requirement to provide pre-test counselling has been identified as an obstacle to implementing named testing and to obtaining high uptakes. Counselling implies a client- or patient-centred, non-directive approach, and a specialist counsellor. The counsellor allows the patient to express her beliefs, concerns and expectations. She helps her to identify the priorities and issues, to consider the risks and benefits of testing, and to explore the options available. The patient can then make an informed decision. This process can be time-consuming, expensive, and may not always yield a high acceptance rate from women (Gill et al., 1989; Simpson et al., 1998).

In response to these drawbacks, institutions have recommended a modi-fied approach to pre-test discussion. For example, the UK Intercollegiate Working Party for enhancing voluntary confidential HIV testing in preg-nancy (1998) recommends universal pre-test discussion by *general* staff, and a *directive* rather than non-directive approach. The health professional *rec-ommends*, rather than simply offers, the test. This approach is favoured, as it is believed to save time and resources, and yield a higher uptake. It is more 'cost-effective'. 'Recently a more pragmatic approach has been advocated, in which a focused testing regime – taking less than a third of the time – is used to encourage normalization of the test' (Madge and Singh, 1998).

But can consent remain truly 'voluntary' in the context of universal 'routine' testing? Although the guidelines state that the woman must give her explicit consent, this may be hard to achieve in practice. The reasons for this include the following:
- 'high status coercion' by professionals (see below);
- imposed targets, placing health professionals under duress to maximize uptake;
- multiple tests, creating confusion;
- lack of time and resources to allow a discussion sufficiently detailed for women to understand the nature and purpose of the test.

Health professionals set the agenda with universal or routine testing. Prenatal testing for HIV (and for that matter, other infections and conditions) might well be low down on the list of priorities for women attending the booking clinic.

A health professional occupies a position of authority, and if he or she recommends a test, many women would feel that it is not within their rights to refuse. This is particularly true of women from some ethnic groups (Sherr et al., 1998/99). Sherr (1999: p. 47) defines this as 'high status coercion' which may 'persuade women to accept any number of tests in the belief that her [sic] care may be jeopardised if she refuses'. Brody (1992) highlights the importance of power in the health professional–patient relationship. It is not *what* the midwives tell the women, but *how* they tell them. The strongest factor influencing uptake, excluding the direct offer of a test, has generally been the individual midwife interviewing the woman (Jones et al., 1998; Simpson et al., 1998). Paradoxically, there may be an *inverse* association with women's knowledge of HIV and transmission (Duffy et al., 1998a; Sherr et al., 1998/99). Studies in South Africa (Karim et al., 1998) showed that many women being recruited for therapeutic trials believed that if they refused testing, they would be deprived of antenatal care, or receive substandard care.

These findings reinforce the hypothesis that consent is driven by the health professional's agenda, and that routine testing may not always be fully voluntary. Women most at risk (aside from intravenous drug users) are from high-prevalence areas, particularly from sub-Saharan Africa, and their first language is not English or any other Western language. They are likely to encounter difficulties with language and communication in western countries.

Schott and Henley (1996) quote studies that show that women who speak little or no English are given fewer choices and less information, and that health professionals tend to be paternalistic and insensitive towards them, concluding that: 'They cannot give genuinely informed consent' (Schott and Henley, 1996: p. 78). Sherr et al. (1998/99) showed that ethnic minority women in London, who were sufficiently fluent in English to answer a questionnaire, were significantly less likely to feel that they could refuse the test or to be able to cope with a positive result. Instead they were more likely to feel overwhelmed by the number of tests.

Health professionals should also take into account that individual autonomy is an unknown concept in some cultures. The individual is seen as an integral part of the family or community and a woman has to consult her spouse, or other members of the family, and even elders, before consenting to medical or surgical procedures (Schott and Henley, 1996; Nuffield Council on Bioethics, 1999; de Zulueta, 2001).

The drive to achieve a high uptake places a considerable burden on the midwives to gain consent for testing from the pregnant women. Some health authorities will not provide funding unless specific uptake targets are met (Phillips et al., 1997). In the UK, an uptake of 90 per cent by the year 2002 has been set as a target. But some clinics have had difficulty achieving up-takes of greater than 40 per cent, *despite* a robust universal policy (Duffy et al., 1998b).

Cost-effectiveness studies recommend or rely on short times for pre-test discussion. For example, Ades et al. (1999) suggest an allocation of two to three minutes. Sherr (1999) and Simpson et al. (1999) describe studies in which the time taken for pre-test discussion was less than three minutes. There are no clear guidelines for how long pre-test discussion should take, but it seems unlikely that all the issues referred to can be discussed in such a short time span. For example, the UK guidelines recommend that the following are included in the pre-test discussion: 'This discussion should ensure that the woman understands the purpose of the test, what it deter-mines, the benefits and problems for herself, her partner and her unborn child of having a test, when the results will be available and that these results are confidential' (Department of Health, 1994: p. 2). The CDC guidelines recommend discussion of these and other issues (CDC, 1995). American authors (e.g. Phillips et al., 1997) also question the likelihood of all the relevant issues being adequately discussed in less than five minutes. They point out the conflicts for the health professionals in providing an 'ideal' pre-test counselling practice with 'the time and cost constraints of busy practices and managed care plans'. These constraints provide the underlying rationale for shorter and shorter time allowed for pre-test briefing or coun-selling.

In the UK, and elsewhere, HIV testing is done in the booking clinic alongside several other prenatal tests, such as testing for syphilis, indicators for Down's syndrome, and early ultrasound scans. The sheer volume of issues to consider is likely to cause confusion. Some tests, for example, for Down's syndrome, are done with the implicit understanding that if they prove positive, the mother is expected to have an abortion. Women who are against abortion may decide against HIV testing for this reason, not realizing that the option of treatment is available (Schott and Henley, 1996).

Macquart-Moulin et al. (1995) point out how testing only women for HIV diverges from the approach usually taken in clinical genetics, where testing for a genetic condition is requested by a couple, both of whom are present during the consultation. They suggest following the latter practice, as the fetus is also placed at risk if the mother's partner is infected.

The greatest ethical difficulty with a routine universal testing policy is that women may believe that they have not got the choice to refuse. The empirical studies highlight the difficulty for the health professionals in delivering a culturally sensitive policy, whilst not depriving an at-risk group of advice which may be of particular value and relevance. Voluntary testing can easily slide into mandatory or near-mandatory testing. Translating policy into practice may distort the process of consent and disempower patients. Indeed Bennett believes that 'routine testing clearly involves a certain amount of coercion' (Bennett, 1999: p. 230).

Some would question how much the individual's right to make a choice should be respected if this autonomy jeopardizes the future of the next generation. It can be argued that the women are hiding their heads in the sand, for sooner or later the disease will manifest itself, and they will have lost opportunities for themselves and their offspring. But, as I have shown, for some women at high risk, the immediate threats may be more compelling, and for some women at low risk, HIV testing may be a fraught domain that they do not wish to enter. 'Doctors give medical guidance as to the optimal course of action but must also recognise that patients' responses will not be formed solely on the basis of clinical data but by their circumstances, needs, rational conclusions and irrational emotions' (British Medical Association, Ethics, Science and Information Division, 1993: p. 3). Women should be allowed to balance the harms and benefits, and not be steamrollered into accepting. A balance needs to be struck (de Zulueta and Sheikh, 1999).

Confidentiality and disclosure to third parties

The UK guidelines strongly recommend that confidentiality issues 'must be strictly maintained' (UK Intercollegiate Working Party, 1998) and that ante-natal clinics must have in place a confidentiality policy, particularly as obstetric notes are hand-held and may be accessible to other family members. Respecting confidentiality flows from the principle of respecting autonomy – allowing individuals to control disclosure of personal information.

The guidelines, however, do not address the dilemma for the health professional if the woman refuses to inform her partner. For some women, disclosure may have very unfortunate consequences, and they may be very reluctant to inform their partners (Temmerman et al., 1995; Schott and Henley, 1996). Men rarely attend for testing (Ryder et al., 1991). Some women have little control over their husbands' behaviour, and indeed over many aspects of their own lives. To respect autonomy is of little relevance – protection from undue harm may be of greater importance.

If a partner is not already HIV-positive, he may be at a significant risk of being infected, particularly as the couple are highly unlikely to be using barrier contraceptives. It can be argued that *his* autonomy is not being respected, as he is being deprived of information material to his future welfare. A simple measure such as the use of condoms could save him from premature death. It may be difficult to hide the secret information from a partner when a woman and her infant are being given antiviral treatment. If he asks why they are receiving it, should the health professionals maintain the deception?

The UK Central Council on Nursing, Health Visiting and Midwifery (UKCC, 1996) and the General Medical Council (GMC) guidelines (GMC, 1997) permit disclosure, but leave it to the health professional's discretion. The health professional may offer confidentiality, but should point out the difficulties in maintaining it, and the risks to the partner. Sometimes he or she will have to choose between duty to the woman or duty to the partner (Boyd, 1992). The woman should be advised if disclosure is planned.

Therapeutic research in pregnancy: ethical issues in placebo-controlled trials

The 1994 ACTG 076 trial was followed by a number of randomized placebo-controlled trials with pregnant women from developing countries. This research initiative has engendered a major controversy and a deep division in the research community. Angry accusations have been rebutted by equally vehement justifications. Both sides have been accused of 'ethical imperialism'. Perhaps the most disturbing outcome has been the proposal to revise the international codes and guidelines for research.

The randomized controlled trial (RCT) is still considered to be the gold standard for the assessment of effectiveness of a drug or an intervention (Chalmers, 1998), although it has been recognized that other statistical methods, for example that of Bayes, may sometimes be used (Sox et al., 1988). The ethical problems associated with the methodology of the RCT have been extensively discussed (Schafer, 1982; Charlton 1991; Sarah et al., 1998). For a trial to be ethical the researchers must be in a position of equipoise: they do not know which therapy will be the most effective (Freedman, 1987). There must also be valid consent. The patient must not only understand the process of randomization, but also the risks and benefits of treatment and non-treatment, and the treatments currently available.

The ACTG 076 regimen is expensive and relatively cumbersome to use. It is a three-part prophylactic regimen that involves giving oral AZT to the pregnant woman several weeks prior to birth, intravenous AZT during labour and delivery, and an AZT syrup to the infant daily for six weeks after delivery. The regime was developed in France and the USA. It is clearly impractical for use in developing countries, where many women may not present for care until late in pregnancy or even in labour. Birth often does not take place in a medical setting, or even in the presence of trained medical staff. Advanced medical technology is often absent (Graham and Newell, 1999; Mofenson, 1999). In addition, if the treatment is only given to HIV-positive women, then a full-scale HIV testing programme is entailed. This also has serious resource implications. There is clearly a strong rationale to find a shorter, simpler and cheaper (and safe) regimen for universal use in resource-poor countries. Hence the impetus for the controversial placebo-controlled trials.

Lurie and Wolf (1997) identified 15 placebo-controlled trials in developing countries, nine of them sponsored by the US government. They claim that these trials are unethical as they 'seriously disturb the equipoise' (1997: p. 854) and knowingly deprive many infants of potentially life-saving prophylaxis. Lurie and Wolf also argue that the trials contravene existing guidelines – in particular, the Declaration of Helsinki (World Medical Association, 1996) and the international ethical guidelines for biomedical research involving human subjects of the Council for International Organizations of Medical Sciences (1993). They also question the scientific rationale for placebo controls, and suggest equivalency trials, using the best known regimen compared against another: 'We believe that such equivalency studies of alternative antiretroviral regimens will provide even more useful results than placebo-controlled trials, without the deaths of hundreds of newborns that are inevitable if placebo groups are used' (Lurie and Wolf, 1997: p. 854).

Marcia Angell (1997) takes an even more critical stance, comparing some of the placebo-controlled trials to the infamous Tuskegee syphilis experiment (Anonymous, 1992). She maintains, as do Lurie and Wolf, that researchers have an obligation to provide the controls with the best current treatment, rather than the best locally available one. In some countries, the latter may be no treatment at all. To do otherwise, she argues, is to adopt a double standard in research, or an ethical relativism that 'could result in widespread exploitation of vulnerable third world populations for research programmes that could not be carried out in the sponsoring countries' (Angell, 1997: p. 848). She and others challenge the 'slavish adherence to the tenets of clinical trials' (ibid.), whereby subjects are treated merely as a means for the sake of research goals. Even informed consent is insufficient protection, she argues, 'because of the asymmetry of knowledge and authority between researchers and their subjects' (Angell, 1997: p. 847).

The justifications for providing placebo have included the following:
- Firstly, if all the research subjects were treated according to the best standards of care of the USA, this would act as a powerful and coercive incentive for women from poor countries to participate in the trial.
- Secondly, the lack of infrastructure in these countries would prevent the full implementation of the 076 regimen.
- Thirdly, if the criteria are too stringent, those countries in the greatest need are deprived of the benefit – affordable and feasible regimes – arising from the research findings.
- Fourthly, the PACTG 076 trial was undertaken with subjects who did not breast-feed. It is clearly essential to find regimes that are of benefit to women who have to breast-feed for cultural, economic and health-related

reasons (Benatar, 1998; Guay et al., 1999; Wilkinson, Karim and Coovadia, 1999).

- Other more complex arguments centre on the validity and reliability of equivalency studies. (Halsey, 1997; Perinatal HIV Intervention Research in Developing Countries Workshop Participants, 1999), and the risk of anaemia (Halsey, 1997).

In a consensus statement (Perinatal HIV Intervention Research in Developing Countries Workshop, 1999) several researchers – the vast majority from the US – stated: 'Most of us . . . believe that a no-antiretroviral comparison may be ethically justified', in the context where no treatment is available in the country where the research is taking place.

The Nuffield Council on Bioethics, in their discussion paper, proposed an interpretation of principle 11–3 of the Helsinki Declaration (World Medical Association, 1996) such that 'the best proven diagnostic and therapeutic method' is interpreted as meaning 'the best *locally available* diagnostic and therapeutic method' (Nuffield Council on Bioethics, 1999: p. 21). The latter may mean literally nothing in many cases. This proposed interpretation represents more than a mere tinkering at the edges, but a fundamental change.

Yet again we see an abrogation of the duty of care of the physician to the patient. This sits uncomfortably with Article One of the Declaration, which defines the researcher's duty 'to remain the protector of the life and health of that person on whom biomedical research is being carried out'. Permitting subjects to be deprived of benefit may sometimes be justified if the harm is minimal and the benefits commensurably great. But it is hard to extend this justification to the prevention of AIDS in infants, particularly as we are dealing with 'third parties' who cannot consent or protect their own interests. Scientific rigour must always be matched by ethical rigour.

In conclusion, research into the prevention of vertical transmission has engendered a public and acrimonious debate and a schism in the medical profession. Perhaps we are witnessing the clash between an ethic of science firmly rooted in the mechanistic-reductionist or modernist paradigm, and an ethic based on a more humanistic, postmodern worldview. The RCT strives to create order and predictability in a world of chaos and complexity. It can provide us with useful evidence for the benefit of interventions, but, in order to achieve this, it eschews individual concerns, needs and relationships. In other words, it eliminates the 'variables' that make us act as moral agents to one another. The postmodern ethic, on the other hand, allows for the individual voice to be heard and tolerates uncertainty (Bauman, 1993; Hodgkin, 1996; Laugharne, 1999).

The research debate has certainly highlighted the gross inequity in income and health care provision between different countries – 'for reasons not insignificantly related to the exploitative and political policies of powerful nations' (Benatar, 1998: p. 222). Bayer (1994) also makes this point, and speculates whether scientific progress will be matched by compassion from the developed nations. One response to the criticisms – a revision of the research guidelines – may lead to a dangerous shift in the ethical requirements for research, such that research subjects from poor countries could be more readily exploited.

Conclusion

In the process of testing for, researching and treating HIV in pregnancy, a fundamental ethical conflict may arise for professionals between the laudable aim of benefiting the future generation, and the duty to respect women's autonomy and to benefit them as individuals. The violation of this duty may sometimes be justifiable, but at other times it clearly is not. Furthermore, the justifications do not satisfactorily address the importance of trust, intrinsic to the relationship between the health professional and the woman seeking antenatal care.

References

Ades, W.E., Sculpher, M.J., Gibb, D.M. *et al.* (1999). Cost effectiveness analysis of HIV screening in United Kingdom. *British Medical Journal* **319**: 1230–4.

Altman, L.K. (1999). Africa lifts AIDS silence. *International Herald Tribune,* 19 July.

Angell, M. (1997). The ethics of clinical research in the third world. *New England Journal of Medicine* **337**: 847–9.

Anonymous (1988). General Medical Council agrees guidelines on AIDS. *British Medical Journal* **296**: 1613.

Anonymous (1992). Twenty years after: the legacy of the Tuskegee syphilis study. *Hastings Center Report* **22**: 29–40.

Anonymous (1998). AIDS, the unbridgeable gap [Editorial]. *Lancet* **351**: 1825.

Anonymous (1999a). AIDS infects half of all Africa babies. *International Herald Tribune,* 13 September.

Anonymous (1999b). A positive response to perinatal HIV [Editorial]. *Lancet* **353**: 511.

Anonymous (1999c). Making AIDS a business imperative [Editorial]. *Lancet* **354**: 1.

Anonymous (1999d). Infant must have HIV test. *Re C (a child). Bulletin of Medical Ethics* **151**: 7–8.

Anonymous (2000a). Ganging up against AIDS. *International Herald Tribune,* 7 January.

Anonymous (2000b). Politicisation of debate on HIV care in South Africa. *Lancet* **355**: 1473.

Bauman, Z. (1993). *Postmodern Ethics.* Oxford: Blackwell.

Bayer, R. (1994). Ethical challenges posed by zidovudine treatment to reduce vertical transmission of HIV. *New England Journal of Medicine* **331**: 1223–5.

Bayley, A. (2000). Narrowing the gap. *Journal of Medical Ethics* **26**: 51–3.

Benatar, S.R. (1998). Imperialism, research ethics and global health. *Journal of Medical Ethics* **24**: 221–2.

Bennett, R. (1999). Should we routinely test pregnant women for HIV? In *HIV and AIDS, Testing, Screening and Confidentiality,* ed. R. Bennett and C.A. Erin. Oxford: Oxford University Press.

Boyd, K.M. (1990). HIV infection: the ethics of anonymised testing and of testing pregnant women. Institute of Medical Ethics working party report. *Journal of Medical Ethics* **16**: 173–8.

Boyd, K.M. (1992). HIV infection and AIDS: the ethics of medical confidentiality. *Journal of Medical Ethics* **18**: 173–9.

Brazier, M. and Lobjoit, M. (1999). Fiduciary relationship: an ethical approach and a legal concept? In *HIV and AIDS, Testing, Screening and Confidentiality,* ed. R. Bennett and C.A. Erin, pp. 179–99. Oxford: Oxford University Press.

British Medical Association (BMA) (1993). *Medical Ethics Today: Its Practice and Philosophy.* London: BMJ Publishing Group.

Brody, H. (1992). *The Healer's Power.* New Haven: Yale University Press.

Buckman, R. (1996). Talking to patients with cancer. *British Medical Journal,* **313**: 669.

Centres for Disease Control and Prevention (CDC) (1995). U.S. Public Health Service recommendations for human immunodeficiency virus counseling and voluntary testing for pregnant women. *Morbidity and Mortality Weekly Reports* **44**(RR-7): 1–15.

Chalmers, I. (1998). Unbiased, relevant and reliable assessments in health care. *British Medical Journal* **317**: 1167–8.

Charlton, B.G. (1991). Medical practice and the double-blind, randomised controlled trial. *British Journal of General Practice* **41**: 355.

Chatterton v *Gerson* [1981] 1 All ER 257.

Children Act 1989 (U.K.)

Chrystie, I.L., Wolfe, C.D.A., Kennedy, J. *et al.* (1995). Voluntary, named testing for HIV in a community-based antenatal clinic: a pilot study. *British Medical Journal* **311**: 928–31.

Cochrane, J. (2000). Narrowing the gap: access to HIV treatments in developing countries. A pharmaceutical company's perspective. *Journal of Medical Ethics* **26**: 47–50.

Cohn, J.A. (1997). Recent advances: HIV-1 infection. *British Medical Journal* **314**: 487–91.

Connor, E.M., Sperling, R.S., Gelber, R. *et al.* (1994). Reduction of maternal–infant transmission of human immuno-deficiency virus type 1 with zidovudine treatment. *New England Journal of Medicine* **331**: 1173–80.

Corbitt, G. (1999). HIV testing and screening. Current practicalities and future possibilities. In *HIV and AIDS, Testing, Screening and Confidentiality,* ed. R. Bennett and C.A. Erin, pp. 21–38. Oxford: Oxford University Press.

Council for International Organizations of Medical Sciences (CIOMS) (1993). *International Ethical Guidelines for Biomedical Research involving Human Subjects.*

Geneva: World Health Organization.

Dabis, F., Msellati, P., Meda, N. *et al.* (1999). 6-month efficacy, tolerance, and acceptability of a short regimen of oral zidovudine to reduce vertical transmission of HIV in breastfed children in Côte d'Ivoire and Burkina Faso: a double blind placebo-controlled multicentre trial. *Lancet* **353**: 786–92.

de Cock, K.M. (1997). Guidelines for managing HIV infection. *British Medical Journal* **315**: 1–2.

de Cock, K.M. and Johnson, A.M. (1998). From exceptionalism to normalisation: a reappraisal of attitudes and practice around HIV testing. *British Medical Journal* **316**: 290–2.

Department of Health and the Central Office of Information (1989). *If You Are Having a Blood Test...* London: HMSO.

Department of Health (1994). *Guidelines for Offering Voluntary Named HIV Antibody Testing to Women Receiving Antenatal Care.* London: Stationery Office.

Department of Health (1997). *Prevalence of HIV in England and Wales in 1996. Annual Report of the Unlinked Anonymous Prevalence Monitoring Programme.* London: Stationery Office.

Department of Health (1999). *HIV and Infant Feeding. Guidance from the UK Chief Medical Officers' Expert Advisory Group on AIDS.* London: Stationery Office.

de Zulueta, P. (2000a). The ethics of anonymised HIV testing of pregnant women: a reappraisal. *Journal of Medical Ethics* **26**: 16–21.

de Zulueta, P. (2000b). The ethics of anonymised HIV testing of pregnant women: a reappraisal. Reply to commentary. *Journal of Medical Ethics* **26**: 25–6.

de Zulueta, P. (2001). Randomised placebo-controlled trials and HIV-infected pregnant women in developing countries: ethical imperialism or unethical exploitation? *Bioethics* **15**(4): 289–311.

de Zulueta, P. and Sheikh, A. (1999). Antenatal screening for HIV [Letter]. *Journal of the Royal Society of Medicine* **92**: 545,

Duffy, T.A., Wolfe, C.D.A., Varden, C. *et al.* (1998a). Women's knowledge and attitudes, and the acceptability of voluntary antenatal HIV testing. *British Journal of Obstetrics and Gynaecology* **105**: 54.

Duffy, T.A., Wolfe, C.D.A., Varden, C. *et al.* (1998b). Antenatal testing: current problems, future solutions. Survey of uptake in one London hospital. *British Medical Journal* **316**: 270–1.

Duke, L. (1999). Culture contributes to crisis where AIDS is seen as a bewitching. Ignorance expands South Africa epidemic. *International Herald Tribune*, 17 February.

Dunn, D., Newell, M.L., Ades, W.E. and Peckham, C.S. (1992). Risk of human immunodeficiency virus type 1 transmission through breastfeeding. *Lancet* **340**: 585–8.

European Mode of Delivery Collaboration (1999). Elective caesarean section versus vaginal delivery in prevention of vertical HIV-1 transmission: a randomised clinical trial. *Lancet* **353**: 1035–9.

Evans, J.S., Marriage, S.C., Walters, M.D.S. and Levin, M. (1995). Unsuspected HIV infection presenting itself in the first year of life. *British Medical Journal* **310**: 1235–6.

Fawzi, W.W., Msamanga, G.I., Spiegelman, D. *et al.* (1998). Randomised trial of effects of vitamin supplements on pregnancy outcomes and T cell counts in HIV-1-infected women in Tanzania. *Lancet* **351**: 1477–82.

Freedman, B. (1987). Equipoise and the ethics of clinical research. *New England Journal of Medicine* **317**: 141–5.

General Medical Council (GMC) (1997). *Serious Communicable Diseases. Protecting Patients, Guiding Doctors.* London: GMC.

Gibb, D.M., MacDonagh, S.E., Tookey, P.A. *et al.* (1997). Uptake of interventions to reduce mother-to-infant transmission of HIV in the United Kingdom and Ireland. *AIDS* **11**: F53–8.

Gibb, D.M., MacDonagh, S.E., Gupta, R. *et al.* (1998). Factors affecting uptake of antenatal HIV testing in London: results of a multicentre study. *British Medical Journal* **316**: 259–61.

Gill, O.N., Adler, M.W. and Day, N.E. (1989). Regular review: monitoring the prevalence of HIV. *British Medical Journal* **299**: 1295–8.

Graham, W.J. and Newell, M.-L. (1999). Seizing the opportunity: collaborative initiatives to reduce HIV and maternal mortality. *Lancet* **353**: 836–9.

Grimes, R.M., Richards, E.P., Helfgott, A.W. and Eriksen, N.L. (1999). Legal considerations in screening women for human immunodeficiency virus. *American Journal of Obstetrics and Gynaecology* **180**: 259–64.

Grubb, A. and Pearl, D.S. (1990). *HIV Testing and the Law. Blood Testing, AIDS and DNA Profiling. Law and Policy.* Family Law Series. Bristol: Jordan and Sons Ltd.

Guay L.A., Musoke, P., Fleming, T. and Bagenda, D. (1999). Intrapartum and neonatal single-dose nevaripine compared with zidovudine for prevention of mother–child transmission of HIV-1 in Kampala, Uganda: HIVNET 012 randomised trial. *Lancet* **35**: 795–802.

Halsey, N. (1997). Ethics and international research. *British Medical Journal* **315**: 965–6.

Hawken, J., Chard, T., Costeloe, K. *et al.* (1995). Risk identification for HIV infection overlooked on routine antenatal care. *Journal of the Royal Society of Medicine* **88**: 634–6.

Heath, R.W., Grint, P.C.A. and Hardiman, W.E. (1988). Anonymous testing of women attending the antenatal clinics for evidence of infection with HIV. *Lancet* **1**: 1394.

Hodgkin, P. (1996). Medicine, postmodernism and the end of certainty. *British Medical Journal* **313**: 1568–9.

Hudson, C.N., Bergenstroem, A. and Bell, E. (1999). The dilemma of antenatal HIV testing: what goes on in the European Community? *Journal of the Royal Society of Medicine* **92**: 273–6.

Jones, S., Sadler, T., Low, N. *et al.* (1998). Does uptake of antenatal HIV testing depend on the individual midwife? *British Medical Journal* **316**: 272–3.

Kahtan, S. (1993). Anonymous testing misleads patient [Letter]. *British Medical Journal* **306**: 1479.

Karim, Q.W., Karim S.S.W., Coovadia, H.M. and Susser, M. (1998). Informed consent for HIV testing in a South African Hospital: is it truly informed and voluntary? *American Journal of Public Health* **88**: 637–40.

Kennedy, I. and Grubb, A. (1994). *Medical Law Text and Materials,* 2nd edn. London: Butterworths.

Laugharne, R. (1999). Evidence-based medicine, user involvement and the post-modern paradigm. *Psychiatric Bulletin* **23**: 641–3.

Lurie, M.P.H. and Wolfe, S.M. (1997). Unethical trials of interventions to reduce perinatal transmission of human immunodeficiency virus in developing countries. *New England Journal of Medicine* **337**: 853–6.

Lyall, E.G.H., Stainsby, C., Taylor, G.P. and Ait-Khaled, M. (1998). Review of uptake of interventions to reduce mother to child transmission of HIV by women aware of their HIV status. *British Medical Journal* **316**: 268–70.

Madge, S., and Singh, S. (1998). The new imperative to test for HIV in pregnancy. *British Journal of General Practice* **48**: 1127–8.

Malloch Brown, M. (2000). Africa' s AIDS disaster is everybody's problem. *International Herald Tribune,* 12 January.

Manuel, C. (1999). HIV screening: benefits and harms to the individual and the community. In *HIV and AIDS, Testing, Screening and Confidentiality,* ed. R. Bennett and C.A. Erin, pp. 61–74. Oxford: Oxford University Press.

Maquart-Moulin, G., Hairon, D., Auqier, P. and Manuel, C. (1995). Vertical transmission of HIV – a rediscussion of testing. *AIDS Care* **7**: 657–62.

Marjan, R.S.R. and Ruminjo, J.K. (1996). Attitudes to prenatal testing and notification for HIV infection in Nairobi, Kenya. *East African Medical Journal* **17**: 665–9.

Marseille, E., Kahn, J.G., Mmiro, F. *et al.* (1999). Cost effectiveness of single-dose nevirapine regimen for mothers and babies to decrease vertical HIV-1 transmission in sub-Saharan Africa. *Lancet* **354**: 803–9.

McGreal, C. (1999). 'This is worse than Apartheid'. *Guardian,* 16 March.

McCullough, L.B. and Chervanak, F.A. (1994). *Ethics in Obstetrics and Gynaecology.* New York: Oxford University Press.

Mercey, D. (1998). Antenatal HIV testing. *British Medical Journal* **316**: 241–2.

Mofenson, L.M. (1999). Short-course zidovudine for prevention of perinatal infection. *Lancet* **353**: 766–7.

Newell, M-L., Gray, G. and Bryson, Y.J. (1997). Prevention of mother-to-child transmission of HIV-infection. *AIDS* **11** (Suppl. A): 165–72.

Nicoll, A., McGarrigle, C., Brady, A.R. *et al.* (1998). Epidemiology and detection of HIV-1 among pregnant women in the United Kingdom: results from national surveillance. *British Medical Journal* **316**: 253–8.

Nicoll, A. and Peckham, C. (1999). Reducing vertical transmission of HIV in the UK. *British Medical Journal* **319**: 1211–12.

Noone, A. and Goldberg, D. (1997). Antenatal HIV testing: what now? *British Medical Journal* **314**: 1429–30.

Novack, D.H., Plumer, R., Smith, R.I. *et al.* (1979). Changes in physicians' attitudes toward telling the cancer patient. *Journal of the American Medical Association* **2412**: 897–900.

Nuffield Council on Bioethics (1999). *The Ethics of Clinical Research in Developing Countries – A Discussion Paper.* London: Nuffield Council of Bioethics.

Pekham, C.S., Tedder, R.S., Briggs, M. and Ades W.E. (1990). Prevalence of maternal HIV infection based on unlinked anonymous testing of newborn babies. *Lancet,* **335**: 516–19.

Peckham, C. and Gibb, D. (1995). Mother-to-child transmission of the human immunodeficiency virus. *New England Journal of Medicine* **333**: 298–302.

Pellegrino, E.D. and Thomasma, D.C. (1988). *For the Patient's Good. The Restoration of Beneficence in Health Care.* New York: Oxford University Press.

Perinatal HIV Intervention Research in Developing Countries Workshop Participants (1999). Science, ethics and the future of research into maternal infant transmission of HIV-1. Consensus statement. *Lancet* **353**: 832–5.

Phillips K.A., Morrison, K.I., Sonnad, S.S. and Bleeker, T. (1997). HIV counseling and testing of pregnant women and women of childbearing age by primary care providers: self-reported beliefs and practices. *Journal of Acquired Immune Deficiency Syndromes and Human Retrovirology* **14**: 174–8.

Pinching, A.J. (2000). The ethics of anonymised HIV testing of pregnant women: a reappraisal. Commentary. *Journal of Medical Ethics* **26**: 22–4.

Postma, M.J., Beck, E.J., Mandalia, S. *et al.* (1999). Universal HIV screening of pregnant women in England: cost effectiveness analysis. *British Medical Journal* **318**: 1656–60.

Richards, E.P. III. (1999). HIV testing, screening, and confidentiality: an American perspective. In *HIV and AIDS, Testing, Screening and Confidentiality*, ed. R. Bennett and C.A. Erin, pp. 75–90. Oxford: Oxford University Press.

Richardson, M.P. and Sharland, M. (1998). Late diagnosis of paediatric HIV in south west London. *British Medical Journal* **316**: 271–2.

Ryder, R., Batter, M. and Nsuami, M. (1991). Fertility rates in 239 HIV-1 sero-positive women in Zaire followed for 3 years post-partum. *AIDS* **5**: 1521–7.

Sarah, J.L., Edwards, R.J., Lilford, J. and Hewison, J. (1998). The ethics of randomised controlled trials from the perspectives of patients, the public and healthcare professionals. *British Medical Journal* **317**: 1209–12.

Scarlatti, G. (1996). Paediatric HIV infection. *Lancet* **348**: 863–7.

Schafer, A. (1982). The ethics of the randomised clinical trial. *New England Journal of Medicine* **307**: 719–24.

Schott, J. and Henley, A. (1996). *Culture, Religion and Childbearing in a Multiracial Society. A Handbook for Health Professionals.* Oxford: Butterworth-Heinemann.

Sherr, L. (1999). Counselling and HIV testing: ethical dilemmas. In *HIV and AIDS, Testing, Screening and Confidentiality*, ed. R. Bennett and C.A. Erin, 39–60. Oxford: Oxford University Press.

Sherr, L., Bergenstroem A., Bell, E. *et al.* (1998/99). The dilemma of antenatal testing: what goes on in the European Community? *Health Trends* **30**: 115–19.

Simpson, W., Johnstone, F., Boyd, F.M. *et al.* (1998). Uptake and acceptability of antenatal testing: randomised controlled trial of different methods of offering the test. *British Medical Journal* **316**: 262–7.

Simpson, W., Johnstone, F.D., Goldberg, D.J. *et al.* (1999). Antenatal testing: assessment of a routine voluntary approach. *British Medical Journal* **318**: 1660–1.

Soderland N., Zwi, K., Kinghorn, A. and Gray, G. (1999). Prevention of vertical transmission of HIV: analysis of cost effectiveness options available in South Africa. *British Medical Journal* **318**: 1650–6.

Sox, H.C. Blatt, M.A., Higgins, M.C. and Marton, K.I. (1988). *Medical Decision Making.* Boston: Butterworth-Heineman.

Temmerman M., Ndinya-Achola J., Amabani, J. and Piot, P. (1995). The right not to know HIV test results. *Lancet* **345**: 969–70.

Thorne, C., Newell, M.-L., Dunn, D. and Peckham, C. (1996). Characteristics of pregnant HIV-infected women in Europe. European Collaborative Study. *AIDS Care* **8**: 33–42.

Tudor-Williams, G. and Lyall, E.G.H. (1999). Mother to infant transmission of HIV. *Current Opinion in Infectious Diseases* **12**: 21–6.

UK Intercollegiate Working Party for Enhancing Voluntary Confidential HIV Testing in Pregnancy (1998). *Reducing Mother to Child Transmission of HIV Infection in the United Kingdom*. London: Royal College of Paediatrics and Child Health.

United Kingdom Central Council for Nursing, Midwifery and Health Visiting (UKCC) (1996). *Guidelines for Professional Practice*. London: UKCC.

UNAIDS (1998a). *Report on the Global HIV/AIDS Epidemic*. Geneva: United Nations.

UNAIDS (1998b). *HIV and Infant Feeding*. Geneva: UN Children's Fund and World Health Organization.

UNAIDS. (1999). *Report on the Global HIV/AIDS Epidemic*. Geneva: United Nations.

Verkaik, R. (1999). Judge orders baby to be HIV tested. *Independent*, 4 September.

Wade, N.A., Birkhead, G.S., Warren, W.L. *et al.* (1998). Abbreviated regimens of zidovudine prophylaxis and perinatal transmission of HIV. *New England Journal of Medicine* **339**: 1409–14.

Wiktor, S.Z., Ekpini, E., Karon, J.M., Nkensagong, J. *et al.* (1999). Short-course oral zidovudine for prevention of mother-to-child transmission of HIV-1 in Abidjan, Cote d'Ivoire: a randomised trial. *Lancet* **353**: 781–5.

Wilkinson, D., Karim, S.S.A. and Coovadia, H.M. (1999). Short course antiretroviral regimens to reduce maternal transmission of HIV. *British Medical Journal* **318**: 479–50.

World Medical Association (1996). *World Medical Association Declaration of Helsinki: Recommendations Guiding Physicians in Biomedical Research involving Human Subjects*. Adopted by the 18th World Medical Assembly, Helsinki, Finland, June 1964. Amended by the 29th World Medical Assembly, Tokyo, Japan, October 1975; 35th World Medical Assembly, Venice, Italy, October 1983; 41st World Medical Assembly, Hong Kong, September 1989 and the 48th World Medical Assembly, Somerset West, Republic of South Africa, October 1996. Reproduced in *Journal of the American Medical Association* **277**: 925–6.

5

Genetic screening: should parents seek to perfect their children genetically?

Rosemarie Tong

Department of Philosophy. University of North Carolina at Charlotte, Charlotte, USA

As the Human Genome Project nears completion, our knowledge about genes linked to human diseases and defects is growing at a dramatic rate. It is already possible to test embryos for several conditions at the pre-implantation stage (through pre-embryo biopsy) and to test fetuses for even more conditions during the course of their gestation (through amniocentesis, chorionic villus sampling and umbilical cord blood sampling) (Robertson, 1994: pp. 155–60). At present, pre-implantation and prenatal screenings focus on severe genetic diseases (Strong, 1997: p. 137). In the near future, however, there will be increased ability to test for mild diseases, late-onset diseases, treatable diseases, propensities for common diseases, and even non-disease characteristics such as longevity, height and body-build (Strong, 1997: p. 137).

Although genetic knowledge of this type may strike us as an unalloyed blessing, ethicists worry that such information might fuel parents' increasing desire for perfect progeny. Up until very recently, parents could not do much to guarantee for themselves the child of their dreams. At most, if their moral views permitted, they could discard a pre-embryo or abort a fetus that tested positive for a relatively small range of genetic maladies, such as Tay–Sachs disease, Down's syndrome and Fragile X (Robertson, 1996). However, as soon as safe, effective and beneficial genetic therapies for embryos and fetuses are developed, parents will have the option of repairing or changing rather than destroying their progeny, an option bound to please those who believe that human life should be protected from the moment of conception onwards (Mehlman and Botkin, 1998: pp. 55–87). But the availability of gene therapy will produce in its wake a new set of ethical issues, no less serious than the ones currently preoccupying us. Some people will not want to use gene therapy for any reason whatsoever, claiming it is too risky, unpredictable or 'unnatural'. Others will argue that gene therapy should be used, but for *therapeutic* purposes only (i.e. for the elimination of genetic diseases and defects). Still others will insist that provided it works well, gene therapy should be available for *non-therapeutic* or enhancement purposes (i.e. for the 'engineering' of a better-than-normal child) as well as for therapeutic purposes (Parens, 1998).

Since it is the position of this last group of people that most concerns us, the question I wish to pose is this. Assuming the successful development of a wide range of safe and efficacious genetic therapies, should parents be encouraged to perfect their children through genetic means – as well as traditional environmental means such as education? To this query many people will, I suppose, answer with an immediate 'yes'. They will reason that parents should do everything in their power to enhance their children. Specifically, parents should begin by striving to create the best possible uterine environment for their progeny. In particular, pregnant women should refrain from drinking alcohol, smoking tobacco and ingesting a wide range of illicit and licit drugs during pregnancy (Matthieu, 1996: pp. 9–11). As prenatal gene therapies develop, pregnant women should also permit physicians to penetrate their bodies, more or less invasively, in order to treat their fetuses' genetic maladies or simply to improve upon their genetic endowments. Finally, parents should provide their children with as many safe, effective and beneficial postnatal genetic and environmental enhancement therapies as they can reasonably afford. After all, isn't it only right for parents to provide their children with such opportunities?

Conceding that the above line of reasoning sounds level-headed and enlightened, I none the less fear its darker side. Do parents really have a right and duty to 'perfect' their children genetically, including their already normal children? For that matter, do parents really have a right and duty to 'perfect' their children environmentally? In this chapter, I will argue that although parents have a limited right to enhance their already normal children genetically, and, conceivably, also a limited duty to do so, they should not be encouraged to do so. Indeed, society should actively discourage parents' quests to 'make' perfect babies (Kass, 1985). It should do so, however, not through legal bans or prohibitions on the development of genetic therapies, but through: (1) the development of practice guidelines for health care researchers and practitioners specializing in genetic screening, testing, diagnosis, counselling and therapy; and, even more importantly, (2) the creation of democratic fora designed to achieve some sort of public consensus about the extent of parents' procreative and rearing rights.

Do parents have a right to enhance their children genetically?

The US lawyer John A. Robertson has analysed in great detail parents' *rights* to select their offspring's characteristics (Robertson, 1994: p. 152). As Robertson sees it, the specific right to select offspring characteristics is linked to two more general rights: (1) a parent's right *not to procreate* children because of the more or less burdensome aspects (physical, psychological and social) of reproduction; and (2) a parent's right *to procreate* a child with particular characteristics (e.g., a child who will resemble his or her parents, or a 'normal' child). This second right derives from 'the great importance to individuals of having biologic offspring – personal meaning in one's life, connection with future generations, and the pleasures of child rearing' (Robertson, 1994: p. 153). Since negative selection activities (carrier screening, pre-implantation screening, prenatal screening and abortion) and positive selection activities (therapeutic ex utero or in utero genetic manipulation) enable parents to select offspring traits, Robert-son views these activities as protected by a person's procreative liberty.

Robertson notes, however, that like all rights, procreative rights are limited. They protect 'only actions designed to enable a couple to have *normal, healthy* offspring whom they intend to rear' (Robertson, 1994: p. 166). Actions that aim to produce offspring who are supernormal (enhancement), subnormal (intentional diminution) or clones, says Robertson, 'deviate too far from the experiences that make reproduction a valued experience' to be protected by procreation liberty rights. However, some of these non-therapeutic actions – those aimed at enhancement – might be viewed as part of 'parental discretion in rearing offspring' (Robertson, 1994: p. 167). Parents presently seek to improve their children in a variety of ways. For example, many parents send their children to the best schools, give them music, art and drama lessons, have their teeth straightened, and so on. Some parents go much farther than this, however. In the name of 'bettering' their children, parents submit their children to sex-alignment operations, certain cosmetic surgeries, growth-hormone treatments, Ritalin therapy and multiple doses of Prozac. So long as parents can show that such interventions are safe, effective and beneficial, state authorities will not interfere with parents' child-rearing activities. Given that this is the case, Robertson reasons that state authorities are not likely to interfere with genetic *enhancement* interventions, although they would be likely to interfere with genetic *diminution* interventions.

Implicit in Robertson's view is the idea that, ordinarily, enhancement of a fetus is beneficial, but that diminution of a fetus is harmful. Robertson's ideas about what constitutes a harm seem to be roughly equivalent to those of Norman Daniels, who views as harmful any actions that detract from so-called species-typical functioning (Daniels, 1986: p. 28). If it is typical for the human species that its members be able to hear and see, for example, deliberately deafening or blinding a fetus is harmful to the fetus. But the question remains whether, according to Daniels's view, actions that *add* to species-typical functioning are also harmful. My reading of Daniels's arguments suggests that, on the contrary, he would view such actions as beneficial. So long as every member of the species can do what is typical for the species reasonably well, it matters not that some members of the species can do it exceptionally well. In fact, it might be a good thing if every member of the species could be a 'peak performer'.

Given the reasonability of Robertson's and Daniels's implied positions on enhancement, it is difficult to identify what might, in the end, be harmful about enhancing one's progeny. Interestingly, in the course of explaining why it would be wrong for deaf parents, who view deafness as a valuable culture rather than a disability, to use genetic therapy prenatally to ensure deaf children for themselves, the lawyer Dena Davis (1997) provides some clues. Davis concedes that since people have different ideas about what counts as an enhancement and what counts as a diminution, deaf parents, wishing to ensure deaf children for themselves, might reasonably argue that the lifestyle in the deaf community is a good one for children – indeed, according to Lennard Davis (1995), a better one than the lifestyle for children in the non-deaf community. In essence, deaf parents might argue in the manner Amish parents argue when they defend their practice of limiting their children to an elementary school education on the grounds that further formal education interferes with the Amish system of home-based vocational training – i.e. learning from your parents how to live a simple, 'God-fearing, agrarian life' (*Wisconsin* v. *Yoder*, 1972).

Although the majority of US society believes that it is the prerogative of parents to shape the values and lives of their children, comments Dena Davis, they still think that it is wrong for Amish parents, for example, to confine their children to the Amish community before these children are mature enough to decide for themselves whether such a small world is the best world for themselves. Davis notes that by depriving their children of the opportunity to secure a high-school diploma, Amish parents virtually ensure 'that their children will remain housewives and agricultural laborers' (Davis, D., 1997: p. 565). An Amish child who rebels against the Amish way of life for one reason or another will find himself or herself without the basic education he or she needs to be anything other than an agricultural labourer or housewife. In Davis's estimation, the parents of this child will have *harmed* him or her by substantially limiting their child's presumed right to control the course of his or her own destiny. Davis then reasons that if Amish parents harm their children by denying them educational opportunities, the lack of which will set them back considerably in the larger, non-Amish community should they decide to enter it, deaf parents would even more egregiously harm their children by using genetic diminution therapies to deprive them permanently of their ability to hear. Davis (1997: pp. 569–70) comments:

[D]eliberately creating a child who will be forced irreversibly into the parents' notion of 'the good life' violates the Kantian principle of treating each person as an end in herself and never as a means only. All parenthood exists as a balance between fulfilment of parental hopes and values and the individual flowering of the actual child in his or her own direction... Parental practices which close exits virtually forever are insufficiently attentive to the child as an end in herself. By closing off the child's right to an open future, they deprive the child as an entity who exists to fulfill parental hopes and dreams, not his own.

Although Davis's arguments are directed against the practice of genetic diminution, the crucial question to ask for our purposes is whether genetically enhancing a child 'closes' or 'opens' doors for him or her. On the one hand, it seems that an enhanced child might have a more open future than a 'normal' child. For example, a person with exceptional intellectual capabilities has the opportunity to pursue a much wider range of career options than a person with minimal intellectual capabilities. On the other hand, an enhanced child might have a future more closed than a 'normal' child if, for example, his parents enhanced his intellectual and rational capacities to such a degree that his physical and emotional capacities shrivelled. There is historical precedent for such a concern. Using simply environmental means (education), John Stuart Mill's father, for example, overdeveloped his son's rational and philosophical talents, and underdeveloped his son's emotional and poetic talents. As a result, John Stuart Mill suffered a mental breakdown as a young adult (Mill, 1956). Clearly, as in the case of parents who argue that they have a right to discipline, educate and medically treat their children as they see fit, parents who argue that they have a right to alter their children genetically as they see fit are subject to state interference if their actions prove harmful to their offspring. Parents do not have a right to harm their children, whether this harm consists in physical or psychological abuse, or in using genetic therapy to determine their children's future.

Do parents have a duty to enhance their children genetically?

The fact that parents have a limited right to enhance their children genetically does not mean they have a duty to do so, unless the term 'enhancement' is interpreted to include not only instances of making normal children better than normal, but also instances of making less-than-normal children normal (Juengst, 1998). Specifically, if the necessary gene therapies were available, parents might have a limited duty to provide their offspring with what LeRoy Walters and Julie Gage Palmer term 'health-related' physical, intellectual and moral genetic enhancements, but not also with 'non-health-related' ones (Walters and Palmer, 1997: pp. 109–11). Among those health-related enhancements listed by Walters and Palmer are eliminating the genes associated with deleterious physical, intellectual and psychiatric conditions. Since health-related enhancements are calculated to bring abnormal individuals up to species-typical functioning only, they are, according to Walters and Palmer, to be distinguished from non-health-related genetic enhancements intended to improve normal individuals who already meet the criteria for species-typical physical, intellectual and psychiatric functioning. Among these non-health-related enhancements, Walters and Palmer include gene-mediated growth hormone treatment for short-statured children who are not growth hormone deficient, increasing the efficiency of long-term memory and otherwise improving the cognitive functioning of people who already fall in normal intelligence ranges, and, as a matter of speculation, stimulation of 'friendliness' genes in non-sociopathic persons. Whether Walters and Palmer have drawn the line between health-related and non-health-related enhancements correctly is not the issue here, since some such division is plausible enough (Frankford, 1998). Here, the issue is whether parents really have a duty to use gene therapy to make their less-than-normal children normal. One way to approach this issue is to reflect on the debate between those who think that parents have a duty to use contraceptives, sterilization procedures or abortion to prevent the birth of a so-called defective child and those who do not.

Proponents of *not* procreating persons who fall substantially short of 'species-typical functioning' argue that it can be emotionally and economically draining to raise less-than-normal children, especially if they have a serious genetic disease. Furthermore, they argue it is not in the best interests of such children that they should be brought into existence. In this connection, the feminist philosopher Laura Purdy (1996: p. 58) has stated:

When I look into my heart to see what it says about this matter, I see, I admit, emotions I would rather not feel – reluctance to face the burdens society must bear, unease in the presence of some disabled persons. But most of all, what I see there are demands of love: to love someone is to care desperately about their welfare and to want for them only *good* things. The thought that I might bring to life a child with serious mental problems when I could, by doing something different, bring forth one without them, is utterly incomprehensible to me.

Purdy believes it can be wrong to bring into the world a child with a serious genetic disease or defect. She would prefer, however, that this type of child should never be conceived rather than it should be aborted subsequent to conception. Purdy argues, first, that since a non-existent entity can neither be harmed nor deprived of the kind of rights only existent entities have, it is not wrong to prevent its conception. Second, she argues that people ought to have children only if they can provide them with a normal opportunity for a good life. Thus, Purdy concludes that because of what most people presumably desire – namely, to nurture and love children who will flourish and live so-called good lives – carriers for genetic disorders which preclude a normal opportunity for a good life should not procreate with their own gametes.

Critics of Purdy's statement express concern that her view reinforces the view of those who long for a society in which only perfect or nearly perfect people are tolerated, precisely the kind of society which the 'imperfects' among us should fear. The fact that our society is routinizing and normalizing genetic screening is, according to these critics, a sign that our society might have eugenic aspirations after all. Although in the past, clinicians recommended prenatal screening only for women over 35 years of age, women or couples carrying genes for genetic disorders, and women or couples who had previously procreated a child with a genetic disorder, they now offer amniocentesis to women under 35 upon request (Asch, 1995: p. 387). Increasingly, pregnant women feel that they have not simply a right to this kind of information, but a duty to get it and seriously to consider aborting their fetus in the event of serious genetic disease.

The bioethicist Adrienne Asch is worried about society's growing tendency to view not only genetic disabilities such as anencephaly, Tay–Sachs disease, Hunter's syndrome and certain other conditions that cause degeneration and death within the first months or years of life (Asch, 1995: p. 386), but also non-fatal genetic maladies such as Down's syndrome, spina bifida, cystic fibrosis and muscular dystrophy, as reasons to terminate a pregnancy. Asch believes that women should think long and hard before deciding to abort their less-than-normal fetuses. She claims that there is no significant moral difference between a woman deciding to abort her fetus because the man with whom she planned to rear the child has suddenly decided to divorce her, and a woman deciding to abort her fetus because it has a limb deformity. In other words, as Asch sees it, it is one thing to abort one's fetus because of something 'wrong' with one's own life circumstances, and quite another to abort one's fetus because of something 'wrong' about it. Asch also claims that if it is unacceptable to abort a normal fetus simply because it is the 'wrong' sex, for example, it is also unacceptable to abort a less-than-normal fetus simply because it has a genetic malady. Asch insists if it is wrong to abort a normal fetus solely because it is female, because doing so sends to women and girls the message that they are not valued as highly as males, then it is also wrong to abort a fetus solely on account of its genetic malady, because doing so sends to persons with genetic maladies the message that they are not valued as highly as persons without genetic maladies. Ableism, says Asch, is no less harmful than sexism.

Since it is all too easy to cross the line that supposedly separates the 'bad' eugenics of the past from the 'good' genomics of the present (Pernick, 1996: pp. 159–66), I am inclined to agree with the view that parents have no moral duty to *abort* their less-than-normal fetuses unless their fetuses' genetic maladies are incompatible with leading a meaningful life – i.e. a reasonably happy and productive life. Nevertheless, I am also inclined to think that should gene therapies be developed for conditions such as Down's syndrome, for example, parents would have a moral duty to use them to treat a fetus or child affected with Down's. Parents who would not avail themselves of such an opportunity would have a difficult time justifying their omission as being in the best interests of their progeny. Disability is not a good in itself. Rather, it is something with which all human beings, to a greater or lesser degree, must cope, so that they can discover or shape meaning for themselves within its limitations.

But even if it is reasonable to argue that parents might have a duty to provide their less-than-normal fetuses and children with genetic therapies intended to make them normal, I do not think it is also reasonable to argue that parents have an equivalent duty to provide their already normal fetuses and children with genetic therapies intended to make them supernormal or extraordinary. Although society praises parents who take care of their children, it does not believe that parents have an obligation to lavish all of their resources on their children to the extent of 'spoiling' their children with too many of society's goods and services. On the contrary, society believes that parents have a right to spend or not spend their resources on their children, so long as they do not abuse or neglect their children. Thus, it is not wrong for a mother to spend money on dancing lessons for herself instead of for her child, so long as she does not, for example, spend the family's entire food, clothing, rent and health care budget at the Arthur Murray Dance Studio. It is wrong for a mother to spend money on luxuries for herself, if by doing so, she deprives her children of basic necessities. A similar line of reasoning would fit the case of genetic therapies intended to make one's already normal children somehow 'perfect'. Parents would not be obligated to use their resources to improve on their already normal children, if the parents wished to use these resources for other purposes

Should parents genetically enhance their children?

Assuming, as concluded in the two previous sections, that although parents do not have a duty to use genetic therapy to improve their already normal children, they have a limited right to do so – should parents be encouraged to exercise this right? To this query the lawyer John Robertson answers that if parents are bent on improving their children, it might be preferable to allow them to do so at the genetic rather than the environmental level. He comments (Robertson, 1994: p. 167) that:

If special tutors and camps, training programs, even the administration of growth hormone to add a few inches to height are within parental rearing discretion, why should genetic interventions to enhance normal offspring traits be any less legitimate? As long as they are safe, effective, and likely to benefit offspring, they would no more impermissibly objectify or commodify offspring than postnatal enhancement efforts do. Indeed, prenatal enhancement might turn out to be preferable because an existing child will not be the immediate object of the effort.

Rather than subjecting an existing child to cosmetic surgery to straighten his or her 'ugly' nose, why not make sure instead that the child is born with an appropriately-shaped nose so that he or she never has to feel badly about his or her 'ugly' nose?

Robertson's point is not to equate all prenatal and postnatal enhancements, nor to imply, for example, that since using Prozac to enhance a child's personality is morally acceptable, then using gene therapy to stimulate a hypothetical 'friendliness' or 'liveliness' gene would also be morally acceptable. Rather, Robertson's point is that pre- and post-birth enhancements should be judged by the same criteria. It remains an open question for Robertson whether parents should try to enhance their children at all, be it at the prenatal or postnatal stage. The crucial issue is the nature and function of the proposed intervention and not its timing. It may be just as wrong or right to use Prozac as a postnatal personality pill as it is to alter a gene for shyness or unfriendliness prenatally.

Among the bioethicists who agree with Robertson that prenatal and postnatal enhancements aimed at one's offspring need to be scrutinized with the same lens is the philosopher Glenn McGee. He makes the case (McGee, 1997: p. 117):

that reproductive genetic enhancement can best be understood within a wider range of other, more mundane parental decisions. The basic choices parents make about schools and nutrition and our ambitions for our offspring are inevitable and appropriate enhancement decisions. The question is not whether but how to enhance the lives and character of our children. All parental enhancements ... are subject to some dangers common to our cultural experiences of parenting. Paying attention to these takes us half the way to understanding why many genetic enhancements may turn out to be a mixed blessing indeed.

McGee (1997: pp. 123–33) claims that parents intent on enhancing their children are prone to sins such as 'calculativeness', 'being overbearing', 'short-sightedness' and 'hasty judgement'. Parents might, for example, choose to enhance traits in their children which society suddenly views as undesirable instead of desirable; or they might become so systematic and rational about improving their children that they deprive themselves and their children of a genuinely *human* parent–child relationship; or they might put so much faith in the power of genetics that they forget the strong role which environment plays in human development; or they might find themselves with a child who, despite all their interventions, still falls short of their expectations. Although such sins are 'not-so-deadly', says McGee, they should nonetheless be avoided by an 'intelligent' and 'cautious' approach to genetic enhancement. Society should, he insists, 'work toward developing protocols and therapies [for genetic enhancement] *experimentally* and *gradually*' (McGee, 1997: p. 132).

Some of McGee's points are reinforced by feminists, such as the philosopher Maggie Little. She worries that parents might be tempted to use genetic therapies as well as environmental therapies, like cosmetic surgery, in order to shape their offspring to fit societal standards of perfection, a largely media-driven set of criteria for human value, and one which reflects some of the worst features of a society that remains racist, sexist, homophobic, ableist, and so on. For example, in a worst-case scenario, African–American parents might request lighter skin for their children, or parents of any race might request thin bodies and blond hair for their daughters. Little views such requests as morally disturbing because 'the norms of appearance at issue are grounded in or get life from a broader system of attitudes and actions that are in fact *unjust*' (Little, 1998: p. 166). For African–Americans to want their children to look more white than black is probably not 'some aesthetic whimsical preference' (Little, 1998). It is more likely a function of a racist history in which being black is devalued and being white is valorized. Similarly, for parents to want their daughters to look like fashion models or movie stars is probably not some aesthetic whimsical preference either, but more likely, a function of a sexist history in which being an obese woman is penalized economically and emotionally, and being a thin woman is re-warded. Rather than welcoming and encouraging diversity and change, many genetic enhancement activities would, in Little's estimation, aim instead for homogeneity and the further ossification of the unjust status quo.

Concerns about justice also occupy Maxwell Mehlman and Jeffrey Botkin in their analyses of genetic technologies, including those aimed at enhancement. As they see it, most of these technologies, but particularly enhancement therapies, will be accessible only to those parents who have insurance coverage, or who can afford to pay for them out-of-pocket. Mehlman and Botkin (1998: p. 99) speculate that, as a result of this situation, society will be divided into two classes: a 'genetic aristocracy' and a 'genetic underclass.' They comment that the former group 'would be virtually free of inherited disorders, would receive powerful genetic therapies for acquired diseases, and would be engineered with superior physical and mental abilities' and that the latter group 'would continue to suffer from genetic illnesses and would have to content itself with less effective, conventional medical treatments. Its members would be able to improve their mental and physical traits only through comparatively laborious traditional methods of self-improvement' (Mehlman and Botkin, 1998).

As bad as the consequences of this divide would be for the individuals in the genetic underclass, Mehlman and Botkin think that the worst consequence of this state of affairs would be the destruction of democratic society. As they see it, a genetically stratified society would undermine social equality in three ways. First, it would increase *actual inequality* by enabling the genetic aristocracy to secure greater genetic health and talent than the genetic underclass. Second, it would erode the *belief in equality of opportunity* by enabling the genetic aristocracy to make themselves 'the best and the brightest,' and then to pass on their genetic advantages to succeeding generations. Finally, it would destroy the hope for *social mobility* in the genetic underclass, who would become increasingly resentful about their lot in life (Mehlman and Botkin, 1998: p. 102).

Mehlman and Botkin consider the possibility of banning genetic therapies, particularly non-therapeutic enhancement interventions, but come to the conclusion that legal bans, and even health care practitioners' treatment refusals, will not work in the long run. Convinced that most people will want to use as much safe, effective and arguably beneficial gene therapy as they can afford, Mehlman and Botkin predict that legislators and judges will succumb to citizens' pressures and that physicians and researchers will meet their patients' demands. As the demand for therapeutic and non-therapeutic genetic intervention increases, claim Mehlman and Botkin, there will only be two possible ways to save democracy: (1) creation of a system of genetic handicapping for the genetically non-enhanced; or (2) a genetic lottery, open to all citizens for no cost, in which the prize is a complete package of genetic services. The latter option is the remedy Mehlman and Botkin favour, on the grounds that the former option will not work for several reasons (Mehlman and Botkin, 1998: pp. 124–8).

In particular, creation of a system of genetic handicapping 'would require us to ignore actual performance differences between individuals' (Mehlman and Botkin, 1998: p. 122). Unlike standard affirmative action, which is based on the claim that there are no relevant performance differences between the person who is given a preference and the person who is not, genetic handicapping is based on the understanding that there are relevant performance differences between persons with genetic disabilities and persons without genetic disabilities. When something 'important is at stake', like airline passengers' safety, ask Mehlman and Botkin, would we really want 'a pilot who had been hired over someone with better eyesight, or stamina, or quicker reflexes, simply in order to level the social playing field?'(Mehlman and Botkin, 1998: pp. 122–3).

Whatever the ultimate merits of a genetic lottery, for now it strikes me as better to resist the tide of demand for genetic enhancement, and to ask health care practitioners to take the lead in doing so. Mehlman and Botkin imply that the major reason health care practitioners cannot resist their patients' demands for intellectually, physically and even morally enhanced offspring for long is that there is no end or aim of medicine with which to counter these demands. Medicine, it has been argued, is simply a set of techniques and tools that can be used to attain whatever ends people have; and physicians and other health care practitioners are simply technicians who exist to please their customers or clients, and to take from them whatever they can afford to pay

(Kass, 1985: pp. 157–86). Such an abdication of meaning as well as responsibility on the part of the medical community strikes me as premature. Caution suggests that, until it becomes untenable, physicians and other health care practitioners should struggle to distinguish between health-related and non-health-related genetic therapies, and that they should provide to their patients only *health-related* genetic therapies, including safe, effective and beneficial health-related enhancement interventions such as genetically engineered immunizations against infectious diseases (Walters and Palmer: 1997, p. 110).

Rather than arguing that it should also be permissible for health care practitioners to provide non-health-related genetic therapies to patients because it is already permissible, for example, for them to provide elective cosmetic surgery to patients, perhaps we should argue instead that both these kinds of interventions fall outside the scope of the moral practice of medicine. Admittedly, just because members of the US medical community refuse to provide non-health-related genetic therapies does not mean that some other group of persons won't. For example, the philosopher James Lindeman Nelson describes a group of persons who may not rely on insurance reimbursement for compensation, but provide direct services to paying customers who seek any and all enhancements; these 'professionals' may not be interested in the goals of medicine, only in their own profits (Lindeman Nelson, in Parens, 1998: s14). However, such rivals to the expertise of physicians and other health care practitioners are not likely to succeed unless large numbers of physicians and health care practitioners break ranks and join their company, a defection not likely in the immediate future.

Assuming that the medical community will remain loyal to its best ideals, it will be important for doctors to try to make health-related genetic therapies available to as many people as possible. Listening to concerns such as those raised by Mehlman and Botkin, the American Medical Association has already stated that health-related genetic therapies should be permitted only if there is equal access to them, 'irrespective of income or other socio-economic considerations' (American Medical Association, 1994: pp. 633, 640–1). To be sure, if citizen and patient demands for non-health-related genetic therapies, particularly therapies that promise to parents not simply normal children but the best, brightest and most beautiful offspring, increase to the point that they can no longer be resisted by physicians, perhaps it will be time to distribute the dice for a genetic lottery.

For now, I hope the public has the courage to answer honestly the question of *why* so many parents want to have 'perfect' babies. It strikes me that the quest for the 'perfect' child is, at root, not a quest to make sure that all children have an equal opportunity to lead a normal and meaningful life, but a quest to guarantee that one's own child will have what it takes to get more pieces of the pie than one's neighbour's child. In other words, the quest for the perfect child aims to increase the gap between the 'haves' and the 'have-nots', and as such should be abandoned by anyone who claims to embrace democratic values. Rather than spending our limited health care resources on designing gene therapies to provide wealthy Westerners with the means to have children designed to suit their whims, we should spend our money instead on developing affordable treatments for the innumerable diseases – some of them genetic, but most of them environmental – which kill hundreds of thousands of children and infants annually throughout the world.

Children's genes are not their entire destiny. Much depends on how much and what kind of health care, education, housing, food and love they are provided. After all, no matter how genetically perfect a child is born, if that supernormal child is put into an uncaring environment, she or he will probably not develop nearly as well as a normal or even less-than-normal child reared in a caring environment. Our task is to create a just society in which imperfect children can thrive, for if we succeed in this task, we may no longer feel a need for perfect children – so satisfied will we be with our world and the opportunities it offers to all human beings equally.

References

American Medical Association, Council on Ethical and Judicial Affairs (1994). Ethical issues related to prenatal genetic testing. *Archives of Family Medicine* **3**: 633–41.

Asch, A. (1995). Can aborting 'imperfect' children be immoral? In *Ethical Issues in Modern Medicine*, ed. J.D. Arras and B. Steinbock, pp. 385–92. Mountain View, CA: Mayfield Publishing Company.

Daniels, N. (1986). *Just Health Care.* New York: Cambridge University Press.

Davis, D.S. (1997). Genetic dilemmas and the child's right to an open future. *Rutgers Law Journal* **28**: 549–92.

Davis, L.J. (1995). *Enforcing Normalcy: Disability, Deafness and the Body.* New York: Verso.

Frankford, D.M. (1998). The treatment/enhancement distinction as an armament in the policy wars. In *Enhancing Human Traits: Ethical and Social Implications*, ed. E. Parens, pp. 70–94. Washington, DC: Georgetown University Press.

Juengst, E.T. (1998). What does *enhancement* mean? In *Enhancing Human Traits: Ethical and Social Implications*, ed. E. Parens, pp. 29–47. Washington, DC: Georgetown University Press.

Kass, L.R. (1985). *Toward a More Natural Science: Biology and Human Affairs*, pp. 80–99. New York: The Free Press.

Little, M.O. (1998). Cosmetic surgery, suspect norms, and the ethics of complicity. In *Enhancing Human Traits: Ethical and Social Implications*, ed. E. Parens, pp. 162–76. Washington, DC: Georgetown University Press.

Matthieu, D. (1996). *Preventing Prenatal Harm: Should the State Intervene?* Washington, DC: Georgetown University Press.

McGee, G. (1997). *The Perfect Child: A Pragmatic Approach to Genetics*. Lanham, MD: Rowman and Littlefield Publishers, Inc.

Mehlman, M.J. and Botkin J.R. (1998). *Access to the Genome: The Challenge to Equality*. Washington, DC: Georgetown University Press.

Mill, J.S. (1956). *On Liberty*. Indianapolis: Bobbs-Merrill.

Parens, E. (1998). Is better always good? *Hastings Center Report* **28**(1): S1–S17.

Pernick, M.S. (1996). *The Black Stork: Eugenics and the Death of 'Defective' Babies in American Medicine and Motion Pictures Since 1935*. New York: Oxford University Press.

Purdy, L.M. (1996). Loving future people. In *Reproducing Persons: Issues in Feminist Bioethics*, ed. L. M. Purdy, pp. 50–74. Ithaca: Cornell University Press.

Robertson, J.A. (1994). *Children of Choice: Freedom and the New Reproductive Technologies*. Princeton: Princeton University Press.

Robertson, J.A. (1996). Genetic selection of offspring characteristics. *Boston University Law Review* **76**(3): 444–8.

Strong, C. (1997). *Ethics in Reproductive and Prenatal Medicine*. New Haven: Yale University Press.

Walters, L. and Palmer, J.G. (1997). *The Ethics of Human Gene Therapy*. New York: Oxford University Press.

Wisconsin v. *Yoder*, 406 U.S. 205, 207 (1972).

6

Is there a duty not to reproduce?

Jean McHale

Faculty of Law, University of Leicester, Leicester, UK

Much of the language used in the debates concerning reproduction sur-rounds the concepts of rights and of choice: the woman's right to reproduce; her right to choose; her right to marry and found a family. Yet there is another rhetoric, one which has arisen again in recent years, that of respon-sible parenting, controlled choice. The argument has been advanced that individuals are not entitled to reproduce in all situations. In fact, that there may rather be certain situations in which they should not reproduce, and even that they may be required *not* to reproduce. It is an uncomfortable language for many in that it harks back to the eugenics debates. This paper explores the extent to which persons can ever be regarded as being under a duty not to reproduce and whether such a duty can be legally enforced. First, when might such a 'duty' arise? Secondly, what considerations would militate against the recognition of such a duty? Thirdly, if such a duty were recog-nized, then how could it actually be enforced in law? As we shall see in a moment, these are very uncomfortable questions, but new technological developments suggest that increasingly they will have to be addressed.

New reproductive technologies provide a means of controlling access to reproductive services. The clinicians act as gatekeepers in the selection of those who will have access to services. In such a situation individuals may be limited in the reproductive choices they make already through state-imposed criteria. In the UK, for example, in the context of the Human Fertilisation and Embryology Authority (HFEA) Revised Code of Practice (1998), which provides that:

Para 3.17. Where people seek licensed treatment, centres should bear in mind the following factors:
(a) their commitment to having and bringing up a child or children;
(b) their ability to provide a stable and supportive environment for any child produced as a result of treatment;
(c) their medical histories and the medical histories of their families;
(d) their health and consequent future ability to look after or provide for a child's needs;
(e) their ages and likely future ability to look after or provide for a child's needs;
(f) their ability to meet the needs of any child or children who may be born as a result of treatment, including the implications of any possible multiple births;

(g) any risk of harm to the child or children who may be born, including the risk of inherited disorders or transmissible diseases, problems during pregnancy and of neglect or abuse; and

(h) the effect of a new baby or babies upon any existing child of the family.

In many respects, Codes of Practice such as that of the HFEA itself and guidelines issued by individual infertility clinics can be regarded as rationing tools in relation to National Health Service (NHS) resources. They reflect also the background to treatment services provided under the legislation, which may take several years and ultimately still be unsuccessful. It is also a controlled reproductive situation. Conception outside the walls of the infertility clinic in the UK is not presently subject to such limitations. Using such criteria in a general regulation of potential parents in this manner must surely be ludicrous in practice? None the less, with the technological developments such as screening during pregnancy that we have today, far more information is now available as to the health/viability of the fetus. It is inevitably the case that the volume of such information will increase in the future. But is it and can it be rightly said that prospective parents are under a duty not to reproduce?

The 'harms' of reproduction

Why talk of a duty not to reproduce? An obvious explanation is that such a duty should be imposed in a situation in which, were reproduction to take place, the resultant child would suffer some form of demonstrable harm after birth, and that such a 'harm' should be avoided. What, though, do we mean in this type of situation by a 'harm'? One possibility is that the 'harm' here is that the child will have some form of physical or mental disorder. The direct 'harm' in the form of a disability which falls upon the child may also be accompanied by further harms, for example, the parents may be affected by the birth of the child. The couple may not be able to cope with the strain of a severely handicapped child, and relationship breakdown may be the result.

Take the example of a couple who discover that they are at a very high risk of passing on a degenerative incurable disorder but who want to go ahead and try to conceive a child. They may have the option of the use of pre-implantation genetic screening, enabling them to select a healthy embryo for implantation. This option is likely to be increasingly available in the future, as evidenced in the report on prenatal genetic testing of the Advisory Committee on Genetic Testing (2000).

But the couple may object to this – for example, they may have ethical/religious objections to the destruction of the embryo or they may want to simply take the risk of going ahead in the hope that in their particular case this risk does not materialize. Should they be told that they are wrong both morally and legally to reproduce without having screening? What of a situation in which they are aware of the risk that 'harm' may arise, but they argue that the disorder is a late-onset disorder, as a consequence not manifesting itself for many years. Again, should they be held to be under a duty not to reproduce?

Laura Purdy has strongly argued that it is wrong to reproduce when we know that there is a high risk of transmitting a genetic disease/defect. She argues that persons who develop a condition such as Huntington's disease are unlikely to have what she terms 'minimally satisfying lives'. As a result, if someone is at risk of passing on the condition, they should not have genetically related children. She admits that there are difficulties in attempting to define a 'minimally satisfying life':

> Conceptions of a minimally satisfying life vary tremendously among societies and within them. *De rigueur* in some circles are private music lessons and trips to Europe, whereas in others providing eight years of schooling is a major accomplishment. But there is no need to consider this complication at length here because we are concerned only with health as a prerequisite for a minimally satisfying life.
>
> (Purdy, 1996: p. 43.)

A more limited claim may be that parents should try to secure something like normal health for their children. While this may be regarded as an unsatisfactory criterion in that in some cultures debilitating conditions may be the norm, Purdy suggests that this objection can be circumvented by saying that parents ought to try to provide for their children health that is normal for that culture, even though it may be inadequate if judged by some outside standard. She states that such a position would still justify efforts to avoid the birth of children at risk for Huntington's disease and other serious genetic diseases in all societies (Purdy, 1996: p. 46). (See also chapters 13, 19, and 20.)

The 'costs' of reproduction

Another reason why some may seek to impose a duty not to reproduce is that of the resultant 'costs' which may result from that reproduction. If the couple at risk of bearing a severely handicapped child make the decision to go ahead, then who precisely will bear the cost of care and of medical treatment if the risks attendant upon handicap materialize? The 'welfare' mother may decide to go ahead and have a child, but the consequent costs of bringing the child into the world are likely to fall upon the State in such a situation – housing, medical treatment and the fact that the woman may be unable to enter the workforce, at least for some time, due to child-care commitments. There has been considerable criticism of such women by governments in the UK, both past and present; in the US, this group has been subject to the targeting of the use of the injectable contraceptive Norplant (Robertson, 1994).

Does harm/cost = duty not to reproduce?

While some 'harms' and some 'costs' may be identified, does this lead us inexorably to the conclusion that persons should be held to be under a duty not to reproduce? Some may think that conception and birth where there is a risk of those harms/costs arising may be undesirable, but does this ever really equate with imposing a duty not to reproduce, and in particular, backing that duty up through some recognition of legal liability?

Robertson (1994) has argued that many of these harms/costs do not legitimate limiting reproductive choices. First, he suggests that few of those conditions would make the life of a child so horrible that its interests would have been better served had that child never been born. Secondly, Robertson argues that because a woman's reproductive interest is generally very strong, there would need to be compelling criteria to override it, and factors such as saving money would not generally be adequate. He takes as examples whether there is a case for compulsory contraception (e.g. Norplant implants) to prevent the birth of offspring with congenital disease or persons who are HIV-positive. Robertson says that both groups have substantial interests in reproduction.

The risk of a handicapped child will ordinarily be one in four. Preventing the birth of a handicapped child would also prevent the greater likelihood that the offspring would not have the disease in question. Avoiding the birth of a handicapped child may also require pre-natal testing and abortion to which the parents are opposed. Similarly women with HIV may still find procreation immensely meaningful, both because it is a prime source of meaning and validation in their social-cultural context and because it meets their need for continuity after the death looming over them.

(Robertson, 1994: p. 84.)

Others, such as Purdy, are less convinced by arguments derived from procreative liberty. She suggests that there are other ways in which reproductive desires may be satisfied, including adoption and the use of new reproductive technologies. She comments that other arguments for having children, such as wanting the genetic line to be continued, are not particularly rational when it brings a sinister legacy of illness and death. She also states that while a desire to bear children who physically resemble oneself is understandable although basically narcissistic, its fulfilment cannot be guaranteed even by normal reproduction. Children also do not necessarily either prove adulthood or cement marriages. Having children on economic grounds as the cushion for old age may not, she argues, provide the expected economic benefit if they are ill; indeed, 'expected economic benefit is, in many cases, a morally questionable reason for having children' (Purdy, 1996: p. 48).

A qualified reproductive right?

A 'duty' not to reproduce may be seen as being in conflict with other recognized 'rights'. It could be argued, however, that some of those persons whose opportunity to conceive naturally was, prima facie, limited by a duty not to reproduce, could still conceive through the use of artificial reproductive technologies. Consider the couple, discussed above, who do not want to avail themselves of the new screening technologies. One alternative is to say to such a couple, 'You will be penalized if you reproduce naturally and the "harm" in the form of the disability materializes. However, you do have the option of pre-implantation genetic diagnosis, and this offers you an alternative; therefore we are not limiting your reproductive choices, your procreative liberty, to any great extent at all. Take the screening which is offered and set your mind at rest.'

But the initial attractions of such an approach pall considerably on further consideration. Before we go down this road we need to address serious and fundamental questions, not simply about an individual's choice, but also about society's attitude to the disabled members of our community. As the Nuffield Council on Bioethics (1995: p. 77, para 8.11) noted,

[i]t has been argued that the availability of prenatal screening and diagnosis, together with the termination of seriously affected pregnancies, both reflect and reinforce the negative attitudes of our society towards those with disabilities. Indeed medical genetics may add a new dimension if genetic disorder came to be seen as a matter of choice rather than fate.

There is also the prospect of the 'slippery slope' to eugenics looming into view (Glover, 1998). Furthermore, the recognition of a duty not to reproduce may be regarded as unacceptable because it may mean that a person will in effect be virtually forced to discover their genetic status should they want to reproduce. This may itself have other consequences with regards to the use of that genetic information – for example, with regards to insurance and employment prospects in years to come. It may also infringe an individual's 'right not to know' (Chadwick et al., 1997). It is worth noting that the Council of Europe (1996), in the Convention for the Protection of Human Rights and Dignity of the Human Being with Regard to the Application of Biology and Medicine, provides that:

Everyone is entitled to know any information collected about his or her health. However, the wishes of individuals not to be so informed shall be observed.

Enforcing a duty not to reproduce – the role of the law?

Just for argument's sake, however, consider what would happen if the objections stated above could be satisfactorily overcome. Say that there are certain, perhaps very limited, situations in which individuals may be wrong in seeking to reproduce – so wrong that they should actually be held to be under a *duty*. In the context of a discussion of the use of Norplant for compulsory contraception, even Robertson (1994: p. 86) goes on to say that his conclusions may differ in certain situations:

If they [the women] lack capacity or interest in rearing, will institutionalise the child at birth, or face a short life span due to their own illness, required contraception would not violate as significant a reproductive interest as if they intended to rear for long periods. If the bodily intrusion associated with compulsory contraception is relatively minor, it may be that compelled contraception in rare cases could be justified, though such policies would be highly controversial.

But this, of course, brings us on to another important issue – namely, to what extent is recognition of such a duty at all practical in law? Some would argue that the a moral duty may be recognizable, but as Robertson has noted, that 'does not mean that those duties should have legal standing' (Robertson, 1994: p. 177).

The first point is whether such a duty would be legally sustainable. To hold a woman or a couple liable for their decision to have a child, despite what are substantial warnings regarding the risks of such a course of action, might also constitute a breach of the European Convention on Human Rights – for example, of Article 12, the right to marry and found a family. There are fundamental questions regarding the privacy of the individual in relation to their home and family life under Article 8 which would arise in such a situation. It should also be noted that the Council of Europe Convention on Human Rights and Biomedicine provides in Article 11 that 'Any form of non-discrimination against a person on grounds of his or her genetic heritage is prohibited'. We need of course to bear this in mind, particularly in view of the fact that those provisions of the European Convention of Human Rights are now justiciable in the English courts since the Human Rights Act 1988 came into force in October 2000. In fact it is likely that there will be challenges brought in the future by those who have been refused access to IVF treatment under just these provisions in the English courts.

Secondly, would this be a duty involving state sanctions, enforceable, for example, through the criminal law or will it be limited to civil liability, perhaps in the form of an action brought by the child consequent upon birth? Take first the State-imposed 'duty'. How do you inform people that they are under such a legal duty, and that if they reproduce without finding out their genetic status, there may be legal consequences? They will need to know that the law has changed in this area. Should there be a nationwide television campaign? Do we have to put up notices in railway stations, general medical practitioners' surgeries and night clubs warning people that if they conceive unwittingly, some form of legal liability may result?

Secondly, how should such a duty be practically enforced in the courts without bringing the whole concept into disrepute? The first possibility is that I might be held liable in criminal law in such a situation. But on what basis? Could there be a special offence of intentionally conceiving, or would this extend to reckless/negligent conception? Would the sanctions be imposed to avert the harm prior to conception itself occurring? Thus in the case of the 'welfare mother' we have already the examples in the US of the use of compulsory contraception – but then presumably the only way in which this could be achieved would be through compulsory testing for the whole population. Would the effect of this be that people would have to have regular tests throughout their lives?

There are very few certainties in the world. In the case of genetic diseases we are talking about probabilities. I may pass on a genetic disease, but also I may not. The probability level obviously differs with regard to the disease in question. Do I then have to simply take the risk, knowing that I may be branded a criminal? It may be possible for certain medical conditions to be cured or at the very least alleviated thanks to developments in medical technology. Could, and indeed should, individuals be allowed to 'wait and see'? After all, with the pace of technological developments such as gene therapy, the serious degenerative late-onset disorder may be curable by the time that infant reaches adulthood. When then would the prosecution take place – 25 years after the event perhaps? If I am prosecuted, just what sanctions will be imposed on me? A prison sentence? I may be told that I could have avoided any legal liability, because I had the opportunity to abort, but what if I am violently opposed to abortion? Or it is the case that I would be told if this condition emerged?

It is also the case that the practical difficulties of recognizing such a duty may also collide with another set of legal principles, namely, membership of the European Union. The imposition of a duty not to reproduce would surely offend against the notion of free movement principles in the European Union (Hervey, 1998). The ability to travel to another nation to bear a child – something which older mothers who have been denied NHS infertility treatment have done, and something which Diane Blood did to enable her to be inseminated with her deceased husband's sperm – would undoubtedly come into play in such a situation (*R* v. *Human Fertilisation and Embryology Authority ex parte Blood*, 1997). Cases such as that of Blood send out a powerful message – European regulation is changing the face of health care today, and single jurisdiction regulation may indeed be inadequate in health care law.

Repaying the state

An alternative is to say to the individual/couple: 'Yes, you may reproduce in a "risky" situation, but if the "harm" does arise and, as a consequence, the state incurs costs, then you will be liable to pay that cost'. This solution, however, can be seen as undesirable, in that at the very least it is discriminatory between those with financial resources and those without. Those with such resources may decide to go ahead and know that whatever happens, they have the resources to care for the children. Disabled children may thus be born, but only to the wealthier members of society. Such a discriminatory provision is not only divisive but again would almost certainly be the subject of challenge on human rights grounds.

Civil law liability

Another option would be to hold the parent/parents accountable in civil law. But by whom? Firstly, there could be a state action in relation to the recovery of costs incidental to NHS treatment for the care of a disabled child. Secondly, an action could be brought by the child, for example, claiming that the parents' actions resulted in their birth in a disadvantaged or disabled condition.

There are a number of difficulties in such a course of action. First, would the parents be worth suing? Are they insured against legal costs? At present the potential for such actions in civil law is limited. The Congenital Disabilities Civil Liability Act 1976 provides that an action may be brought by a child born with a disability as a result of an occurrence which affects either of its parents in their ability to have a normal healthy child, or an occurrence which affects the mother during pregnancy and either mother and child during birth. The child's claim under this statute, however, is limited because it derives from breaches of duty owed to the parent of the child. While there is the possibility that fathers may be sued under the Congenital Disabilities Civil Liability Act 1976, the mother is excluded from liability with the exception of the situation where she has been involved in a road traffic accident. Limiting actions under the 1976 Act could be seen in terms of limited notions of paternal misconduct. However, as Brazier (1998: p. 268) notes, today medical science makes everything so much more complex:

Some of the practical grounds for exempting mothers from liability for parental liability for prenatal injury need to re-examined in relation to fathers too. Questions as to what constitutes reasonable parental conduct, what good suing a parent does the disabled child, may apply with equal force to both parent.

Alternatively a child may seek to bring an action at common law, claiming that they should have never been born. This is known as a 'wrongful life' action. The existence of such an action in English law was rejected in *McKay* v *Essex AHA* (1982). Mary McKay was born in 1975. She had been infected, whilst in the womb, with rubella and as a consequence was partially blind and deaf. The allegation was made that one doctor had acted negligently in failing to treat rubella infection. Also it was claimed that another doctor had either negligently mislaid a blood sample or had failed to interpret the results of such tests. The real issue in the case was, however, the claim by Mary McKay that the doctor owed her a duty of care when she was in utero, which involved advising her mother as to the desirability of having an abortion, which advice the mother said she would have accepted.

In the Court of Appeal the claim was rejected on a number of grounds. First, if the duty of care to the fetus involved imposing a duty on the doctor – albeit indirectly – to prevent the child's birth, the child would have a cause of action against her mother if she refused to have an abortion. The fact that a doctor can lawfully terminate life did not mean that the child had a right to die. To recognize such a right would be contrary to public policy. Secondly, the Law Commission in their Report on Injuries to Unborn Children (1974), which had rejected the wrongful life claim, had been of the view that such a claim would impose intolerable burdens on the medical profession, because of subconscious pressure to advise abortion in doubtful cases through fear of action for damages. Interestingly one of the members of the Court of Appeal, Griffith LJ, did not see this as a tenable ground. He was of the view that provided that the defendants gave a balanced explanation of risks involved in alleged pregnancy, including risk of injury to the fetus, the doctor could not be expected to do more. But that may only exonerate the doctor; what of the mother?

Thirdly, the Court of Appeal was unhappy regarding the evaluation of damages. How could a court attempt to evaluate non-existence – to compare non-existence and the value of existence in a disabled state? The only duty of care which can be recognized was one that could be assessed in monetary terms. Stephenson LJ, for example, noted the rejection of a wrongful life claim in the 1967 US case of *Gleitman* v *Cosgrave,* where the court had said that in assessing damages the problem was the question of whether X would have been better off not being born at all, 'A man who knows nothing of death or nothingness cannot possibly know whether that is so' (227 A 2d 689 at 711).

Finally, the Court of Appeal held that section 4(5) of the Congenital Disabilities (Civil Liability) Act 1976 excluded liability in wrongful life claims, a point on which all the members of the Court of Appeal in this case agreed. Section 4(5) of the 1975 Act provides that the Act applies to all births after its passing, and in respect of any such birth, it replaces any law in force before its passage whereby a person could be held liable to a child in respect of disabilities with which it might be born.

The rejection of wrongful life actions is itself a controversial area, one which goes considerably beyond the scope of this chapter, and much has been written on the issue (Harris, 1998). The policy arguments against their acceptance, as outlined in relation to the judgments of the Court of Appeal in this case, have been echoed by academic commentators (Lee, 1989; Fortin, 1987). An alternative approach which has been suggested is to change the terminology used. For example, Mason and McCall Smith have suggested that 'we favour abandoning the principle of "wrongful life" in favour of diminished life; we can then look not at a comparison, whether it be between the neonate's current existence and non-existence or with normality, but rather at the actual suffering that has been caused' (Mason and McCall Smith, 1999: p. 165). They comment further that, 'This carries the practical advantage that the courts can understand and accommodate this form of damage, which allows for a distinction to be made between the serious and slight defect' (Mason and McCall Smith, 1999: p. 165–6), although presumably the difficulty with this approach is to ascertain what precisely constitutes the actual suffering caused. At the present time, however, recognition of such an action appears unlikely in English civil law.

Even if such an action were recognized in principle, establishing it could prove difficult. What of fathers? Should civil law liability apply only where the individual is in an established relationship? What of the woman who becomes accidentally pregnant? Does this mean that the concept of parental liability extends beyond the scope of the Child Support Agency to civil law liability? What if genetic tests are undertaken which, while they appear clear, are actually faulty? Presumably in this situation the couple would not be liable, but here an action may then be brought against the clinician, precisely the type of action rejected in *McKay*. What happens if it is some time since the couple was tested, but they conceive and then discover that the fetus is handicapped? Are they held to be not liable in law as long as they have taken 'reasonable steps' to discover their risk of transmitting disease/defect?

The difficulties that arise in the context of the competent adult are magnified still further when we consider mentally incompetent persons and the teenage pregnancy. Do we penalize teenagers whether or not they know of the risk which they may be under with regards to conception? What about the overlap with abortion once a woman discovers, during pregnancy, that she is carrying a handicapped fetus?

The consequences of a duty not to reproduce are such that it is unlikely that the courts would be willing to impose such a duty, at present, upon the parents. None the less the possibility does remain, given the enhanced availability of genetic knowledge, that this situation may change. Attitudes regarding individuals taking responsibility for their own health and that of others may indeed have a bearing here.

Concluding thoughts

Enforcing a duty not to reproduce may seem unrealistic and even perhaps ludicrous at present, but as technology develops and the increasing emphasis in our society on the birth of the 'perfect child' continues, this is a matter that will undoubtedly arise in the future. Comparisons can be drawn with the way in which pregnancy over the last decade has become policed by those who advocate responsible motherhood. This has on occasions, as we have seen in relation to enforced Caesarean sections, led to an area of private life being increasingly subject to regulation. While the English courts have now affirmed, for example, the right of the pregnant woman to refuse a Caesarean section, this debate is still ongoing (*Re MB*, 1997; *St George's NHS Trust* v *S*, 1998; Bailey Harris, 1998; Wells, 1998). (See Chapter 17.) Again, while behaviour during pregnancy is not explicitly regulated in English law (*Re F*, 1988) in the way in which it has been in many US states, leading to criminal sanctions being placed upon women whose behaviour may place the fetus at risk of harm, the pressure placed upon pregnant women to behave 'responsibly' has definitely heightened (Roth, 1999). (See Chapter 7.) As more widespread genetic information becomes available, it is likely to render us increasingly critical of those who make what we regard as being the 'wrong' decision in relation to reproduction. What that wrong decision is remains of course to be seen. Choosing to avert a handicap may be one such decision, but acting on preferences about height/eye colour and indeed intelligence may be others.

Any restrictions are likely to meet challenges on human rights grounds and the Human Rights Act 1998 would undoubtedly be used in this context. The rights of the fetus, and of the woman, are likely to lead to heated debates. None the less, while these are uncomfortable arguments, and while there are considerable problems in the legal enforcement of such duties, there is no doubt that the changing face of genetics will force us to address them. What is important is that such arguments should be addressed in advance by clinicians, lawyers and philosophers alike, rather than allowing ourselves to be precipitated into dealing with them in the courtroom.

References

Advisory Committee on Genetic Testing. (2000). *Prenatal Genetic Testing*. London: Department of Health.

Bailey Harris, R. (1998). Pregnancy, autonomy and refusal of medical treatment. *Law Quarterly Review*, **144**: 550.

Brazier, M. (1998) Parental responsibilities, foetal welfare and children's health.' In *Family Law into the Millennium*, ed. C. Bridge, pp. 266–293. London: Butterworths.

Chadwick, R., Shickle, D., and Levitt, M. (eds) (1997). *The Right to Know and the Right Not to Know*. Aldershot: Ashgate.

Council of Europe (1996). *Convention for the Protection of Human Rights and Dignity of the Human Being with Regard to the Application of Biology and Medicine: Bioethics Conventions*. Strasburg: Dir/Jur(96)2.

Fortin, J. (1987). Is the wrongful life action really dead?' *Journal of Social Welfare Law*, p. 306.

Gleitman v *Cosgrave* (1967) 227 A. 2d 689.

Glover, J. (1998). Eugenics: some lessons from the Nazi experience. In *The Future of Human Reproduction*, ed. J. Harris and S. Holm, p. 55–65. Oxford: Oxford University Press.

Harris, J. (1998). *Clones, Genes and Immortality* Oxford: Oxford University Press.

Hervey, T. (1998). *European Social Law and Policy*. London: Longmans.

Human Fertilisation and Embryology Authority (1998). *Code of Practice*, 4th edn. London: Stationery Office.

Lee, R. (1989). To be or not to be, is that the question: the claim of wrongful life. In *Birthrights*, ed. R. Lee and R. Morgan. London: Routledge.

McKay v *Essex* AHA [1982] 2 All ER 771.

Mason, J.K., and McCall Smith, R.A. (1999). *Law and Medical Ethics*. London: Butterworths, 5th edn.

Nuffield Council on Bioethics. (1995). *Genetic Screening*. London: Nuffield Council on Bioethics.

Purdy, L. (1996). *Reproducing Persons: Issues in Feminist Bioethics*. Ithaca, NY: Cornell University Press.

R v *Human Fertilisation and Embryology Authority ex parte Blood* [1997] 2 All ER 687.

Re F (in utero) [1988] 2 All ER 193.

Re MB [1997] 8 Med LR 217.

Robertson, J. (1994). *Children of Choice; Freedom and the New Reproductive Technologies* Princeton; Princeton University Press.

Roth, R. (1999). *Making Women Pay: The Hidden Costs of Fetal Rights*. Ithaca, NY: Cornell University Press.

St Georges Healthcare NHS Trust v *S* [1998] 3 All ER 673.

Wells, C. (1998) On the outside looking in: perspectives on enforced caesareans. In *Feminist Perspectives on Health Care Law*, ed. S. Sheldon and M. Thomson. London: Cavendish.

7

Between fathers and fetuses: the social construction of male reproduction and the politics of fetal harm

Cynthia R. Daniels

Political Science Department, Rutger University, New Brunswick, USA

In contemporary American political discourse 'crack babies' have been treated as *filius nullius* – as if they had no biological fathers. With no link between fathers and fetuses, no inheritance of harm could be attributed to the father's use of drugs. The absence of fathers in debates over drug addiction and fetal harm has had profound consequences for women, for it has dictated that women alone bear the burden and blame for the production of 'crack babies'.

Since at least the late 1980s, and in some cases far earlier, studies have shown a clear link between paternal exposures to drugs, alcohol, smoking, environmental and occupational toxins, and fetal health problems. Yet men have been spared the retribution aimed at women. In fact, while women are targeted as the primary source of fetal health problems, reports of male reproductive harm often place sperm at the centre of discourse as the 'littlest ones' victimized by reproductive toxins, somehow without involving their male makers as responsible agents.

Scientific research linking reproductive toxins to fetal health problems reflects deeply embedded assumptions about men and women's relation to reproductive biology. Critical analysis of the nature of fetal risks thus requires not only examination of the biology of risk, but also assessment of what Evelyn Fox Keller has called the 'collective consciousness' that fundamentally shapes scientific inquiry on gender difference – a consciousness that is constituted by 'a set of beliefs given existence by language rather than by bodies' (Keller, 1992: p. 25).

In debates over fetal harm, the production of this collective consciousness takes place in many social locations: in science laboratories, where the priorities of research are defined; in editorial rooms, where reporters decide which news warrants coverage and what slant to take on stories; and in courts and legislatures, where decisions are made regarding the definition of and culpability for social problems.

This chapter examines the cultural characterizations of sperm and male reproduction in science, news stories and public policy, all of which have shielded men from culpability for fetal health problems. (A more detailed discussion of the rise of the concept of fetal rights and fetal protectionism can be found in Daniels, 1993.) After a brief discussion of the social construction of maternity and paternity, I analyse the symbols of the 'crack baby', 'pregnant addict' and 'absent father' as central to public discourse on fetal harm, particularly in the US. Finally, I explore the range of complex questions about biological gender difference generated by the politics of fetal risks, and the problematic nature of the idea of individual causality in discussions of fetal harm.

Social constructions of maternity and paternity

In Western industrial cultures, notions of masculinity have been historically associated with the denial of men's physical vulnerabilities and bodily needs, which are instead projected onto the maternal body. Debates over fetal harm have been constituted by the analytically distinct and antithetical categories of male virility and vulnerability. Men were assumed either to be invulnerable to harm from the toxicity of drugs, alcohol and environmental and occupational hazards, or to be rendered completely infertile by any vulnerability to risk. In particular, sperm that crossed the line from virile to vulnerable by being damaged by reproductive toxins were assumed to be incapable of fertilization. And the converse operated as well – men not rendered infertile by their toxic exposures were assumed to be immune from any other form of reproductive risk (such as genetic damage).

Social constructions of maternity, by contrast, have been firmly aligned with assumptions of women's vulnerability. The science of reproductive risks historically developed in response to women's occupational exposures, where it was assumed that the physical stress and toxic exposures of the workplace would result in the degeneration of women's reproductive systems. Protective labour law selectively exaggerated the vulnerabilities of white women to occupational hazards and virtually ignored risks to working women of colour (Baer, 1978; Kessler-Harris, 1982; Lehrer, 1987; Daniels, 1991, 1993). Until well into the twentieth century, science, policy and law deeply reflected the association of maternity with vulnerability.

The cultural associations of paternity with virility and maternity with vulnerability formed the context within which the symbols of the 'crack baby', 'pregnant addict' and 'absent father' emerged at the center of debate over fetal hazards. (A more detailed analysis of the social and political construction of these concepts can be found in my longer treatment of this issue in Daniels, 1993, where I analyse the science, media, policy and law discourses surrounding the emergence of the ideas of fetal protectionism and fetal rights.)

'Crack babies' and 'pregnant addicts'

By now, the images of the crack baby and addicted mother are familiar to anyone who has read news reports of pregnancy and addiction. In the US, media attention began to focus in 1988 on babies affected by maternal drug use, with the release of a study by Dr. Ira Chasnoff, director of the National Association for Perinatal Addiction Research and Education (NAPARE), which reported that 375 000 babies were born every year 'exposed to illicit drugs in the womb' (Chasnoff, 1989: pp. 208–10). The study was fundamentally flawed in a number of ways. Chasnoff's sample was biased by the fact that 34 of the 36 hospitals surveyed were public inner-city hospitals. The study made no distinction between a single use of illegal drugs and chronic drug addiction during pregnancy; nor did it document the actual effects of drug use on newborn infants.

The limitations of the study were never reported. Instead, the press picked up and exaggerated Chasnoff's findings, often reporting that 375 000 babies were born every year 'addicted to cocaine' (Brody, 1988: p. 1; Stone, 1989: p. 3). As the distinctions between drug use and abuse collapsed, the reported numbers of crack babies exploded. By 1990, news stories reported that one out of every ten children was born 'addicted to crack cocaine' or damaged by women's use of drugs (Daniels, 1993). By 1993, nine influential national daily newspapers in the United States had run more than 197 stories on pregnancy and cocaine addiction alone (including the *New York Times, Wall Street Journal, Washington Post, Christian Science Monitor, Los Angeles Times, Chicago Tribune, Boston Globe, Atlanta Constitution/Atlanta Journal* and *USA Today*).

The mindset created by this public discourse encouraged physicians, nurses and social workers to attribute many serious problems experienced by infants at birth to the use of drugs or alcohol by the child's mother, particularly in low-income inner-city neighbourhoods.

Symptoms associated with 'crack babies' ranged from very specific conditions that could, in fact, be tied to maternal drug use (such as drug withdrawal symptoms) to low birth weight, small head circumference, irritability, respiratory problems, gastrointestinal problems and diarrhoea – conditions that could easily be caused by poor nutrition or a host of environmental factors. (For a complete discussion of the symptoms associated with fetal cocaine exposure, see Zuckerman, 1991: pp. 26–35.) More highly controlled studies estimated that approximately 41 000 babies were born annually in the US with clear symptoms of drug-related health problems (such as drug withdrawal symptoms), a far cry from the 375 000, presented by NAPARE, as exposed to drugs in the womb (Dicker and Leighton, 1990). The results of these studies were never reported by the national press, just as the press rarely reports research showing little or no association between moderate drug and alcohol use and fetal health problems (Koren and Klein, 1991). There are two stages to the 'screening' process by which research makes it into the press. First, science journals review, accept or reject reports of findings. Koren at el. (1989) found that professional scientific journals were predisposed against reporting negative or 'null' associations between drug use and fetal risks. Once scientific reports did begin to appear in journals, Koren and Klein (1991) found a similar predisposition in the press against reporting negative findings.

The sense of social distress created by images of addicted babies wired to tubes in hospital incubators fed a profound need to blame. Public concern over crack babies contains all of the characteristics of a response to plague – fuelling the impulse of privileged populations to locate, target and contain one group as the primary source of contamination and risk (Mack, 1991). As Linda Singer has observed in relation to the spread of AIDS, the epidemic 'provides an occasion and rationale for multiplying points of intervention into the lives and bodies of populations' (Singer, 1993: p. 117). The policy response to the plague narrative was to find a target population to blame, and poor inner-city women were the most obvious targets. Newspaper stories contributed to this impulse by presenting images of African–American women as virtual monsters, snorting cocaine on the way to the delivery room and abandoning horribly damaged babies in hospitals. In some instances, drug use was characterized as a form of child abuse *in utero*, where cocaine 'literally batters the developing child' (see Brody, 1988: p. 1; Stone, 1989: p. 3).

Criminal prosecutors responded to the sense of crisis by targeting pregnant women for prosecution. By 1993, between 200 and 400 women had been charged with fetal drug delivery, fetal abuse or manslaughter (in cases where the pregnancy had ended in a stillbirth). Despite the fact that nearly every case challenged in the courts has resulted in the dismissal or acquittal of charges against women, prosecutors continue to bring criminal charges against women they suspect of drug or alcohol use during pregnancy. To date, almost all of these cases have been brought against African–American women (Paltrow, 1992). (However, it is difficult to calculate total numbers, since so many women are charged by local prosecutors who do not report their cases to any central national source.)

What has been the response of state and federal public health agencies to women and fetal health? Public health departments have produced warning labels on wine, beer, and liquor bottles and cigarette packages, together with an avalanche of public notices about pregnancy and alcohol consumption in restaurants and bars. Such labels stigmatize women by perpetuating assumptions that only women are vulnerable to risk and that women, therefore, are the primary source of fetal harm. Men are left entirely out of the frame as social attention focuses exclusively on the maternal–fetal nexus.

By implying women's ignorance or ill intentions, public health warnings aimed at pregnant women legitimate an atmosphere that encourages public retribution against women, by focusing exclusively on individual behaviour and not on the social and political causes of low birth weight, fetal birth defects or other health problems. Retribution is invited by the fact that public health warnings aimed at men (e.g. for heart disease, high blood pressure, cigarette smoking and steroid use) focus on behaviours that cause harm to *self*, whereas messages aimed at women focus exclusively on women's harm to *others* (the fetus).

One New Jersey public health advertisement displays an image of a pregnant woman holding a drink and warns, 'A pregnant woman never drinks alone' (N.J. Perinatal Cooperative, 1993). Yet a pregnant woman also never drinks in isolation from the effects of her home, her job and her physical, social and political environment. Even symptoms specific to drug or alcohol abuse, such as drug withdrawal symptoms or fetal alcohol syndrome, are complicated by simple factors such as poor nutrition. For instance, one study of pregnancy and alcohol use (controlling for age, smoking, drug abuse, reproductive history, medical problems, socio-economic status and race) found that women who consumed at least three drinks a day but ate balanced diets experienced a rate of fetal alcohol syndrome (FAS) of only 4.5 per cent, while women who drank the same amount and were malnourished had an FAS rate of 71 per cent (Bingol et al., 1987). The study showed that poor nutrition is tied directly to income – FAS is a measure not only of maternal alcoholism but also of economic class. There has been no press coverage of this study.

Public campaigns to 'stem the tide of crack babies' are clearly racialized, primarily targeting women of colour in low-income communities. Scientific research has supported the racialized nature of debate by focusing research heavily on drugs used most commonly in poor inner cities (such as crack) and not on substances most often abused by higher-income women (such as prescription drugs). Public health warnings typically silhouette African–American or Latina women; they are often produced in Spanish and directed at inner-city neighbourhoods.

Counteracting the symbol of the pregnant addict requires breaking the exclusive connection between pregnant women and 'crack babies'. The circle of causality has widened since feminist advocates started influencing media coverage of the issue, and since news stories began suggesting the relation on fetal health of the combined effects of poverty, addiction and exposures to workplace and environmental toxins. The precise causes of fetal health problems are immensely complicated. A woman living in the inner city is likely to have had little health care before she became pregnant, and also poor antenatal care. If she is employed in a hospital, she might be exposed to radiation, chemotherapeutic drugs, viruses or sterilizants such as ethylene oxide. If she works in a laundrette or dry cleaners, she might be exposed to solvents, cleaners or excessive heat. If she works in a factory, she might be required to do heavy lifting, or she might be exposed to toxic chemicals and the dust of heavy metals. If she lives in a low-income neighbourhood, she is likely to be exposed to lead from outdated plumbing or in the dust from old paint (Massachusetts Coalition for Occupational Safety and Health, 1992).

But drawing fathers into the circle of causality, essential to a deconstruction of the symbol of the pregnant addict, has proved more difficult. Both metaphorically and literally, fathers were absent from virtually all of the news stories on fetal health and addiction. The absence of fathers in news reports of crack babies was made easier to believe by the racial subtext of the story: African–American women are often characterized as abandoned, single mothers – women dangerously unconstrained by nuclear family relations. The absent father came to represent not only men's physical distance from the out-of-wedlock child but also men's distance from fetal harm.

Virile fathers and the 'all or nothing' sperm theory

Embedded in scientific research and newspaper and magazine stories were further assumptions about male reproduction that posed serious barriers to the father/fetal connection. Scientific literature on reproductive toxicity has traditionally dismissed the links between paternal use of drugs and alcohol (or exposure to occupational or environmental toxins) and harm to fetal health, because it was assumed that damaged sperm were incapable of fertilizing eggs. Indeed, male reproductive success was *defined* as the ability to penetrate an egg. Because penetration was the measure of normality, those sperm that succeeded were assumed to be healthy. By defining male reproductive health along the principles of this 'all or nothing' theory, most scientific studies until the late 1980s dismissed the possibility that defective sperm could contribute to fetal health problems. The 'all or nothing' theory was based on certain culturally imbued assumptions about the reproductive process. As Emily Martin has so well documented, scientists characterized the egg as the passive recipient and the sperm as conqueror in the process of fertilization (Martin, 1991).

The assumption that men harmed by toxic exposures would be rendered infertile deflected research away from the connections between fathers and fetal harm. As a result of the 'virile sperm' theory of conception, scientific studies, until the late 1980s, focused almost exclusively on infertility as the primary outcome of hazardous exposures and the main source of reproductive problems for men. Male reproductive health was defined by 'total sperm ejaculate', and healthy reproductive function was measured by 'ejaculatory performance' – measures of volume, sperm concentration and number, sperm velocity and motility, sperm swimming characteristics, and sperm morphology, shape and size (Burger et al., 1989).

Scientists who did try to pursue the father–fetal connection, such as Gladys Friedler at Boston University – who was the first to document a link in mice between paternal exposure to morphine and birth defects in their offspring in the 1970s – had difficulty funding their research or publishing their work. The significance of Friedler's work is that she found mutagenic effects from paternal exposures not only in the progeny of male mice exposed to morphine and alcohol, but also in the second generation or 'grandchildren' of exposed mice. In all cases, she controlled for maternal exposures so that causality could be more clearly linked to paternal exposures (Friedler and Wheeling, 1979; Friedler, 1985, Friedler, 1987–8).

A number of social and political events generated the first studies linking environmental exposures to male reproductive harm. The cultural construction of male reproduction was particularly evident in these early studies.

In 1979, scientific concern was raised by a study in Florida that documented a 40 per cent overall drop in sperm count for men over the past 50 years. Scientists responded with 'a flurry of sperm-count studies' about 'the big drop' (Castleman, 1993). By 1990, researchers at the University of Copenhagen had examined 61 sperm-count studies and determined that there had, in fact, been a 42 per cent decline in sperm count over the past 50 years, from 113 to 66 million per millilitre of semen (Carlsen et al., 1992). While this was far from the 20 million generally assumed to be the minimum for male fertility, it raised concern lest the downward trend should continue. Remarkably, in searching for a cause, scientists first focused on the fashion shift from boxer shorts to jockey shorts. Heat kills sperm, and because jockey shorts hold the testicles close to the body, they might decrease sperm production. The researchers also suspected increased sexual activity. Men who engage in frequent sex have lower sperm counts than men who wait a number of days between sexual encounters. After controlling for both promiscuity levels and discounting the 'jockey shorts' thesis, the Copenhagen researchers found an association between the increase in testicular cancer in key countries and substantial sperm-count declines. They speculated that the aetiology of both could be found in exposures to environmental toxins (Carlsen et al., 1992). Although still concentrating on male fertility, rather than on potential links between paternal exposure and fetal harm, the Copenhagen study did suggest that sperm might be more vulnerable to hazards than previously assumed, and that more research was needed on the potential links between toxic exposures and male reproductive health problems. But the links between paternal exposures and fetal health problems would not fully emerge until the assumption that damaged sperm were incapable of fertilization was thrown into question by a larger shift in the dominant paradigm of fertility and reproduction, a shift generated by the development of the 'seductive egg' theory.

The 'seductive egg' theory

The 'seductive egg' theory originated from research on sea urchins. Unlike mammalian reproduction, sea urchins engage in 'external fertilization' – sperm are released into the ocean, where they must locate eggs floating free in the sea. Scientists explained sperm's ability to find eggs of the same species by postulating that eggs release a substance or 'chemical signal' that attracts sperm (Shapiro, 1997: p. 293). This process of sperm 'chemotaxis' was then extended to research on human reproduction.

In 1991, research confirmed that sperm swam toward the fluid surrounding the egg when isolated in test tubes (Ralt et al., 1991). Major science magazines reported the news with titles such as 'Does Egg Beckon Sperm When Time Is Right?' (*Science*, April 1991), 'Eggs Urge Sperm to Swim Up and See Them' (*New Scientist*, April 1991) and 'Do Sperm Find Eggs Attractive?' (*Nature*, May 1991). As *Science News* recharacterized the process of fertilization, 'A human egg cell does not idle languidly in the female reproductive tract, like some Sleeping Beauty waiting for a sperm Prince Charming to come along and awaken it for fertilization. Instead, new research indicates that most eggs actively beckon to would-be partners, releasing an as-yet-unidentified chemical to lure sperm cells' (Ezzell, 1991: p. 214).

Emily Martin has noted that scientists confronted with this new evidence in the late 1980s vacillated between a model that emphasized the egg as seductress and the more mutual paradigm of sperm–egg fusion (Martin, 1991). In either case, the sperm takes on a less aggressive role in the process of fertilization. The fusion model is devoid of (most of) the human agency imparted to eggs and sperm in traditional descriptions, opting instead for a characterization that relies on a simple chemical process.

Changing characterizations of the process of fertilization thus created a new context (valid or not) for research supporting the link between paternal exposures and fetal harm. Yet a mutual picture of procreation did not necessarily lessen women's culpability for fetal harm. In the 'aggressive egg' model, women were once again at fault for seducing if not 'bad men', then at least 'bad sperm.' While potentially drawing men into the circle of causality with women, cultural constructions embedded in scientific magazines and newspaper stories continued to lay the blame at women's door. Yet by 1991, growing evidence had clearly implicated men in fetal health problems.

The evidence of male-mediated developmental toxicology

Male reproductive exposures are now strongly suspected of causing not only infertility but also miscarriage, low birth weight, congenital abnormalities, cancer, neurological illness and other childhood health problems (Davis et al., 1992: p. 289). Studies of male reproductive health and toxicity have concentrated primarily on the effects of occupational and environmental exposures of men and less on the effects of what scientists refer to as men's 'lifestyle factors', such as drinking, smoking, or drug use (Davis et al., 1992; Colie, 1993; Friedler, 1993; Olshan and Faustman, 1993).

Because adult males continuously produce sperm throughout their lives, the germ cells from which sperm originate are continuously dividing and developing. Sperm take approximately 72 days to develop to maturity, and then move for another 12 days through the duct called the epididymis, where they acquire the ability to fertilize an egg. During this developmental process, sperm may be particularly susceptible to damage from toxins because cells that are dividing are more vulnerable to toxicity than cells that are fully developed and at rest, as are eggs in the female reproductive system. Abnormal sperm may still be capable of fertilizing an egg because speed may be more important than size or shape, as was suggested in the earliest article on this subject (Moore, 1989).

Some of the earliest epidemiological research studied the effects of radiation exposures on the children born to men who survived the atomic bombs at Nagasaki and Hiroshima. However, few associations were found between paternal exposures and childhood health problems, possibly due to the fact that so few men conceived children in the six months after the bombing, when the exposure effects of radiation were at their strongest (Yoshimoto, 1990; Olshan and Faustman, 1993). A number of events triggered studies of male reproduction during the 1970s and 1980s. Vietnam veterans concerned about the effects of the herbicide Agent Orange called for studies on links between male exposures during the war and childhood diseases of their offspring. A 1980 study of more than 500 men indicated that men who showed signs of toxic exposure to dioxin (TCDD) in Agent Orange had twice the incidence of children with congenital anomalies than men without symptoms (Stellman and Stellman, 1980: p. 444). Other studies also showed increased rates of spinal malformation, spina bifida, congenital heart defects and facial clefting in the children of Vietnam veterans. Later studies, however, failed to confirm these findings. Controversy persists over the paternal–fetal effects of the herbicide, no doubt fuelled in part by the legitimacy and liability implications of positive associations for the US government (Colie, 1993: p. 6).

In 1977, men working at an Occidental Chemical plant in Lathrop, California noticed a pattern of sterility among their co-workers. In the 1950s, the company had actually funded research on the carcinogenicity and reproductive effects of the pesticide produced there, DBCP (dibromochloropropane), but had quietly shelved the research after findings demonstrated associations between DBCP exposures and reproductive effects in laboratory animals (Robinson, 1991: pp. xiii–xv). Later studies confirmed that the men's sterility was linked to their DBCP exposure, and the chemical was banned from further use in the US. By 1980, researchers had documented not only sterility but also increases in spontaneous abortion resulting from paternal exposure to DBCP (Kharrazi, Patashnik, and Goldsmith, 1980). Seventeen studies have now evaluated the impact of pesticides and herbicides on male reproduction and paternal–fetal health (Olshan and Faustman, 1993: p. 195).

Other studies have analysed the effects of occupational exposures on paternal–fetal health, with many finding significant associations between paternal exposures and fetal health problems. Toluene, xylene, benzene, TCE, vinyl chloride, lead, and mercury have all been associated with spontaneous abortion. Paints, solvents, metals, dyes and hydrocarbons have been associated with childhood leukaemia and childhood brain tumours (summarized in Olshan and Faustman, 1993: p. 196). In analyses by occupation, janitors, mechanics, farm workers and metal workers have been reported to have an excess number of children with Down's syndrome (Olshan and Faustman, 1993: p. 196). One study of 727 children born with anencephaly found correlations for paternal employment as painters (Colie, 1993: p. 7). Painters and workers exposed to hydrocarbons have also been shown to have higher rates of children with childhood leukaemia and brain tumours (Savitz and Chen, 1990). More than 30 studies have examined the relationship between paternal occupation and childhood cancer (Olshan and Faustman 1993: p. 197).

There are problems with many of these studies, although the difficulties apply to both men and women. It is difficult, for instance, to specify the nature of exposures to toxic substances at work. It is also difficult to get a sample size large enough to provide conclusive results, especially for conditions that are typically rare in children. And, as in all epidemiological studies, it is difficult to control for confounding factors, such as the effects of multiple chemical exposures and alcohol or drug use. However, whilst the problem of confounding variables is common to all epidemiological studies of reproductive toxicity, for cultural reasons scientists are more acutely aware of methodological caveats when studying men. For instance, studies of paternal effects are routinely criticized for not controlling for maternal exposures, while studies on women virtually never control for the exposures of fathers. Studies on men's occupational and environmental exposures rarely control for men's use of drugs or alcohol. Studies that do focus on the effects of lifestyle factors on men's reproduction are criticized for not controlling for men's workplace exposures, while studies of women and drug use do not control for women's occupational exposures.

The biological processes of male-mediated teratogenicity have also been examined through clinical studies on animals and studies of the effect of toxic exposures directly on sperm. All of the problems of confounding variables associated with epidemiological research can be avoided by conducting animal studies. The earliest studies of the effects of illicit drugs, for instance, were conducted on mice. Even given the limitations of scientific knowledge, it is clear that men can pass on genetic defects to children. Down's syndrome and Prader Willi syndrome have been passed to children through the paternal germ cell. The question is whether similar processes can occur when environmental exposures cause genetic mutations in sperm (Colie, 1993). What is the evidence of paternal–fetal effects of drugs, alcohol and cigarette smoking?

In a study of more than 14 000 birth records in San Francisco, researchers found associations between paternal smoking and various birth defects, including cleft lip, cleft palate and hydrocephalus (Savitz, Schwingle and Keels, 1991). Significant associations have also been found between paternal smoking and brain cancer in children, and between paternal smoking and low birth weight – a difference of up to 238 grams (*c.* 8.4 ounces) if a father smoked two packs of cigarettes a day (Savitz and Sandler, 1991: pp. 123–32; Davis, 1991: p. 123; Merewood, 1992: p. 8). In addition, cotinine, a metabolite of nicotine, has been found in seminal fluid, although researchers are unsure what effect this might have on fetal health (Davis et al., 1992: p. 290; Davis, 1991: p. 123). Bruce Ames of the University of California, Berkeley, has suggested that the link between smoking and birth defects could be due to smokers' low levels of vitamin C. Vitamin C helps to protect sperm from the genetic damage caused by oxidants in the body, but the vitamin is depleted in the body of cigarette smokers. Ames found that men with low levels of the vitamin experienced double the oxidation damage to the DNA in their sperm (Schmidt, 1992: p. 92).

Paternal alcohol use has been found to produce low birth weight and an increased risk of birth defects. In animal studies, paternal exposure to ethanol produced behavioural abnormalities in offspring. Alcoholism in men is known to produce testicular atrophy. Case reports suggest an association between paternal drinking and 'malformations and cognitive deficiencies' in the children of alcoholic men (Little and Sing, 1987; Colie, 1993: p. 59; Friedler, 1993; Olshan and Faustman, 1993: p. 197).

Cocaine has been found to increase the number of abnormal sperm and to decrease sperm motility. Ricardo Yazigi, Randall Odem and Kenneth Polakoski discovered that cocaine could bind to sperm and thereby be transmitted to the egg during fertilization. Reports of cocaine 'piggybacking' on sperm have led to controversy in the scientific community over whether this phenomenon could contribute to birth defects (Brachen et al., 1990; Yazigi, Odem and Polakoski, 1991). In animal studies, opiates (such as morphine and methadone) administered to fathers, but not to mothers, have produced birth defects and behavioural abnormalities in the first *and* second generations of the father's offspring (Friedler and Wheeling 1979; Friedler, 1985). Drug addiction in men using hashish, opium or heroin has been shown to cause structural defects in sperm (El-Gothamy and El-Samahy, 1992). Despite the limitations of scientific research on male reproduction, few scientists question that biological mechanisms exist for establishing links between paternal and fetal health.

Press coverage of male-mediated harm

The scientific evidence on male-mediated risks has generated quite different stories in popular magazines and newspapers than it has for women. Whilst images of crack babies and irresponsible mothers prevail in stories about maternal exposures to drugs, visual images in popular science magazines and news stories about male reproduction place sperm in the centre of focus as the tiniest victims of toxicity. Such narratives and images helped to frame the public response to research on men. Even in newspaper stories that address the connection between paternal exposures and fetal health, certain patterns of reporting emerge that function to reduce male culpability for fetal harm.

First, while men are absent from stories on maternal–fetal harm, *women are always present* in news stories on paternally-mediated risks. In all of the stories that draw connections between paternal exposures and fetal harm, maternal exposure was also mentioned as a possible source of harm. In this way, male responsibility is always *shared* with women. The presence of the pregnant woman means that the father is never cast as the sole source of harm. No article suggests or implies that 'drug-clean' women may produce harmed babies as a result of their partner's drug use.

Second, *maternally mediated fetal risks are assumed to be certain and known.* Evidence of male-mediated risks are often prefaced with statements such as, 'While doctors are well aware of the effects that maternal smoking, drinking and exposure to certain drugs can have on the fetus, far less is known about the father's role in producing healthy offspring' (Merewood, 1992: p. 8). *U.S. News and World Report* began an article on paternal–fetal harm in these terms, 'It is common wisdom that mothers-to-be should steer clear of toxic chemicals that could cause birth defects... Now similar precautions are being urged on fathers-to-be' (Schmidt, 1992: p. 92).

Third, research on men is always *qualified and limited.* A *Chicago Tribune* story, for instance, stated, 'Research like this [on men] may sound convincing, but Dr. David Savitz ... warns that it's far too early to panic. "We have no documented evidence that certain exposures cause certain birth defects," he says' (Merewood, 1992: p. 8). A *New York Times* story (on toxicity to sperm) (Blakeslee, 1991: p. A1) summarized the reservations of one researcher, '[E]pidemiological studies cannot prove cause and effect, said Dr. John Peters... In real life, people are exposed sporadically to combinations of substances that might interact... To show more dramatic associations, he said, scientists would need to study *hundreds of thousands of people over many years*' (emphasis mine). Yet there appear to be no such reservations about studies on women.

Fourth, paternal exposures to illegal drugs are *always* contextualized by *reference to 'involuntary' environmental and workplace exposures*, thereby reducing men's culpability for harm. These are precisely the kinds of complicating exposures absent from reporting on maternal drug use.

Fifth, *the language and images of harmed children and 'crack babies' are absent from stories on men*. A sterile scientific terminology is used to describe studies on paternal exposures, with the rhetoric of 'suffering crack babies' replaced by 'damaged DNA', 'abnormal offspring' and 'genetic anomalies'. One *New York Times* (1992: p. C12) story linking vitamin C deficiencies (produced by male cigarette smoking) with fetal damage reported, 'The study demonstrated a direct relationship between a diet low in vitamin C and increased DNA damage in sperm cells... Any damage to this genetic structure may predispose a man to having children with genetic anomalies'. After reporting that children of fathers who smoke have been found to be at increased risk for leukaemia and lymphoma, the article ends with the recommendation of a physician that men who smoke 'either modify their diets to include fruits and vegetables or take a vitamin C supplement each day'. While sperm 'delivers', 'transports' or 'carries' the drug to the egg in such stories, it never 'assaults' the fetus, as stories on drug use and women imply. When the sperm is not presented as itself a victim, it acts as a shield for men – deflecting or capturing the blame that might otherwise be placed on the father. One news story entitled 'Sperm Under Siege', presented an image of sperm at the centre of a target, menaced by bottles of alcohol and chemicals (Merewood, 1991). Another presented a cartoon image of a man and his sperm huddled under an umbrella whilst packets of cigarettes, martini glasses and canisters of toxins rained down upon them (Black and Moore, 1992). Indeed, in newspapers the only images to accompany these stories were photographs or cartoon images of sperm – never of fathers. Yet of the 853 column inches dedicated to pregnancy, alcohol and drug abuse by the *New York Times* in one two-year period, almost 200 column inches were taken up by photographic images of crack babies and their drug-addicted mothers (Schroedel and Peretz, 1993).

The biological mechanism of paternal–fetal harm have been made invisible not by science itself, but by the lens through which scientific evidence is perceived. A shift in research – and in its wake, scientific reporting – thus requires the transformation of the gendered lens through which evidence is perceived. Even when research implicates men, this lens may obscure the full effects of paternal–fetal exposures. As Evelyn Fox Keller has observed, unarticulated gender assumptions affect not only the questions and methodologies of scientific research but also 'what counts as an acceptable answer or a satisfying explanation' (Keller, 1992: p. 31). For this reason, scientists who have engaged in research on paternal–fetal hazards have met with scepticism from colleagues, editors and newspaper reporters alike.

Paternal effects and 'political correctness'

Evidence of paternal–fetal harm has generated, at best, virtual silence from public health authorities and the courts, or, at worst, active hostility. An editorial in *Reproductive Toxicology* (Scialli, 1993) argued that the impulse to link paternal exposures with fetal effects is a result not of science but of 'political correctness', 'There has been no quarrel that testicular toxicants can produce fertility impairment, but paternally mediated effects on conceived pregnancies is [*sic*] a different matter altogether'. The article concedes that 'several' studies on paternally mediated effects have been 'nicely performed and reported', but taken as a whole they are 'difficult to interpret' (Scialli, 1993: p. 189). Of those who defend the evidence for paternal/fetal links, the editorial (Scialli, 1993) concludes:

The people who make these accusations appear to believe that paternally mediated effects *must* occur in humans, for the sake of fairness... It is argued that because father and mother make equal genetic contributions to the *conceptus*, they must have equal opportunity to transmit toxic effects. Students of developmental biology understand that there is nothing equal about male and female contributions to development... There are several million unequivocal examples of children damaged by intrauterine exposure to toxicants encountered by the mother during gestation. There are no unequivocal examples for paternal exposures.

Yet except for those rare and tragic cases where women are exposed to substances such as thalidomide which cause severe, visible deformities, the question of causality remains profoundly complicated for both women and men. The fact that even the chronic abuse of drugs and alcohol by men has been dismissed, whilst so much attention has focused on even the occasional use of drugs and alcohol by pregnant women, points to the clear ways in which gendered constructions shape both the science and policy of risk.

Even researchers who accept the validity of evidence on male-mediated fetal risks are led to quite different social and political conclusions. The most direct recommendation comes from Ames of the University of California, Berkeley, who, rather than advocating altering male behaviour or printing warning signs on cigarette packages, recommends that the US government raise the standard for minimum daily requirements for vitamin C for all Americans to account for the reproductive effects of paternal smoking (Wright, 1993: p. 10). This is quite a mild remedy, and one that applies equally to men and women, of course. Even in cases where men are exposed to known reproductive hazards, scientists have been remarkably reluctant to recommend the most simple restrictions on men. At the first major medical meeting on male-mediated developmental toxins at the University of Pittsburgh in 1992, men were given 'conflicting advice' about whether to postpone procreation during cancer treatment (or 'bank' sperm before treatment). The journal *Human Reproduction* published a recommendation stating that sperm saved in the early stages of chemotherapy was safe 'based on the belief that since the drugs did not kill sperm ... the sperm were healthy', but others argued that sperm that survive therapy may be more likely to carry genetic defects (Miller, 1992: p. 5).

It is not just the nature of the risk but also the symbolic construction of the population targeted that has determined the public response to fetal risks. The evidence that does now exist suggests that men's actions can have a profound effect on fetal health – both before conception and throughout pregnancy. Yet preventative measures focus almost exclusively on maternally mediated harm. While the mechanisms of harm may not be identical, given the additional avenues of harm that can be delivered through the female body during gestation, it is clear that paternal exposures to toxins can affect both male reproductive health and fetal health.

Science and media representations shaped by gendered constructs of vulnerability and virility have led not just to the negative targeting of women, but also the systematic neglect of men's health needs. Recognition of male vulnerability is thus essential to the protection of male health, as well as the prevention of fetal harm. Ultimately, talk about individual causality for either men or women, whilst important, directs attention away from the more profound social determinants of parental and fetal health – good nutrition, good health care and a clean and safe environment.

References

Baer, J.A. (1978). *The Chains of Protection: The Judicial Response to Women's Labor Legislation.* Westport, CT: Greenwood.

Bingol, N., Schuster, C. and Fuchs, M. et al. (1987). The influence of socioeconomic factors on the occurrence of fetal alcohol syndrome. *Advances in Alcohol and Substance Abuse* **6**: 105–18.

Black, R. and Moore, P. (1992). The myth of the macho sperm. *Parenting* **6**: 29–31.

Blakeslee, S. (1991). Research on birth defects shifts to flaws in sperm. *New York Times* (January):A1.

Brachen, M.B., Eshenazi, B., Sachse, K. et. al. (1990). Association of cocaine use with sperm concentration, motility and morphology. *Fertility and Sterility* **53**: 315–22.

Brody, J.E. (1988). Widespread abuse of drugs by pregnant women is found. *New York Times* (August 30):1.

Burger, E.J., Jr., Tardiff, R.G., Scialli, A.R. and Zenick, H. (Eds) (1989). *Sperm Measures and Reproductive Success.* New York: Alan R. Liss.

Carlsen, E., Giwercman, A., Keiding, M. and Skakkebaek, M.E. (1992). Evidence for decreasing quality of semen during past fifty years. *British Medical Journal* **305**: 609–12.

Castleman, M. (1993). The big drop. *Sierra* (March/April): 36–8.

Chasnoff, I. (1989). Drug use and women: establishing a standard of care. *Annals of the New York Academy of Science* **562**: 208–10.

Colie, C.F. (1993). Male mediated teratogenesis. *Reproductive Toxicology* 7: 3–9.

Daniels, C.R. (1991). Competing gender paradigms: gender difference, fetal rights and the case of Johnson Controls. *Policy Studies Review* 10: 51–68.

Daniels, C.R. (1993). *At Women's Expense: State Power and the Politics of Fetal Rights.* Cambridge, MA: Harvard University Press.

Davis, D.L. (1991). Paternal smoking and fetal health. *Lancet* 337: 123.

Davis, D.L., Friedler, G., Mattison, D. and Morris, R. (1992). Male-mediated teratogenesis and other reproductive effects: biological and epidemiologic findings and a plea for clinical research. *Reproductive Toxicology* 6: 289–92.

Dicker, M. and Leighton, E. (1990). Trends in diagnosed drug problems among newborns: United States, 1979–1987. Paper presented at the annual meeting of the American Public Health Association, New York City, November.

El-Gothamy, Z. and El-Samahy, M. (1992). Ultrastructure sperm defects in addicts. *Fertility and Sterility* 57: 699–702.

Ezzell, C. (1991). Eggs not silent partners in conception. *Science News* 139: 214.

Friedler, G. (1985). Effects of limited paternal exposure to xenobiotic agents on the development of progeny. *Neurobehavioral Toxicology and Teratology* 7: 739–43.

Friedler, G. (1987–88). Effects on future generations of paternal exposure to alcohol and other drugs. *Alcohol Health and Research World* (Winter):126–9.

Friedler, G. (1993). Developmental toxicology: male-mediated effects. In *Occupational and Environmental Reproductive Hazards*, ed. M. Paul, pp. 52–9. Baltimore: Williams & Wilkins.

Friedler, G. and Wheeling, H.S. (1979). Behavioral effects in offspring of male mice injected with opioids prior to mating. In *Protracted Effects of Perinatal Drug Dependence*, vol. II, *Pharmacology, Biochemistry and Behavior*, pp. S23–S28. Fayetteville, NY: ANKHO International.

Keller, E.F. (1992). *Secrets of Life, Secrets of Death.* New York: Routledge.

Kessler-Harris, A. (1982). *Out to Work.* New York: Oxford University Press.

Kharrazi, M., Patashnik, G. and Goldsmith, J.R. (1980). Reproductive effects of Dibromochloropropane. *Israel Journal of Medical Science* 6: 403–6.

Koren, G., Graham, K. and Shear, H. (1989). Bias against the null hypothesis. *Lancet* 2: 1440–2.

Koren, G. and Klein, N. (1991). Bias against negative studies in newspaper reports of medical research. *Journal of the American Medical Association* 266: 1824–6.

Lehrer, S. (1987). *Origins of Protective Labor Legislation.* Albany, NY: SUNY Press.

Little, R.E. and Sing, C.F. (1987). Father's drinking and infant birth weight: report of an association. *Teratology* 36: 59–65.

Mack, A. (Ed.) (1991). *In Time of Plague.* New York: New York University Press.

Martin, E. (1987). *The Woman in the Body.* Boston: Beacon Press.

Martin, E. (1991). The egg and the sperm: how science has constructed a romance based on stereotypical male–female roles. *Signs: Journal of Women in Culture and Society* 16: 485–501.

Massachusetts Coalition for Occupational Safety and Health (1992). *Confronting Reproductive Hazards on the Job.* Boston: MassCosh.

Merewood, A. (1991). Sperm under siege. *Health* (April): 53–76.

Merewood, A. (1992). Studies reveal men's role in producing healthy babies. *Chicago Tribune*, (January 12): 8.

Miller, S.K. (1992). Can children be damaged by fathers' cancer therapy? *New Scientist* No. 135: 5.

Moore, H. M. (1989). Sperm you can count on. *New Scientist* (June 10): 38–91.

New York Times (1992). Vitamin C deficiency in a man's diet might cause problems for offspring. February 12: C12.

Olshan, A.F. and Faustman, E.M. (1993). Male-mediated developmental toxicity. *Reproductive Toxicology* 7: 191–202.

Paltrow, L. (1992). Criminal prosecutions against pregnant women: national update and overview. New York: Center for Reproductive Law and Policy.

Ralt, D., Eisenbach, M., Mashiach, S., Thompson, D. and Garbers, D. (1991). Sperm attraction to a follicular factor(s) correlates with human egg fertilizability. *Proceedings of the National Academy of Sciences* 88: 2840–4.

Robinson, J.C. (1991). *Toils and Toxics: Workplace Struggles and Political Strategies for Occupational Health.* Berkeley: University of California Press.

Savitz, D. and Chen, J. (1990). Parental occupation and childhood cancer: review of epidemiological studies. *Environmental Health Perspectives* 88: 325–37.

Savitz, D. and. Sandler, D.P. (1991). Prenatal exposure to parents' smoking and childhood cancer. *American Journal of Epidemiology,* 133: 123–32.

Savitz, D., Schwingle, P.J. and Keels, M.A. (1991). Influence of paternal age, smoking and alcohol consumption on congenital anomalies. *Teratology* 44: 429–40.

Schmidt, K.F. (1992). The dark legacy of fatherhood. *U.S. News and World Report* (December 14): 92.

Schroedel, J.R. and Peretz, P. (1993). A gender analysis of policy formation: the case of fetal abuse. Unpublished paper, Western Political Science Association meeting, Pasadena, California, March 18–20.

Scialli, A. (1993). Paternally mediated effects and political correctness. *Reproductive Toxicology* 7: 189–90.

Shapiro, B. (1997). The existential decision of a sperm. *Cell* 49: 293–4.

Singer, L. (1993). *Erotic Welfare.* New York: Routledge.

Stellman, S. and Stellman, J. (1980). Health problems among 535 Vietnam veterans potentially exposed to herbicides. *American Journal of Epidemiology* 112: 444.

Stone, A. (1989). It's 'tip of the iceberg' in protecting infants. *USA Today* (August 25): 3.

Wright, B. (1993). Smokers' sperm spell trouble for future generations. *New Scientist* (March 6): 10.

Yazigi, R.A., Odem, R.R. and Polakoski, K.L. (1991). Demonstration of specific binding of cocaine to human spermatozoa. *Journal of the American Medical Association* 266: 1956–9.

Yoshimoto, Y. (1990). Cancer risk among children of atomic bomb survivors: a review of RERF epidemiologic studies. *Journal of the American Medical Association* 264: 596–600.

Zuckerman, B. (1991). Drug-exposed infants: understanding the medical risk. *The Future of Children* 1 (Spring): 26–35.

8

Restricting the freedom of pregnant women

Susan Bewley

Women's Health Services, Guy's and St. Thomas' Hospitals Trust, London, UK

Introduction

In an aggressive response to the dangers of drug-taking in pregnancy, women have been jailed during pregnancy for taking illicit drugs and immediately following delivery if newborn drug tests prove positive (Paltrow, 1990; Berger, 1991). Court judgments have claimed that 'a child has a legal right to begin life with a sound mind and body' (*Smith* v *Brennan*, 1960). The argument appears to be that pregnant drug addicts should stop, as it is wrong to harm fetuses (who will become babies who have a right to be born of sound mind and body). If mothers do not stop, other actions are justified on this view – even those involving force or coercion (Logli, 1990; Nolan, 1990).

However, there are many ways in which mothers put fetuses at risk, apart from taking illegal drugs (such as heroin or cocaine). Examples include taking legal drugs (such as alcohol or cigarettes), failing to attend for antenatal care, inhaling environmental pollutants or even skiing. Actions against pregnant drug takers are taking place within a wider programme of legal enforcement of women's ethical obligations to their fetuses (Kolder et al, 1987; Nelson and Milliken, 1989; *Re S*, 1992).

This chapter examines moral arguments used to justify society acting against pregnant women on behalf of their unborn children. I have used the drug-taker as a 'hard case' and constructed a framework to examine any action against pregnant women (see Figure 8.1).

The moral relationship of mother and fetus

A necessary condition before limiting a pregnant woman's freedom is that a moral relationship exists between mother and fetus. The claims of those wishing to limit pregnant women's freedom are firstly, that a fetus has full rights, and, secondly, that the right to life (Kluge, 1988) or prenatal care (Keyserlingk, 1984) overrides the mother's right to autonomy or inviolability.

Although counter-arguments may be made that the unborn fetus has no moral status (Harris, 1985), or that the right of a woman to control her body

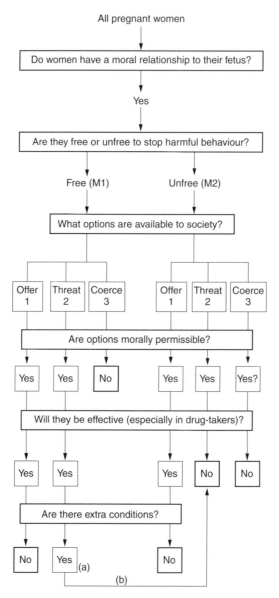

Key: (a) Offers should be tried first. Threats should only be used if offers fail.
A real and serious risk of harm to the fetus must exist; as restrictions on liberty increase, so must the justification; there should be no less drastic method for achieving the same end; the harm prevented should be less than that caused; and compensation might have to be considered for limits on freedom.
(b) The existence of threats aimed at M1 (for whom they are effective) affects M2 (for whom they will be ineffective or even counter-productive).

Figure 8.1. Limiting pregnant women's freedom – the logic of the argument.

is absolute (Thomson, 1974), these are derived from the abortion debate and are inadequate. The issue is the harming of a future person rather than killing. The moral status of the embryo (so important in the abortion debate) is irrelevant to the existence of obligations with respect to harming a future person who indisputably has moral status (Gillon, 1988).

I assume: (1) A fetus has some, even full, moral status; (2) A woman does not have an absolute right to control her body; (3) In general, people have a basic human right not to be interfered with (Hart, 1955); and (4) If a mother has obligations to her fetus, then so has society.

Although (3) may be overridden by another moral consideration, the existence of this right means that a powerful justification must exist if a pregnant woman's freedom is to be limited. The existence of a duty of a mother not to harm her fetus may provide a good reason to apply a restraint, but the burden of proof is on those who wish to restrict freedom.

Do fetuses have rights? This question will be answered differently by rights-based, duty-based or goal-based moralists (Dworkin, 1977). Rights-based moralists who ground rights in autonomy would consider a right as something that can only be enjoyed by autonomous agents, since rights, on this view, protect choice (Hart, 1985). Hart conceives of rights as a kind of property that can be possessed or owned by individuals, and, by analogy, can be given away. One characteristic of rights is that they are capable of being waived. Thus the capacity to alienate or waive rights is central to having them. A non-autonomous fetus cannot have rights, unless the rights it possesses in the future impose duties on us now to care for it so as to ensure that it may achieve this personhood later. But this would mean that the adult physically disabled by thalidomide had a right not to be born of unsound body, whereas the severely brain-damaged individual whose mother took poisonous drugs did not. Taking drugs that inhibit autonomy might become permissible if autonomy is the central moral value. Thus I would rather consider maternal duties towards her fetus due to its intrinsic value.

It is possible to distinguish the claim that a fetus has a right to be born of sound mind and body from the right not to be damaged (implying being made worse off than some previous state, for example by a pregnancy disease) and from the right not to be deliberately or negligently harmed. If a conceptus with a serious chromosomal disorder implants and grows without interference, it will be born unhealthy (without a sound mind and body) but undamaged or unharmed by anyone else.

If the maternal duty is to ensure that her fetus is born *in good health,* then a mother fails in her duty if the fetus is not born in good health. She fails whether her baby has a withdrawal syndrome or Down's syndrome. Does this mean that ensuring the fetus is not born at all would be a fulfilment of the duty? If abortion is tolerated, then one way to fulfil the duty is to abort the unhealthy fetus. Glover (1977: p. 146) states that, 'If aborting the abnormal fetus can be followed by having another, normal one, it will be wrong not to do this'. If abortion is not tolerated, then a mother on drugs who stops can fulfil her duty, whereas a woman carrying a Down's syndrome baby automatically fails. It would be an odd obligation that led to moral failure following chromosomal accidents.

What about ensuring that a fetus is born in *the best possible health*? A positive duty of this sort would entail doing everything possible to avoid harms. However, a lapse or omission would be a failure even if it occurred through ignorance. A mother who did not take all possible steps to read and scan the Internet about dangers in pregnancy would be culpable if a harm then resulted. With the ever-increasing knowledge of influences on pregnancy, such a positive duty is terribly onerous, and ultimately impossible to fulfil. A pregnant woman's life would become a nightmare, devoting herself entirely to protecting her fetus's well-being (Annas, 1986).

The maternal duty might be expressed as taking *reasonable steps to ensure her fetus is born in good health*. A complex weighing is needed to assess what is reasonable, including the size of benefit expected (or harm avoided) and the amount of discomfort the mother will endure. A comparison with the expectation of behaviour judged reasonable in a parent of a small child might be helpful. Parents do not have to be perfect, just 'good enough'. For example, it is not considered a moral failing (nor appropriate to take legal action) if parents occasionally shout at children, leave them with childminders, or quieten them with chocolate, even if, in excess, these things are harmful.

However, pregnant women have a unique disadvantage, compared to parents, as they cannot be separated from their fetuses. Nobody can directly help the fetus, or relieve the pregnant woman of her obligation, even temporarily. Should this intimacy increase her obligation, if she is doing everything reasonable by the standards of a parent of a newborn child? For example, if smoking in the presence of a fetus or newborn had an identical risk of harm to growth, should a pregnant mother suffer more discomfort for them both to be acting equally reasonably? The addicted mother of a newborn has the option to smoke in another room. She should not put cigarettes in the child's mouth, and would be commended if she did not smoke in the child's presence, but giving up entirely would not be the minimum reasonable behaviour. These three actions are not separable in pregnancy. Pregnant women would have to achieve supreme control over their behaviour, which is not expected of new parents.

It seems unjust to have a minimum standard of behaviour that is markedly different to that expected of parents of newborns, especially when it is only applicable to the mother. However, it might be argued that extra duties (beyond reasonable steps) are incurred because a pregnant woman has a *different relationship* from that of a mother of a newborn, though both are in a special relationship with their offspring.

Do pregnant women have a different special relationship? For example, kidney donations between mother and child are not enforced. Why should a mother-to-be have more obligations than the mother-that-is? Most special relationships are entered into willingly. Although many people choose to have children, this is not always so – for example, when unplanned or the result of rape. In such a case, either the maternal obligation is less (which seems unjust to the unplanned fetus, who is less protected by maternal duty than the planned one), or we accept that special relationships thrust more than reasonable obligations even upon raped women, against their will. Interestingly, the only special relationship which is never chosen is that of a child to its parents! Maybe a pregnant woman's duty, without being as much as doing everything possible, is still more than doing what is reasonable? Because the relationship of one inside another is unique, so there is a unique special relationship and extra duties are incurred. But is one being inside the other actually morally relevant? What is at stake is the way the fetus is dependent on the mother and can be damaged by her actions. Conversely, the mother alone shoulders these obligations and the burdens of pregnancy.

Special relationships do not usually demand an unreasonable sacrifice, or supererogatory behaviour, as the minimum required to have fulfilled the duty. For example, no one else has an obligation to have their bodily integrity violated to save the life of another (*McFall* v *Shimp*, 1978), and yet this was the basis for enforced Caesarean section orders before their legal validity was overturned (Kluge, 1988). Philippa Foot draws a powerful distinction between justice and charity in cases of failure to save life (Foot, 1977). A mother might not have an obligation to have her bodily integrity violated (or to take more than reasonable steps) for her fetus, but she would be uncharitable if she did not. A parallel can be drawn with the pregnancy cases where the mother fails to protect her baby from harm (rather than fails to save its life by Caesarean section). It would seem unjust that pregnant women have a different standard by which to measure fulfilment of the obligation to fetuses than is found in any other special relationship.

In addition, being unique (the situation of one inside another) does not adequately explain why maternal duties should be uniquely onerous. It cannot be just because the fetus is particularly vulnerable, as a parent's obligation to a child does not change when the vulnerability changes. Parents of a sick child may be expected to do more than when the child is well, but the standard, of doing what is reasonable (given the situation), does not change.

Pregnant women are discomforted by pregnancy and undergo direct risks to their health and life. Treatments in pregnancy vary in discomfort. Some might require taking a short course of drugs (for example antibiotics); others might require long hospital admission for rest, and separation from other children who might also suffer (for example, for recurrent stillbirth). Few parents die through caring for their small infants (although it may make them exhausted) though many women become ill and die in pregnancy. As many as one per cent of UK women have a 'near-miss' life-threatening event in childbirth, and half a million women worldwide die annually in childbirth. Even in the developed world one woman in 10 000 dies as a direct result of pregnancy. Perhaps this illuminates how much pregnant women generally do beyond the reasonable minimum. By giving up smoking, alcohol, sports or certain foods, attending frequently for health checks, or classes, evincing tremendous interest and concern, and submitting themselves to invasive tests, procedures and hospitalization, women perform daily acts on behalf of their fetuses that are well beyond the reasonable minimum (thus beyond the call of duty, or supererogatory) (Department of Health, 1998).

Society's response and the permissibility of different strategies to stop a mother harming her fetus

If children are not their parents' property, but rather future members of society, then society has a legitimate interest in their welfare. If pregnant women fail to fulfil their obligations, and serious harms occur, society must respond on behalf of the unborn, as it too has an obligation to its future members to take reasonable steps to ensure that they are born in good health. A variety of strategies are available to influence a pregnant woman's behaviour, voluntarily or by force.

Let us compare in two parts methods of influencing and encouraging people to fulfil their moral obligations. What is effective (with regard to stopping the harmful behaviour and damaged babies)? And what is permissible? Society's aim could be: (1) to stop drug-taking in pregnancy; (2) to make women fulfil their obligations; or (3) to minimize preventable harms to babies. If the three outcomes were indistinguishable, it would not matter; but (3) must be the aim. If the goals overlapped but were not identical, society would be able to tolerate a situation where babies were healthy despite the persistence of drug-taking and mothers who failed to fulfil their obligations.

Offers and threats

The difference between a proposal that contains an offer or a threat is that, in the former, the receiver is no worse off than before by rejecting the offer, whereas, in the latter, she is worse off if she does not comply with the threat. Many proposals are bipolar, containing both an offer and a threat. Whereas offers do not usually require justification, as there is no proposal to harm anyone (by making their situation worse), threats do. To illustrate this, a simple unipolar offer might be 'If you get off drugs, you will be given a medal'. This incentive does not require justification (although it may not be effective). A unipolar threat would be 'If you do not get off drugs, your name will be published for public condemnation'. By contrast with the offer, this threat requires a justification (such as the benefit of preventing fetal damage outweighing the humiliation and harm caused to women). If the two uni-polar strategies are equally effective, the choice of the threat strategy rather than the offer one is not justifiable, because nothing now weighs against the harms caused through threatening people. Offers are thus morally preferable to threats when they are equally effective. To opt for a threat, if an offer is available, requires firstly, that it is more effective and secondly, that the difference in effectiveness is itself justified. If 1000 drug addicts stop before or after having their names publicized, as opposed to 999 with the medal option, it has to be argued that the one extra drug-free baby justifies 1000 women being threatened with ostracism by their neighbours.

Different types of threat to pregnant women can be identified: to imprison during pregnancy; to punish after delivery; or to separate the mother and baby after birth (by imprisoning the mother or taking the baby away). Some threats materialize immediately, some materialize later. Offers can be made without needing a justification, whereas threats cannot. It is worth noting that both are pointless if women are not free to respond.

Let us examine the specific threat to separate mother and baby if she continues to take drugs. If women know that they will be jailed or their babies taken away on the basis of a blood or urine test on the newborn, this is a threat operating during the antenatal period to persuade them to stop drugs. It relies on an assumption that the woman wants to keep her baby (which may be correct in most cases). But if a woman did not care for her baby, it might have the opposite effect, and become an incentive to continue drugs. Secondly, the baby has become an instrument of society's will towards its mother's behaviour. It is used as a means to threaten its mother rather than being treated as an end in itself, which seems inconsistent with the concern for fetal and neonatal well-being from which the threat sprang. Enactment of the threat is inherently an admission of its failure or ineffectiveness. If drug-taking during pregnancy is a form of 'fetal abuse' (Landwith, 1987), once the baby is born the abuse stops, as the drug no longer crosses the placenta. Birth corrects the abuse. In addition, the intention of a drug addict is not necessarily to hurt the fetus. Once her baby is born the identical action, of injecting herself, would not count as child abuse. If society wanted to prevent so-called 'fetal abuse' to an individual fetus, taking the post-birth action against the mother is too late. A post-birth action is appropriate for punishment but not prevention, except that it might deter the next woman. Effective threats should be preferred. Separation has now taken on the character of punishment, with the newborn baby being used as a means to punish its mother. The threat to separate a mother from her baby merely because there is evidence she continued to take drugs during pregnancy is not morally justifiable.

Use of the Mental Health Act could also be seen as a threat to pregnant women, except that it is correctly applied only to enforce non-consensual treatments for psychiatric illnesses. If a woman is mentally incompetent through such an illness, decisions about interventions can be made (such as consent for Caesarean section) in her 'best interests', but abuse of this provision is not to be encouraged. (A fuller discussion of this issue in the context of recent UK case law is provided by Wendy Savage, Chapter 17.)

Coercion

Coercion has two different senses: (1) to prevent a person from doing as she or he chooses; and (2) to make a choice less eligible by threats. There is a point where the second becomes the first, where there is no real choice, as it has become meaningless because of the severity of the threat. Coercion is the most extreme form of threat, and it is in this stronger sense that it will be used. Coercion is prima facie wrong because it removes liberty, the freedom to do as one chooses, and thus violates autonomy.

If a woman can give up drugs freely, it is not justifiable to coerce her, though non-coercive threats to encourage her may be justified. If it is ever permissible to use coercion, it will only be when a woman cannot stop her harmful behaviour by herself. This might be illustrated using two infectious diseases that harm others. If a woman had Lassa fever (often fatal and highly infectious through airborne passage) it would be justified to quarantine her (and override her right of liberty) as she is presenting a serious danger to others and cannot voluntarily stop breathing. A man with Hepatitis B (often fatal though not highly infectious, and transmitted only through close contact with bodily fluids) presents a danger to others only if he engages in certain activities (such as sex or blood donation). He is free to choose whether to have unprotected sex or donate blood, and is culpable when he does. But it would not be justified to quarantine him because he might engage in a dangerous activity over which he has control. Indeed, this is the situation in English law. It is possible to detain a person under the Public Health (Control of Diseases) Act 1984, but not to forcibly treat him or her. Diseases such as cholera, plague, relapsing fever, smallpox and typhoid are included, but not conditions such as HIV or AIDS. Quarantine might be used as a last resort only if many people with Hepatitis B neglected their obligations to others, and would wrong those who would not have put others at risk.

If society could increase the likelihood of a drug-taker stopping with offers or non-coercive threats, but does not, then if she continues to take drugs she is less reprehensible than if she had rejected such offers or threats, although she is not guiltless. The presence or absence of incentives, such as free antenatal care and drug treatment programmes, changes the degree of culpability. Offers and non-coercive threats have to be reserved for those women who can stop taking drugs. If a person can stop, she should be allowed and encouraged to do so; otherwise her autonomy is violated. Coercion should be reserved for those cases where women cannot stop their harmful behaviour.

Punishment for reckless endangerment

Is drug-taking in pregnancy necessarily reckless? Bonnie Steinbock argues that drink-driving is always immoral despite the fact that many of the drivers caught are alcoholics, who cannot stop drinking. They are not compelled to drive, unlike their craving for alcohol which has to be satisfied. To drive a car after having drunk alcohol is reckless behaviour. She claims that drunk drivers who cause death are indeed murdering through recklessness (Steinbock, 1985). The analogy is useful for the distinction that can be drawn. Unlike the alcoholic driver, the pregnant alcoholic cannot separate taking alcohol from the effect on the fetus – although she could avoid other additional reckless behaviour, such as driving when intoxicated, she cannot avoid giving the fetus a dose of the drug as she satisfies her craving. The two behaviours, satisfying the craving and delivering alcohol to the fetus, cannot be separated, even if she would like to do one but not the other. So, delivering drugs to the fetus is not reckless like drink-driving. The equivalent reckless behaviour is not taking drugs when pregnant, but rather, knowingly getting pregnant when addicted to dangerous drugs. Thus, the reckless behaviour to be punished would be getting pregnant, rather than taking drugs. It is difficult to know what to make of this conclusion except to note that it must be impossible to determine which pregnancies are conceived recklessly, and what would be an appropriate punishment.

If a mother has a positive urine drug test, she has failed to respond to threats made earlier in pregnancy. If one woman cannot respond to the threat, and another can but did not, both will have positive urine tests but only one persists in intentional wrongdoing. Both may be jailed, a punishment, for having failed to respond to the threat, not for intentional or reckless wrongdoing. If punishment should be reserved for wrong acts performed freely, then it would be wrong to punish merely for failure to respond to a threat (as this includes both women who can and cannot stop their harmful behaviour).

Punishment should be limited to those cases in which harm has been caused by the behaviour which was freely performed, and where there was intent to cause harm. Punishment does not undo harm nor prevent it, as it can only be used after a wrongdoing, and therefore must be the least preferred option in terms of changing behaviour. However, the existence of punishment after birth might act as a deterrent against harmful behaviours earlier in pregnancy, and thus it joins the array of threats available to society to influence behaviour. It can be used as a threat during pregnancy, even if it only materializes after birth.

Moral ranking of different strategies

The order of preference of strategies to influence behaviour is: (1) offers (or incentives) over threats; (2) non-coercive means over coercive means; with (3) physical force and punishment being the least preferable. They need not be mutually exclusive (though some are, such as the promise of medical confidentiality and the revealing of urine sample results to the police).

It is permissible to use offers and non-coercive threats when women can stop harmful behaviour (although threats need extra justification over offer), whereas coercion is only permissible, if at all, when women cannot stop freely. It thus becomes crucial which drug-takers are or are not free.

The will of a drug-taker

Frankfurt's account of freedom reflects well the complexity of autonomy, and presents a way to unravel the drug addict's intent. He describes what distinguishes us as human beings as our 'ability to form second-order desires' (Frankfurt, 1971) – only human beings can want to want something. Although a woman might have conflicting first-order wants, it is the identification with a second-order desire that determines the kind of person she is. For example, a pregnant woman might want both to take drugs and not to be dependent on this desire. A second-order desire is 'I want to want to give up drugs'. It cannot be assumed that because a woman takes drugs she intends to do harm, or that she does not care for her fetus. It can only be said that the desire to take drugs outweighed any desire to help the fetus. What she does, a result of the first-order conflicts, does not tell us what she really wants, her second-order desire. A woman who cannot give up drugs, despite her best intent, does not have a free will. Her first-order desire to take drugs overwhelms another first-order desire to do the best for her fetus, and possibly a second-order desire to be a drug-free woman. This is a double tragedy, as she harms her fetus, against her will, and her will is not free and autonomous.

Although some women stop taking drugs in pregnancy, this does not mean that others did not try to give them up or wanted to stay on them. Real life may be more complicated, as the first- and second-order desires of an addict might change throughout the day, as the cravings wax and wane, or throughout the pregnancy, as the fetus grows and interacts. Women experience different degrees of difficulty in stopping. Let us imagine two pregnant women: M1, who can modify her behaviour; and M2, who cannot stop harmful behaviour voluntarily, whatever her will. M1 may stop taking drugs either because she is mindful of her duty and does not wish to harm her baby, or because she is reluctantly goaded into stopping. M1 can be told that if she attends antenatal clinic and gets off drugs, she has an increased chance of an unharmed baby. When a mother wishes to do the best for her baby, the result of this offer corresponds to one part of her will and her interests. Alternatively, she could respond to a threat such as going to jail if she does not get off drugs. The realization of the threat is against her interests (as she goes to jail) and that of the child (who will be separated from its mother). Women who were indifferent to the fate of their babies might be uninterested in an offer, but still responsive to a threat. There may be women who want to take drugs for whom only threats work. For these women who are not compelled to take drugs, the threat of going to prison or being punished if their urine tests are positive may work. A 'recreational' user, who takes drugs occasionally for the pleasant effect, might stop in the face of threats. The existence of a future punishment is in itself a present threat, but if it is in society's armamentarium, it acts as a threat to all pregnant women. It is not a threat that can be made selectively. Thus we must consider the effect that threats made to influence M1 might have on M2.

M2 cannot stop taking drugs, whatever her will or second-order desires, because she is compelled to continue. What does it mean to say that a woman is compelled to take drugs? A drug addict who reacts to falling levels or shortage of supply with feelings of severe discomfort (withdrawal syndrome) has no choice but to respond with the reasonable and purposive action of buying or finding more drugs. Thus the drug addict is unfree, as the threat of discomfort means that she is compelled to take a certain action (Greenspan, 1978). We can see that M2's drug taking has become immune to offers or threats. The only way to stop her taking drugs is by force, for example, by incarceration to (hopefully) cut off her supply of drugs, an external coercion corresponding to the inner compulsion to take drugs.

Compulsions might affect our assessment of what is reasonable. What is reasonably expected changes with the amount of discomfort anticipated on stopping the drug. Thus the biological effect of dependence-producing drugs will be critical in making a judgement, not just the damage caused. Some soft cheeses contain the listeriosis bacterium, which can cause miscarriage, fatal intra-uterine infections and premature labour (with all its consequent complications). If eating soft blue cheese and taking heroin had the same adverse effects on fetuses, but an addict's discomfort on stopping heroin was markedly worse, then the mother who continues to eat gorgonzola would be more culpable than the woman who continues to take heroin.

Compulsions also interact with threats and offers. To avoid suffering severe discomfort, by withdrawal of the drug M2 craves and is compelled to take, the rational and reasonable action is to avoid giving a sample of urine, or miss the clinic. If M2 realizes that the clinic staff will be suspicious and send the police to her house, a better tactic would be to conceal the pregnancy. Thus, the combination of the threat and compulsion works against both M2's and society's intention to do the best for her baby. Antenatal care, even in the presence of drug-taking, is of benefit for picking up other diseases of pregnancy, such as diabetes, pre-eclampsia and growth retardation, and it creates the possibility of giving advice, treatment or intervention through a timed delivery. Avoiding the clinic is now a worse outcome, as the fetus is still exposed to drugs and has lost the chance of benefiting from pregnancy care. A 'harm limitation' exercise has the goal of producing the best achievable health in the baby, not the riskier goal of stopping drug-taking entirely. For women who are compelled to take drugs there is the potential to make matters worse by deterring drug addicts from obtaining medical care.

The most attractive incentive would be a safe supply of the drug. Indeed, the policy of British antenatal care and drug maintenance programmes is to stabilize registered addicts on drugs prescribed by licensed doctors. This can be justified simply by being safer than street drugs (which may be con- taminated or given via shared infected needles). If the woman attends the antenatal clinic at the same time, two potential improvements to her baby's health are made even before drug reduction (De Swiet, 1989). Although it may be wrong to tolerate preventable harms to babies, it is assuredly worse to create the conditions in which more harms occur. Like many moral conflicts, it is not a choice between right and wrong, but of the lesser of two evils.

The complexity of judging and influencing maternal behaviour

With this complex model in mind, the drug-taking pregnancy can be viewed not merely as a grave danger to the fetus due to maternal failing, but as an opportunity to offer intervention and improve fetal health. The pregnant drug addict may be harmed, or even die, as a consequence of her drug-taking, and thus the incentive to improve her own health may be added to fetal incentives. She may stabilize her life and improve her circumstances, such that she can care adequately for her child. She may minimize her use of drugs or stop them altogether. If her will is in conflict, as described earlier, she has the opportunity to identify more strongly with that part that wishes to do the best for her fetus, or wishes not to be a drug addict, and thus become more truly an autonomous person. If, without drug treatment programmes for pregnant women (Chavkin, 1990), she misses this opportunity, society fails both to aid her fetus and to help her realize her autonomy and potential. Strategies that threaten her, or that through fear or interaction with her compulsion diminish rational and reflective self-evaluation, reduce her autonomy (already reduced by addiction). Other incentives that might encourage M2 to minimize harm to her fetus, such as public education, free and confidential health care, non-judgemental attitudes and access to social service help, will get drug-takers into clinics. Free contraception and pre- pregnancy counselling are preventative measures that could be available before she becomes pregnant. If society can work with the compulsion, or at least understand its nature, it will be most effective. A pragmatic aim would be to stabilize an addict first, and tackle the drugs later. A threat cannot be carried out at least until a woman is obviously pregnant, or identifies herself as such. Pregnancy is not obvious early on, when the fetus is developing and most vulnerable to harmful substances. It is possible to conceal pregnancy right up to delivery. Offers are the only practical way to influence behaviour in women who are unidentified to society's agents. If society's response has to wait for visible signs of pregnancy, rather than the mother volunteering herself, many vital months are wasted.

Widening the scope

Several more qualifications still have to be considered before limiting pregnant women's freedom: (1) there should be a real and serious risk to a particular fetus; (2) as a woman's freedom is increasingly interfered with, so the justification for the limitation should become stronger; (3) there has to be no less drastic method for achieving the same end; (4) the harm prevented should not be less than any harm caused; and (5) if freedom is limited, women are harmed by interference with their basic right of liberty (albeit justifiably, and thus not wronged) and there is a case for compensation.

Real and serious risk

It is not enough that a risk exists. If the risk is very remote – for example, every millionth pregnant woman walking on icy pavements falls over and suffers a stillbirth – that would not seem to justify keeping pregnant women indoors all winter. If the risk is of trivial harm – let us say that listening to commercial radio made babies respond by smiling to advertising jingles – that would not justify banning pregnant women from listening to the radio. At a minimum, the risk to this fetus must be real and serious.

Increasing restrictions on liberty, increasing justification

An example of justifiable limitation on freedom might be long-distance air travel close to delivery. It seems reasonable to balance the small risk of premature delivery and a great limitation on freedom if women could not travel at all against a higher chance at term and less limitation on freedom. As the limitation lasts only for a few weeks, it is not as restrictive as incarceration for a detoxification programme.

No less drastic method for achieving the same end

A drug that no mother could stop taking voluntarily would be an inhaled environmental pollutant. If there was an escape of the very teratogenic (embryo-deforming) poison gas dioxin blowing towards a city, a justification of forcibly rounding up the pregnant women to transport them away could be based on avoiding harm to their fetuses. However, less drastic measures, such as announcements on public loudspeakers, must be preferred. It would be better still to strengthen regulations on factories to prevent such accidents.

If preventing fetal harm overrides women's rights to freedom, or bodily integrity, it can also be used to override their wishes regarding the continuing of the pregnancy. One problem with using harm prevention arguments to override a woman's right to freedom is the 'slippery slope'. The arguments can boomerang back to argue for enforced abortions (if abortion is justified as the killing of a being without full moral status), when an abortion is a lesser wrong than allowing the continuance of a pregnancy that will lead to a life of suffering. If the wind blew the dioxin cloud too fast, the only way to prevent the harm of damaged fetuses would be to abort them.

Harm prevented should be more than that caused

There should also be good evidence that harm can and will be prevented. There are very many causes of fetal damage, some interacting with one another. When damage occurs before a woman realizes she is pregnant, or before she tells anyone, limitations on her freedom will be too late. For example, alcohol may damage babies through a variety of mechanisms from conception to three months (Pratt, 1984). Only the most draconian measures (such as screening the entire female population for pregnancy) would be able to identify those women whose behaviour in early pregnancy is an avoidable source of harm. There is no evidence that threat strategies prevent harm. What little work there is on substance abuse reporting laws show no change in substance abuse in subsequent pregnancies (Delke et al., 1993).

Compensation for interfering with freedom

Women might claim compensation for interference with their freedom. If a woman cannot work in certain jobs there should be no penalty, such as dismissal, as this would act as a strong disincentive to tell the truth, or even as a pressure towards termination. Maternity leave, maternity pay and sex discrimination laws can be considered as compensations for losses of freedom.

Conclusion

The moral obligation of a pregnant woman is to take reasonable steps to ensure that her fetus is born in good health. Society wishes, rightly, to diminish harmful maternal behaviour during pregnancy. There are a variety of strategies, limited by what is morally justified and what is effective. The pragmatic aim is not narrowly to get women to stop drugs, but to achieve the healthiest possible mothers and babies. The use of incentives is preferable to threats, coercion or punishment. There are good reasons to doubt the efficacy of threats when a mother is addicted to drugs, and it is wrong to punish her for behaviour that is compulsive. One comprehensive strategy might be to have a 'hands-off, offers only' system which should not deter those women who cannot stop drug-taking from seeking health care, but does not tackle indifferent women who only stop under threat. This is the system in the UK, where the fetus has no legal status (Bewley, 1994) and women have free antenatal care, free prescriptions, non-coercive drug treatment programmes and guarantees of medical confidentiality. Women can no longer be forced to undergo Caesarean sections in the fetal interest (*St George's Healthcare NHS Trust* v *R.V. Collins and others, ex parte S*, 1998) and have not been prosecuted for drug-taking in pregnancy or the resulting harms, although children can be taken into care after birth. On the other hand, a threat strategy (such as antenatal urine test results being revealed to the police, jailing for drug-taking in pregnancy and separation on the basis of neonatal testing) may stop drug-taking in women who are not compelled to take drugs, although it risks alienating others who are so compelled from antenatal care altogether.

Both strategies cannot influence all women's behaviour at the same time. There is an unavoidable tension between them. Whichever is chosen, it *inevitably* will fail to prevent all preventable harm. The choice has to be made on the criteria of moral preferability and effectiveness (or 'least overall harm'). The threats strategy is less preferable, morally. Before considering implementation, it must at least be more effective. There is no medical evidence whatsoever for this. It is wrong to limit pregnant, drug-taking women's freedom, in the ways described, especially in the absence of having unsuccessfully tried morally preferable methods.

References

Annas, G. (1986). Pregnant women as fetal containers. *Hastings Center Report* **16**: 13–14.

Berger, M. (1991). Behind bars before birth. *The Sunday Times*, 18th September.

Bewley, S. (1994) Legal frameworks to prevent harm *in utero*. *Medical Law International* **1**: 277–87.

Chavkin, W. (1990). Drug addiction and pregnancy: policy crossroads. *American Journal of Public Health* **80**: 483.

Delke, I., Sanchez-Ramos, L. and Briones, D. (1993). Effects of substance abuse reporting laws on cocaine use in subsequent pregnancies. *American Journal of Obstetrics and Gynecology* **168**: 403.

Department of Health (1998). *Why Mothers Die: Report on Confidential Enquiry into Maternal Deaths in the United Kingdom,* 1st edn. London: HMSO.

De Swiet, M. (1989). *Medical Disorders in Obstetric Practice.* Oxford: Blackwell.

Dworkin, R. (1977). *Taking Rights Seriously.* London: Duckworth.

Foot, P. (1977). Euthanasia. In *The Philosophy and Public Affairs Reader,* pp. 276–303. Princeton: Princeton University Press.

Frankfurt, H.G. (1971). Freedom of the will and the concept of a person. *Journal of Philosophy* **67**: 5–20.

Gillon, R. (1988) Pregnancy, obstetrics and the moral status of the fetus. *Journal of Medical Ethics* **14**: 3–4.

Glover, J. (1977) *Causing Death and Saving Lives,* 1st edn. Harmondsworth: Penguin.

Greenspan, P.S. (1978). Behaviour control and freedom of action. *Philosophical Review* **87**: 225–40.

Harris, J. (1985). *The Value of Life: An Introduction to Medical Ethics.* London: Routledge and Kegan Paul.

Hart, H.L.A. (1955). Are there any natural rights? *Philosophical Review* **64**: 175–91.

Hart, H.L.A. (1985). Are there any natural rights? In *Theories of Rights,* ed. J. Waldron, pp. 77–90. Oxford: Oxford University Press.

Keyserlingk, E.W. (1984). The unborn child's right to prenatal care: a comparative law perspective. *McGill Legal Studies* **5**: 184.

Kluge, E.H. (1988). When Caesarean section operations imposed by a court are justified. *Journal of Medical Ethics* **14**: 206–11.

Kolder, V.E.B., Gallagher, J. and Parsons, M.T. (1987). Court ordered Cesarean sections. *New England Journal of Medicine* **316**: 1192–6.

Landwith, J. (1987). Fetal abuse and neglect: an emerging controversy. *Paediatrics* **79**: 508–14.

Logli, P.A. (1990). Drugs in the womb: the newest battlefield in the war on drugs. *Criminal Justice Ethics,* Winter/Spring: 23–9.

McFall v *Shimp.* (1978) The Court of Common Pleas, Allegheny County, Pennsylvania, order of 26th July.

Nelson, L.J. and Milliken, M. (1989). Compelled medical treatment of pregnant women: life, liberty and law in conflict. *Journal of the American Medical Association* **259**: 1060–6.

Nolan, K. (1990). Protecting fetuses from prenatal hazards: whose crimes? What punishment? *Criminal Justice Ethics* (Winter/Spring): 13–23.

Paltrow, L.M. (1990) When becoming pregnant is a crime. *Criminal Justice and Ethics* (Winter/Spring): 41–7.

Pratt, O.E. (1984). What do we know of the mechanisms of alcohol damage *in utero?* In *Mechanisms of Alcohol Damage in Utero,* CIBA Foundation Symposium, pp. 1–7. London: Pitman.

Re S: law report (1992) *The Independent,* 14th October.

St George's Healthcare NHS Trust v *R.V. Collins and others, ex parte S* (1998) 3 All ER 673.

Smith v *Brennan* (1960). 157 Ad2 497, 503.

Steinbock. B. (1985). Drunk driving. *Philosophy and Public Affairs* **14**: 278–95.

Thomson, J.J. (1974). A defense of abortion. In *The Rights and Wrongs of Abortion,* ed. M. Cohen, T. Nagel and T. Scanlon, pp. 3–22. Princeton: Princeton University Press.

Inception of pregnancy: new reproductive technologies

Ethical issues in embryo interventions and cloning

Françoise Shenfield

Centre for Medical Ethics, UCL Medical School, London, UK

Introduction

Although the first IVF (in vitro fertilization) child has passed the age of majority, ethical dilemmas linked to the field continue to be subject to the world's scrutiny. Arguably, some are 'classical' problems of assisted reproduction, either because they pertain intrinsically to the essence of IVF (as in embryo research), or because they relate to techniques preceding IVF as a means of assisted reproduction (for instance, sperm donation). Another dilemma is that of embryo reduction, itself often a consequence of IVF techniques (although in the UK, since the Human Fertilisation and Embryology Act (1990), most multiple pregnancies of a high order are the consequence of non-licensed ovulation induction). Indeed some Scandinavian countries have either altered their legislation or professional codes of practice recently in order to limit embryo transfer to one or two embryos per cycle and to decrease the rate of multiple pregnancies. Embryo reduction is discussed by Mary Mahowald in Chapter 16 and will, therefore, not be dealt with at length here. Then there is the question of what responsibilities we owe to the children of assisted conception (an issue discussed by Christine Overall in Chapter 19).

The choice of issues to discuss has been narrowed down to newer techniques specifically linked to IVF, and only made possible when IVF itself matured into a more successful and more common treatment. There is necessarily a more acute need to analyse these less 'classical' dilemmas, such as ICSI (intra-cytoplasmic sperm injection), a revolution in the treatment of subfertile men which involves micro-injecting the egg with a single sperm, and pre-implantation diagnosis, a genetic diagnostic technique involving biopsy of the embryo in vitro. As for the even newer issues related to technological advances, such as ovarian tissue freezing or reproductive cloning, their practical application is probably still quite distant. This does not, however, mean that we should not tackle the ethical issues that they raise now.

All these 'micoethical' issues should also be seen in the larger 'macroethical' context, including issues of social justice such as equal access to fertility treatment. These are questions of public policy and funding of the health system. It seems wrong for the patient's chance of appropriate treatment to be dictated by its cost (or cost-effectiveness). However, although we know that health expenses are increasing worldwide, the problem of efficacious spending on health is a political and ethical matter beyond the scope of this chapter. It nevertheless deserves a mention, as 'keeping to budget' has now become a major concern in health care choices all over the world (Hermeren, 1998). In passing, however, it is still puzzling to observe that in our wealthier countries huge sums of money are spent at the end of life, whilst objectors to the whole field of life-creating fertility treatment are still arguing that it is money misspent on a 'non-medical matter' (Shenfield, 1997).

In the final section of this chapter I shall move on to ethical issues in reproductive and therapeutic human cloning, briefly drawing on arguments about difference and identity from the French psychoanalytical feminist Julia Kristeva (1991). Thus the choice in this chapter is necessarily somewhat eclectic – even entire books dedicated to these issues cannot hope to be exhaustive (e.g. Shenfield and Sureau, 1997).

Embryo research and screening

Embryo research is necessary to the continual improvement of assisted reproduction techniques such as IVF; yet it was also one of the most contentious fields when it began. As shown in a three-day meeting held in December 1996 at the Council of Europe on the protection of the human embryo, this essential question is still central. The meeting was held a month after the Committee of Ministers of the Council of Europe had approved the text of the Convention for the Protection of Human Rights and Dignity of the Human Being With Regard to the Application of Biology and Medicine (Convention of Human Rights and Biomedicine; (Council of Europe, 1996)). Controversy over embryo research has been heightened since then by the growing commercial importance of stem cells derived from embryonic and fetal tissue (see Chapter 15).

The famous semantic debate over the term 'pre-embryo' actually obscures the matter even further. Using the term 'pre-embryo' to refer to 'the stage of the conceptus for the interval from the completion of the process of fertilisation until the establishment of biologic individuation' (Jones and Schrader, 1992) aroused suspicion that the embryo's supposed human essence was deliberately ignored or lessened by adding the prefix (Seve, 1994).

On a utilitarian argument, the improvement of success rates in IVF is beneficial to welfare; if IVF is morally acceptable, so is embryo research, the latter being necessary to the improvement of the former. Both the Human Fertilisation and Embryology Act (HFEA) 1990 and the July 1994 *Loi* reflect, in the UK and France, the intensity and breadth of public concern in matters of reproduction. Both avoid qualifying the status of the embryo as such, within the only two categories known in law: '*res*' (thing, property) or person. The HFEA Code of Practice stresses 'that the special status of the embryo is fundamental to the provisions of the Act' without defining this special quality, and French law underlines the respect due to the human body 'as soon as life begins', without defining this precise moment. French legislation, however, makes the creation of embryos purely for research purposes a criminal offence (*Loi* no 94, Article 511, section 18).

Even if this utilitarian argument were accepted as uncontroversial – which it is patently not – two further problems arise: the source of embryos, and their fate. If non-viable embryos are to be preferred on the grounds that no harm is done, less good may result – the results may not be easily applicable to viable embryos. So perhaps abandoned or surplus embryos are to be preferred. The two cases are different – not all surplus embryos will be abandoned. In English law any couple cryopreserving surplus embryos must give consent and choose their fate (donation, research or destruction) when the legal time limit for cryopreservation has elapsed. From May 1996 the HFEA lengthened the statutory limit for cryopreservation of embryos, in-itially five years, to 10 years within specific clinical settings and with consent. The transition from five to 10 years led to a major public debate in 1996 in the UK about the 'abandoned' embryos whose gamete providers could not be traced. May one then use abandoned embryos, for which, by definition, there would not need to be any consent, before they are due to be destroyed? This could arguably be the case in settings where there is as yet no legislation, but it is hard to imagine this within the UK setting, where the ultimate fate of the embryo must be decided in advance by the provider couple at the time of cryopreservation.

In most cases embryos used for research will in fact be destroyed, as the safety of the potential child who might ensue cannot be assured, and it can actually be argued that it would be unethical to replace such embryos *in utero*. The possibility of cryopreservation of embryos since 1984 has enabled couples to have further attempts at embryo transfer from one stimulation IVF cycle. The availability of cryopreservation makes the creation of embryos purely for research purposes even more controversial, but perhaps more necessary – surplus or supernumerary embryos may be frozen for possible later use, and might only be given for research once the couple have become parents.

Once pre-implantation research on the embryo is accepted, it follows that its status as a non-person is implicitly recognized. This is not because its consent cannot be obtained, as parents are entitled in law to give consent on behalf of children below the standards of 'Gillick competence' (*Gillick* v *West Norfolk and Wisbech Area Health Authority*, 1985), but rather because its destruction is necessarily planned, distancing the embryo from full human status. Where parental consent is recognized, the parent is expected to decide in the best interests of the incompetent child; deciding to destroy the embryo is *ipso facto* not in its best interests.

By definition, when the technique researched has proven to be safe and useful, it may become therapeutic or diagnostic. Then the embryo concerned may be allowed to fulfil its potential to become a person, which, in English law, it does not become until born alive.

By contrast, therapeutic or diagnostic interventions may be performed for the benefit of the embryo. ICSI, for example, is one of the techniques that has radically changed the outlook for male infertility – although it was sometimes criticized for being used therapeutically when actually it was still in the research stage. Here the benefit lies in averting the possibility of transmission of sex chromosome anomalies which might in particular threaten the future fertility of the male child of an ICSI couple. Some have even advocated pre-implantation diagnosis following ICSI, but this is arguably too powerful a tool to use for what may be seen as only a moderately severe disability. This leads us to consider the indications for pre-implantation diagnosis, and the notion of 'severe handicap', already used in the terminology of legal termination of pregnancy. Embryo screening is not research, but neither is it necessarily therapeutic, at least so far as the embryo rather than the parents is concerned.

Pre-implantation genetic diagnosis (PGD) triggers the fear of potential genetic manipulation, and is often considered to be on the slippery slope to criminal eugenics (Testard and Sele, 1995). If eugenics is defined as a practice imposed on a population, and not in terms of individual couples' choice to avert possible serious disease (e.g. cystic fibrosis), this accusation founders (Shenfield, 1997). Other fears concern phantasmatic perversions of heredity, or at least poorly controlled intrusions into the genome of germline cells. The most complex ethical question is in fact not so much the current practice of pre-implantation diagnosis, but rather what might be the consequences of its evolving techniques. Will pre-implantation diagnosis lead couples to expect the assurance of a 'perfect' baby?

This very point is alluded to in the joint public consultation document published in November 1999 by the HFEA and the ACGT, spelling out that neither body thinks it 'would be acceptable to test for any social or psychological characteristics, normal physical variations, or any other conditions which are not associated with disability or a serious medical condition'. The questions for consultation centre around, but do not actually mention, the distinction between positive and negative eugenics, perhaps because the terms are so historically tainted (Missa, 1999). Instead the document concentrates on practical issues, within the context of licensing clinics for testing specific inherited conditions and restricting access through guidelines that limit which patients might avail themselves of PGD. Such questions have already been asked in the context of antenatal screening in general. No legislation that allows termination of pregnancy on the grounds of a 'serious' disorder has actually drawn up a list of the conditions that would qualify. It seems appropriate to suggest that PGD could also be called Pre-Gravid Testing, and that it can be compared to other forms of prenatal testing already in place in many countries.

The specific ethical problems of pre-implantation diagnosis are also linked to its particular constraints, especially the need to undergo IVF. It is thus understandable that the more classical approach (prenatal diagnosis, possibly followed by therapeutic termination of pregnancy) may sometimes be preferred by patients. Studies have shown different preferences according to the past experience of the couples concerned and the gender of the potential parent (Chamayou et al., 1998). In practice, it is for the time being a matter of rather restricted choice, as the number of units available worldwide for this technique is extremely limited, making it available only to a few prospective parents. Needless to say, counselling is of great importance in all these decisions. The need for long-term surveillance of this particularly 'precious' offspring in turn entails recording the births and follow-up of the children with their specific dilemmas already described in detail (Milliez and Sureau, 1997).

Another concern in pre-implantation diagnosis is the dilemma between the fundamental principle of confidentiality for the couple and the right to privacy of the potential child, together with the psychological consequences of intrusion for the children. The problem of confidentiality with regards to the child sometimes seems insoluble, as it entails a parental, if not sometimes a state, decision, as is the case with non-anonymity of gamete donors in Sweden. In this context it is useful to stress the responsibility that the adults involved, carers as well as putative parents, have towards the vulnerable future third party – the child to be. Fifteen years after implementation of the law in Sweden, 89 per cent of the parents of sperm donor children still have not informed them of their origins (Gottlieb et al., 2000), perhaps exemplifying the complexity of this dilemma.

Cryopreservation of reproductive tissues

Fragility and vulnerability are also uppermost in issues concerning the cryopreservation of reproductive tissues of adolescents who are suffering from cancer, the treatment of which threatens their future reproductive capacity. This is especially sensitive as reproduction is not a matter which they or their peers are accustomed to considering. They are facing serious disease if not possible death, and are often under the age of majority (although often *Gillick* competent). (It is also generally good practice to involve the parents in these sensitive decisions.) A UK working party is, at the time of writing, about to address the issues with paediatric oncologists, lawyers, psychologists, ethicists and patients' groups. However, we are only now starting to address a problem which can only grow larger in view of the increased ability to store successfully testicular or ovarian tissue for future reproduction.

In this case the intent, that is the conservation of the reproductive ability of children and adolescents, seems prima facie beneficent, but that may primarily be the *parents*' intent, possibly biased by a desire to one day have a grandchild who might remind them of a beloved deceased child. But is this in the adolescent's own best interests? Ovarian biopsy may indeed be a fairly risky procedure in a relatively sick adolescent girl, much more so than sperm donation or testicular biopsy from a boy. Again we face a situation where the intent and the consent of the child or adolescent concerned may not be identical, where one could not be presumed to take place of the other. Could a biopsy be taken, for instance, when the child is unable to consent because he or she is not deemed *Gillick* competent, or when he or she is so seriously ill that therapeutic privilege is invoked? Would the judgment be similar to that in the case of Diane Blood (*R* v *HFEA*, 1997), or would it be different because adults are presumed competent in law whereas young people are not?

Cloning and the human embryo

Cloning and reproduction, especially cloning the human embryo, made the headlines after the report at one of the American Fertility Society meetings, in 1994, of an experiment describing embryo-splitting. This eventually led to federal funds being withheld from embryo research in the US, with the consequence that now it is happening practically solely within the private sector. The principle of the creation of identical human beings is thus not a new subject, but the method described by Wilmut and colleagues certainly is (Wilmut et al., 1997).

The actual birth of the sheep Dolly, after somatic nuclear transfer, renewed the debate about the meaning of human identity. Many objected to the dangers of 'deliberate twinning'. The term deliberate is crucial in more than one sense. A deliberate action implies responsibility for that action, and Hans Jonas's 'responsibility principle' is apposite (Jones and Herr, 1984). Jonas has also stated that the two most awesome kinds of responsibility we may ever face are those of politicians towards society and of parents to their children. This arguably may be extended to future or planned children, the matter which concerns us in assisted reproduction. It is indeed because we are responsible, or moral subjects, that we wish to analyse rationally the arguments for and against cloning for reproductive purposes.

Interestingly, the introduction of the report by the group of advisers to the European Union (European Commission, 1997) states, 'As there is no discrimination against twins per se, it follows that there is no *per se* objection to genetically identical human beings'. This makes it clear that one must find other arguments than the *noumenon* ('thing in itself') of cloning (its 'real existence') in order to counter arguments in favour of human reproductive cloning.

One such counter argument has been rooted in the notion of human dignity, together with others like uniqueness and respect. These qualities appear in the introduction of the first international statement in the field of bioethics, the Universal Declaration on the Human Genome and Human Rights adopted in November 1997 by UNESCO, including a specific article taking the replication of identical human beings as an example of violation of dignity. The UNESCO declaration on the genome places human dignity in the context of uniqueness, whilst the CCNE (French National Ethics Committee) report to the French President (CCNE, 1997) starts with the caveat that personal identity and genetic identity are not to be confused, stressing that human cloning would totally disrupt the relation or balance between genetic and personal identity. The argument of dignity is underlined, using the Kantian categorical precept – 'to treat each and everyone as an end to themselves and not merely as a means to an end'.

Of course we know that a clone obtained by somatic cell nuclear transfer would not be totally identical to the adult donor of the nucleus, because of the recipient cytoplasm bearing the maternal mitochondria; but more importantly, the same argument can be used against reproductive cloning by embryo-splitting and transfer to different surrogate mothers at different times. To quote the report:

It would be absurd to consider that an adult and his clonal duplicate who must necessarily be born much later, and is bound to have a different life history, could be to any degree presented as two copies of a single and identical person. To believe such a thing would be to fall victim to the reductive illusion which is born of the dismal confusion between identity in the physical sense of sameness (*idem*) and in the moral sense of selfness (*ipse*).

The Latin *ipse* is very much nearer to the notion of *identity* (one's self), whereas *idem* relates to the notion of *identical*, at least as seen by others.

The report continues:

[N]evertheless, although to possess the same genome in no way leads two individuals to own the same psyche, reproductive cloning would still inaugurate a fundamental upheaval of the relationship between genetic identity and personal identity in its biological and cultural dimensions. The uniqueness of each human being, which upholds human autonomy and dignity, is immediately expressed by the unique appearance of body and countenance which is the result of the singularity of each genome ... [P]redetermination of all the genetic characteristics of a future human being [is] judged ... an offence against the human condition.

The first problem, therefore, seems to be one of lack of liberty for the future person induced by an increase in genetic determinism. This begs two questions. The first concerns autonomy, a principle described in the CCNE report as 'support(ed) by the uniqueness and dignity of the person'. One of our duties is to respect the autonomy of subjects. The autonomous human being (who may be defined as one who is 'submitted to his or her own laws') may allegedly be threatened in this very quality by facing his or her relatively identical clones. Conversely, relationship as well as autonomy might be threatened by cloning. In the words of the CCNE report, 'reproductive cloning would ... inaugurate a new mode of filiation, ... an individual born by cloning would be both a descendant and a twin of an adult'. The very concept of filiation could become meaningless.

But if human clones are 'born' of a different kind of relationship, does that necessarily make them any less a part of human society? Can we not argue instead that the best way to counteract discrimination is to accept difference as a valuable addition to the rich tapestry of life rather than fear its consequences? Thus, the CCNE concludes that we may recognize 'that persons' singularity and autonomy, ... are ... the two essential elements of the human condition and dignity'. The recognition and acceptance of the differences amongst persons makes the tolerance of our differences even more pertinent. Indeed if dignity has to be defined in any essential manner, as it must be if enshrined in international declarations, it is the unique quality of all human beings, also recognized in their differences, even if there is a degree of sameness, which gives us dignity.

The second question is whether normal, sexual reproduction guarantees freedom for the new individual, in a way that cloning does not. This is obviously absurd, and we have therefore to conclude that even if normal sexual reproduction were a necessary condition for human liberty, it is far from being a sufficient one. However, what about identity rather than liberty? How would the child of cloning develop a sexual identity? Let us say that a somatic cell nucleus from a sterile, azoospermic father is inserted into an enucleated oocyte. It seems reasonable to suppose that the constraints imposed by the father's sexual identity would somehow affect the cloned child; would this be a reduction of the child's liberty? In the US report commissioned by President Clinton (US National Bioethics Advisory Commission, 1997), fears about harms to the children who may be created in this manner, particularly psychological harms associated with a possibly diminished sense of individuality and personal autonomy, belong to the same analysis.

Perhaps feminist psychoanalytical arguments can help us understand the problem of identity – for example, the work of Julia Kristeva (1991) and Luce Irigaray (see Whitford, 1991). Kristeva argues that we cannot respect and accept strangers if we have not accepted our own portion of strangeness, in other words, the stranger within ourselves (Kristeva, 1991). The implication for cloning is that the parent(s) seeking reproductive cloning cannot accept that strangeness carried in the matrix of the gestating mother. In the same analytical vein, one could argue that the fantasy of immortality, or the desire for genetic perpetuation at any cost by those who cannot procreate, seems a more narcissistic venture than the often unconscious choice of a reproductive partner.

In a similarly psychoanalytical fashion, Irigaray begins from the Lacanian account of the mirror stage in identity development, but adds a feminist twist. For men, ego formation depends on coming to see the world as a mirror, on which the male projects his own ego; women are part of the mirror, so that they never see reflections of themselves (Whitford, 1991: p. 34). It might be suggested that seeing one's own cloned, literal double in the mirror threatens the entire process of masculine ego formation.

Whatever the merit of these arguments, they offer a new slant on the debate about cloning. The implication for cloning, after the manner of both Kristeva and Irigaray, is that deeper psychoanalytical forces are at work in popular revulsion at the idea. Because the identity of the subject is shaky, and subjectivity itself something to be constructed rather than a given, cloning poses a threat to our personal identity which we find difficult to tolerate. Another psychoanalytical question concerns the child thus conceived, rather than the parent – how will the child cope with building his or her sexual identity?

Therapeutic cloning (or other applications of cloning technology which do not involve the creation of genetically identical individuals) has led to much less dismay. The European Commission Group of Advisors on the Ethical Implications of Biotechnology (1997) report reiterates in its summary that:

As far as the human applications are concerned, it distinguishes between reproductive and non-reproductive (research), and also nuclear and replacement and embryo splitting limited to the in vitro phase, i.e. as a research tool, as in the possible development of stem cell cultures for repairing organs. As all research, the objective is essential in analysing the ethical quality.

The European report stresses that therapeutic cloning should aim either to throw light on the causes of human disease or to contribute to the alleviation of suffering. The embryo should not be replaced in a uterus. Finally, the report concludes with a clear condemnation of reproductive cloning, and calls for fully informing the public and stimulating debate.

Conclusion

Cloning is only one example, among the many discussed in this chapter, of ethical dilemmas in the new reproductive technologies. All call for wider discussion in the traditional dialectical manner between professionals and patients. Positive steps towards this wider discussion have been taken at international declaratory levels (such as the Bioethics Convention of the Council of Europe) and in national bodies such as the Human Fertilisation and Embryology Authority (HFEA) and Human Genetics Advisory Commission (HGAC) in the UK – for example, in the HFEA consultation documents on sex selection for social reasons, cloning and pre-implantation genetic diagnosis (HGAC and HFEA, 1998). All raise questions about what respect is owed to the embryo, its moral status, as well as about human rights, including the right to reproduce and the right to a family life. To a practising clinician, all these questions are real, but the responsibility we owe to the vulnerable future child is the most awesome.

References

Chamayou, S., Guglielmino, A., Giambona, A., Siciliano, S., Di Stefano, G., Sciblilia, G., Humeau, C., Maggio, A. and Di Leo, S. (1998). Attitudes of potential users in Sicily towards preimplantation genetic diagnosis for beta thalassaemia and aneuploidies. *Human Reproduction* **13**: 1936–44.

Comité Consultatif National d'Ethique pour les Sciences de la Vie et de la Sante (CCNE) (1997). Réponse au President de la République au sujet du clonage reproductif. Paris: Levallois Perret: Biomédition.

Council of Europe (1996). *Convention for the Protection of Human Rights and Dignity of the Human Being with Regard to the Application of Biology and Medicine: Bioethics Convention*. Strasbourg: Dir/Jur (96) 2.

European Commission Group of Advisors on the Ethical Implications of Biotechnology (1997). *Ethical Aspects of Cloning Techniques*. Brussels: European Commission.

Gillick v *West Norfolk and Wisbech Area Health Authority* [1985] 3 All ER 402.

Hermeren, G. (1998). *The Ethics of Health Care Choices: Means and Ends*. European Standing Conference of National Ethics Committees, Council of Europe CBD1/NEC (97) 2. Brussels: Council of Europe.

Gottlieb, C., Lalos, O. and Lindblad, F. (2000). Disclosure of donor insemination to the child: the impact of the Swedish legislation on couples' attitudes. *Human Reproduction* **15**: 2052–6.

Human Genetics Advisory Commission and Human Fertilisation and Embryology Authority (1998). *Cloning Issues in Reproduction: Consultation Document*. London: Office of Science and Technology.

Jonas, H. and Herr, D. (1984). *The Imperative of Responsibility: In Search of an Ethics for the Technological Age*. Chicago: University of Chicago Press.

Jones, H.W. and Schrader, C. (1992). And just what is a pre-embryo? *Fertility and Sterility* **52**: 189–91.

Kristeva, J. (1991). *Strangers to Ourselves.* New York: Columbia University Press.

Loi no 94 654 du 29 Juillet 1994, Relative au Don, Assistance Médicale a la Procréation et Diagnostique Prénatal (1994). Paris: Journal Officiel du 30 Juillet 1994.

Milliez, J. and Sureau, C. (1997). Pre-implantation diagnosis and the eugenic debate: our responsibility to future generations. In *Ethical Dilemmas in Assisted Reproduction*, ed. F. Shenfield and C. Sureau, pp. 51–9. Canthorpe: Parthenon.

Missa, J.N. (1999). Eugenics. *Ethical Dilemmas in Obstetrics and Gynaecology* **13**: 533–41.

R v *Human Fertilisation and Embryology Authority, ex parte Blood* [1997] 2 ALL ER687.

Seve, L. (1994). *Pour une critique de la raison bioéthique.* Paris: éditions Odile Jacob.

Shenfield, F. (1997). Justice and access to fertility treatments. In *Ethical Dilemmas in Assisted Reproduction*, ed. F. Shenfield and C. Sureau, pp. 4–16. Canthorpe: Parthenon.

Shenfield, F. and Sureau, C. (Eds) (1997). *Ethical Dilemmas in Assisted Reproduction.* Canthorpe: Parthenon.

Testard, J. and Sele, B. (1995). Towards an efficient medical eugenics: is the desirable always the feasible? *Human Reproduction* **11**: 3086–90.

UNESCO (1997). *Universal Declaration on the Human Genome.* Paris: UNESCO.

US National Bioethics Advisory Commission (1997). *Report and Recommendations of the US National Bioethics Advisory Commission on the Cloning of Human Beings.* Rockville, Maryland: USNBAC.

Whitford, M. (1991). *Luce Irigaray: Philosophy in the Feminine.* London: Routledge.

Wilmut, I., Schnieke, E., McWhir, J., Kind, A.J. and Campbell, K.H.S. (1997). Viable offspring derived from fetal and adult mammalian cells. *Nature* **385**: 810–13.

10

A case-study in IVF: paternalism and autonomy in a 'high-risk' pregnancy

Gillian M. Lockwood

Midland Fertility Services, Aldridge, UK

Introduction

Renal transplantation, the treatment of choice for patients with end-stage renal failure, can correct the infertility due to chronic ill health, anaemia and tubal damage generally encountered when these patients are managed by renal dialysis. Currently only 1 in 50 women of child-bearing age becomes pregnant following a renal transplant, and it may be that many more would welcome the chance of biological parenthood if their fertility problems could be overcome. The first successful pregnancy, conceived in 1956 following an identical twin renal transplant, was reported in 1963 (Murray et al., 1963).

Until recently, pregnancy had been thought to present considerable hazards to the transplant recipient. However, some reviews (Sturgiss and Davison, 1992; Davison, 1994) have suggested that pregnancy in the graft recipient, unlike the rare pregnancy in patients undergoing dialysis, is usually likely to lead to a live birth, and that pregnancy may have little or no adverse effect on either renal function or blood pressure in the transplant recipient. The current medical consensus is that if, prior to conception, renal function is well preserved, and if the patient does not develop high blood pressure, only a minority of transplant recipients will experience a deterioration of their renal function attributable to pregnancy (Lindheimer and Katz, 1992).

It is inevitable that the rapid return to good health enjoyed by the majority of women following successful renal transplantation should encourage them to consider conception. Although only a small proportion of women with a functioning graft become spontaneously pregnant, modern assisted reproductive technologies (ARTs), especially in vitro fertilization and embryo transfer (IVF-ET), could theoretically increase this proportion to near-normal levels. Pregnancy, especially if ART is required, clearly entails extra risks for the renal transplant recipient, but these are risks that, with appropriate counselling, the patient may be prepared and even eager to take.

In this chapter, I shall discuss the ethical dilemmas involved in counselling renal transplant patients seeking pregnancy but requiring ART. This case concerned a couple with long-standing infertility who were assisted by means of IVF-ET. The wife was a renal transplant recipient whose initial renal failure was due to severe, recurrent pre-eclampsia, a potentially life-threatening condition of late pregnancy causing raised blood pressure and renal complications, which can progress to cause fits and cerebro-vascular accidents (strokes). It is associated with severe growth retardation of the fetus, and often, premature delivery.

A case of high risk pregnancy

A 34-year-old woman (Mrs A) was referred to an IVF unit following eight years of failure to conceive after a reversal-of-sterilization operation had been performed. (Lockwood, Ledger and Barlow, 1995). She had been born with one poorly developed kidney only, but this was not known until, at age 20, she was investigated for very severe pre-eclamptic toxaemia (PET), which she suffered during her first pregnancy. Her baby was born premature at 26 weeks' gestation, and he died shortly after birth from complications of extreme prematurity.

A second pregnancy in the following year was also complicated by severe PET, renal damage, premature delivery at 26 weeks' gestation, and neonatal death. Sterilization by tubal ligation was offered and accepted under these circumstances, in view of the anticipated further deterioration of her renal function with any subsequent pregnancy. There was a significant further advance of her renal disease, necessitating the initiation of haemodialysis (a kidney machine) two years later, and a living, related donor renal transplant (from her mother) was subsequently performed. After the transplant, Mrs A remained well and maintained good kidney function on a combination of anti-rejection drugs, steroids and blood pressure tablets. At age 26, a reversal-of-sterilization operation was performed because she had become so distressed by her childlessness, but hysterosalpingography (a test to check for fallopian tubal patency) two years later, when pregnancy had not occurred, showed that both tubes had once again become blocked.

At the time that Mr and Mrs A were referred to the IVF unit, there were no case reports of successful IVF in women with renal transplants, but specialists were becoming increasingly reluctant to advise women with transplants *against* trying for a baby, as medical care for 'high risk' pregnancies was improving dramatically. Following discussion with the Transplantation Unit and the high-risk pregnancy specialists, the IVF unit felt that an IVF treatment cycle could be offered to Mr and Mrs A as long as the risks of IVF-ET, over and above those attendant upon a spontaneous pregnancy in these circumstances, were understood and accepted by the couple and minimized as far as possible, by the IVF team.

An IVF treatment cycle was started using the normal drug regimen, but the patient was given a much lower dose than usual, with the aim of minimizing the effect of the hormone stimulation on the transplanted kidney. Two oocytes (eggs) were obtained, which fertilized normally in vitro, and the two embryos were transferred to the uterus 54 hours later. Mrs A's pregnancy test was positive 13 days after embryo transfer, and an ultrasound scan performed at eight weeks' gestation showed a viable twin pregnancy.

Throughout the treatment cycle and during pregnancy, the patient's anti-rejection drugs (azathioprine and prednisolone) were continued at maintenance doses. Renal function was monitored closely throughout the treatment cycle and during pregnancy, remaining remarkably stable.

The pregnancy was complicated at 20 weeks' gestation by a right deep vein thrombosis, affecting the femoral and external iliac veins, and anti-coagulation with heparin and warfarin was required. Spontaneous rupture of the membranes, leading to premature delivery, occurred at 29 weeks' gestation; the twins were delivered vaginally and in good condition three hours later. The twin girls were small for dates (at 1.48 and 1.19 kg) but were otherwise well, requiring only minimal resuscitation and respiratory support. After delivery of her babies, Mrs A remained well and her renal graft continued to function normally, with no change in immunosuppressive or antihypertensive (blood pressure) medication required.

Risks to the mother, the fetus and the neonate

Severe pre-eclampsia and eclampsia can result in irreversible damage to the maternal kidney, particularly due to acute renal cortical necrosis. Women who have recurrent pre-eclampsia in several pregnancies or blood pressures that remain elevated in the period following delivery (the puerperium), especially if they have pre-existing renal disease and/or hypertension, have a higher incidence of later cardiovascular disorders and a reduced life expectancy (Chesley, Annitto and Cosgrove, 1989). Pregnancy is recognized to be a privileged immunological state, and therefore episodes of rejection during pregnancy might be expected to be lower than for non-pregnant transplant recipients. Nevertheless, rejection episodes occur in nine per cent of pregnant women, occasionally in women who have had years of stable renal functioning prior to conception. More rarely, rejection episodes occur in the puerperium, when they may represent a rebound effect from the altered immunosuppressiveness of pregancy.

Immunosuppressive (anti-rejection) drugs are theoretically toxic to the developing fetus; however, maternal health and graft function require immunosuppression to be maintained. Women with impaired renal function are recognized to be at risk of giving birth prematurely, often to growth-retarded or small-for-dates babies. A large French study of women with pre-existing renal damage reported a prematurity rate of 17 per cent and a spontaneous abortion rate (miscarriage) of 20 per cent, as compared to prematurity and spontaneous abortion rates of 8 and 12 per cent, respectively, in the normal population (Jungers et al., 1986). However, the long-term health effect of events in utero for the offspring of transplanted mothers is harder to quantify. There is animal evidence of delayed effects of immunosuppressive therapies and intra-uterine growth retardation.

Case discussion

The decision to accept the couple for IVF treatment posed significant dilemmas of both a technical (obstetric and renal) and an ethical nature. Severe pre-eclampsia can present as a progressive condition, tending to occur with greater virulence in successive pregnancies (Campbell and MacGillivrey, 1985). This, after all, had been the rationale behind the original decision to sterilize the patient after the death of her second baby, precipitated by pre-eclampsia and extreme prematurity. The successfully functioning transplanted kidney had been donated by the patient's mother and therefore, as an organ, was 30 years older than the patient herself. Hence there were real concerns that the transplanted kidney could be jeopardized by the strain of a normal pregnancy. The use of donated oocytes, which can permit postmenopausal women of 50 + years to become pregnant through IVF-ET, has demonstrated a significant incidence of pregnancy-associated hypertension and frank pre-eclampsia, suggesting that the aged kidney is less able to withstand the stress of pregnancy.

An editorial review (Davison and Redman, 1997) reported that 35 per cent of all conceptions in renal transplant patients failed to progress beyond the first trimester because of therapeutic (approximately 20 per cent) and spontaneous (approximately 14 per cent) abortions. Problems occur some time after delivery in 11 per cent of all women with transplants, unless the pregnancy was complicated prior to 28 weeks' gestation, in which case remote problems can occur in 24 per cent of pregnancies. However, of the conceptions that continue beyond the first trimester, 94 per cent end successfully, in spite of a 30 per cent chance of developing hypertension, pre-eclampsia, or both. Distinguishing between time-dependent and pregnancy-induced problems is clearly difficult. Davison (1992) cites registry data indicating that 10 per cent of mothers who are transplant recipients die within one to seven years of childbirth.

The technique of IVF-ET also poses additional problems for the renal transplant patient. The hormone drug regime involves supra-physiological levels of oestradiol, which are associated with a higher risk of thrombotic (blood-clotting) episodes than in normal pregnancy. Access to the ovaries may be compounded by the positioning of the transplanted kidney in the pelvis, although ultrasound screening does permit the kidney to be readily visualized. Successful pregnancy rates per embryo transfer in IVF-ET have tended to depend on multiple embryos, but a multiple pregnancy (seen in 25 per cent of all IVF pregnancies following a three-embryo transfer) would exert even greater strain on the kidney than a singleton; is more likely to be associated with the development of pre-eclampsia and carries increased risk of premature delivery of the babies.

In an attempt to mitigate all these medical factors, the IVF unit embarked on a very low-dose stimulation regimen and was content with a lower than usual harvest of eggs at retrieval. It was agreed that only two embryos would be transferred, and minimal post-transfer hormone support was given to minimize the risks.

The ethical aspects of undertaking IVF and embryo transfer in these circumstances are possibly harder to quantify and yet more contentious. It is recognized that even under optimum circumstances, at the most effective units, the probability of a successful pregnancy with a single treatment cycle of IVF-ET is only about 25 per cent. Was it acceptable to expose Mrs A to all the risks of an IVF cycle that was four times as likely to fail as to succeed? Even where the IVF is successful in establishing a pregnancy, there is still the non-negligible risk that renal function may deteriorate. The patient may be safely delivered, but again become dependent upon renal dialysis. The Human Fertilisation and Embryology Act 1990 laid great stress of the importance of obtaining true informed consent from patients undertaking procedures such as IVF; it was particularly important that the patient and her husband were made aware of the risks associated not only with the failure of IVF-ET but also with its success.

Arguments that could be advanced against offering fertility treatment to renal transplant recipients, such as whether it is in the best interests of the patient to be helped to achieve a state as a result of which she may suffer chronic ill health or even early death, have also been advanced against permitting 'old', i.e. post-menopausal, women to become pregnant through the technique of egg-donation IVF. In both instances, one could argue that as long as the risks associated with fertility treatment and pregnancy were thoroughly explained to and accepted by the woman (and her partner), then to refuse treatment on the sole ground that her health may deteriorate is unacceptably paternalistic on the part of the clinicians involved. Mrs A stated that if she had not agreed to the sterilization (which she claimed she had been placed under undue pressure to accept at the time she was diagnosed with renal failure), then she would not only have been able to, but definitely would have tried to, achieve a further pregnancy, as she did after the reversal of sterilization was performed.

The Human Fertilisation and Embryology Act 1990 also places great emphasis on the 'interests of the child' who may be born as a result of procedures such as IVF-ET. This emphasis has been interpreted by some authorities as encouraging fertility units to feel justified in refusing treatment to women with significant health problems (or to post-menopausal women) as it would, so they claim, not be in the 'interests of the child' to be born to a mother with reduced life expectancy due to chronic ill health or comparatively advanced age. Apart from the obvious rejoinders that society happily countenances *men* becoming fathers at an age when their life expectancy is reduced, and the medical profession's heroic efforts to assist women with serious health problems who become pregnant *spontaneously*, it is unquestionably in the interests of the child. After all, the child *will only be born* if his transplanted mother is offered fertility treatment and she *should* be offered such treatment, even if he loses his mother at an early age or has to deal with the consequences of her ill health, as otherwise *he* won't exist!

References

Campbell, D.M. and MacGillivrey, I. (1985). Pre-eclampsia in a second pregnancy. *British Journal of Obstetrics and Gynaecology* **92**: 131–40.

Chesley, L.C., Annitto, J.E. and Cosgrove, R.A. (1989). *The Remote Prognosis of Pregnant Women.*

Davison, J.M. (1992). Renal disease. In *Medical Disorders in Obstetric Practice,* ed. M. Swiet. Oxford: Blackwell Scientific Publications.

Davison, J.M. (1994). Pregnancy in renal allograft recipients: problems, prognosis and practicalities. *Balliere's Clinical Obstetrics and Gynecology* **8**: 501–25.

Davison, J.M. and Redman, C.W.G. (1997). Pregnancy post-transplant. *British Journal of Obstetrics and Gynaecology* **104**: 1106–7.

Jungers, P., Forget, D., Henry-Amar, et al. (1986). Chronic kidney disease and pregnancy. In *Advances in Nephrology Year Book,* ed. J. Grunfeld, M. Maxwell, J. Bach et al., vol. 14, pp. 103–41. Linn, MO: Mosby, Inc.

Lindheimer, M.D. and Katz, A.I. (1992). Pregnancy in the renal transplant patient. *American Journal of Kidney Disease* **19**: 173.

Lockwood, G.M., Ledger, W.L. and Barlow, D.H. (1995). Successful pregnancy outcome in a renal transplant patient following in-vitro fertilization. *Human Reproduction* **10**: 1528–30.

Murray, J.E., Reed, D.E., Harrison, J.H. et al. (1963). Successful pregnancies after human renal transplantation. *New England Journal of Medicine* **269**: 341–3.

Sturgiss, S.N. and Davison, J.M. (1992). Effect of pregnancy on long-term function of renal allografts. *American Journal of Kidney Disease* **19**: 167–72.

11

The ethics of secrecy in donor insemination

Heather Widdows

Centre for the Study of Global Ethics, University of Birmingham, UK

Secrecy has been an integral part of donor insemination (DI) since its beginning (reputedly in 1884) (Daniels and Haimes, 1998). Recently attention has been given to the possible adverse effects of secrecy and, accordingly, the practice of secrecy in DI has been questioned. This chapter will attempt to analyse the reasons that have been given for and against secrecy and will consider the effect which changing the practices of secrecy might have on DI.

Introduction

Many explanations have been put forward for continuing the practice of secrecy in DI. These justifications range from patient confidentiality to social reasons such as the stigma attached to illegitimacy. The supposed stigma of illegitimacy is now vastly reduced to the point of being negligible, as are other historical reasons, such as those cited by Pfeffer (1993), namely the stigmas of adultery and masturbation. Such reasons cannot be regarded as major factors, though they may continue to carry some weight in certain social groups. Secrecy has become, either through time or design, not simply an addendum to DI but part of the structure of the procedure (Nachtigall, 1993). The integral part which secrecy has played in DI makes exploration and analysis of this topic difficult. Not only is DI less in the public eye, and so less discussed than other assisted reproductive technologies; secrecy also 'covers its own tracks', in that little evidence exists regarding the effects of secrecy on families who have used DI to conceive. Parents are unwilling to talk about their use of the procedure, and offspring of DI are unable to as they do not know the manner of their conception.

In this chapter I will explore the issues of secrecy, focusing on two areas: anonymity of donor; and non-disclosure to the child. I will present the arguments used both for and against secrecy and assess their validity. Further, I will claim that if one does support the arguments for openness, then this has far-reaching consequences for the current structure and practice of DI. Other reasons for secrecy, such as protecting patient confidentiality and the more controversial claim that secrecy benefits the doctor, I will not explore. (Secrecy is also believed to protect the doctor, as it prevents thorough examination of the procedure – including doctors' practices of making social decisions about access and donors, which they are not qualified to make (Haimes, 1993).) The rationale for such a selection is simply that I judge the two selected areas to be the most important issues in the justification, and thus continuation, of the culture of secrecy in DI.

Donor anonymity

The ethics of donor anonymity in DI has become prominent over the last two decades, and has been brought into relief by the removal of donor anonymity in certain countries. Sweden was the first country to introduce such a law, in 1985, followed by Austria, which introduced a similar law, in 1992. Such identifying information is also available in New Zealand and Australia. Changes to DI practice in these countries provide a context in which some of the usual justifications for secrecy can be assessed. In addition, recent advances in genetics have strengthened claims that knowing one's genetic parentage is an important part of understanding one's own identity (at least medically). Moreover, such advances have also reduced the likelihood of keeping non-genetic parentage secret. Taken together these factors have led many to re-examine the traditional assumption that donor anonymity is the 'self-evident principle of DI' (Bateman Novaes, 1998: p. 119).

Two main reasons given for keeping the donor anonymous are: first, a practical reason, that anonymity is necessary to ensure that there are willing donors; and second, that anonymity ensures that donors have the 'correct attitude'.

First, the supposition that if donor anonymity were removed, then donors would no longer be willing to donate sperm can now be tested against the evidence which is emerging in countries where anonymity has been removed. The most detailed evidence comes from Sweden. The Swedish legislation (Swedish Law of Artificial Insemination, March 18, 1985, no. 1140/1984) allows the DI 'child' access to identifying information about the donor when she or he reaches maturity. Many predicted that outlawing anonymity and making the donor identifiable would result in a dearth of donors and even the end of DI; for example, two Swedish doctors wrote articles to this effect (Edvinsson et al., 1990, and Hagenfeldt, 1990, cited by Daniels and Lalos, 1995).

However, such predictions proved alarmist. After the introduction of the law the number of donors did initially decrease, as did the number of DI births, and simultaneously the number of couples travelling to other European countries for DI increased (Daniels and Lalos, 1995). At first sight such evidence appears to suggest that both donors and potential parents were uncomfortable with the removal of donor anonymity – donors were less willing to donate and parents were choosing to go to countries which continued the practice of donor anonymity. However, this is not the only explanation, and it is arguable that other factors were at work.

For example, Daniels and Lalos (1995) suggest that one alternative explanation for the decline in donors derives from changes in legislation regarding the screening of semen – namely, the compulsory testing of semen for HIV before and after six months of cryopreservation. These changes resulted in private clinics ceasing to offer DI, which meant that donors were no longer required, and that couples had no choice other than to seek treatment elsewhere. A further possibility is that this increase in couples seeking treatment outside Sweden is an indicator not of dissatisfaction among donors with the removal of anonymity, but of the dissatisfaction of medical advisors, who adopted the practice of 'advising and referring couples to have treatment outside Sweden' (Daniels and Lalos, 1995: p. 1872). However, Daniels and Lalos do note that their view is contested by Bygdeman (cited in Daniels and Lalos, 1995), who argues that both the decline in donors and the trend for couples to seek treatment abroad was a direct reaction to the fact that their anonymity would no longer be protected.

To support the claim that donor anonymity does not stop donors from donating, Daniels and Lalos surveyed the numbers of donors in the eight DI programmes in Sweden between 1989 (the first year that figures were recorded) and 1993. These figures show a steady increase in the number of donors, and an overall increase of 65 per cent (Daniels and Lalos, 1995). Unfortunately, there are no comprehensive figures from before the 1985 legislation. However, Daniels and Lalos conclude that 'despite this limitation, it is clear that the number of available donors is increasing' (Daniels and Lalos, 1995: p. 1873). To support this conclusion they cite statistics from the University Hospital of Northern Sweden, which had collected donor figures both before and after the introduction of the law. These figures show that the number of donors pre- and post-legislation remained static, and later (coinciding with high-profile recruitment campaigns) the number of donors began steadily to increase, thus supporting their claim that despite the removal of anonymity donor numbers are increasing.

From this evidence it can be concluded that removing donor anonymity would not stop donors coming forward, but that it would cause changes to the structure and current practice of DI. The two most notable changes in Sweden were changes in public perceptions of DI, and more crucially to the type of men coming forward to donate sperm. In order to encourage donors to come forward, new strategies were needed and high-profile recruitment campaigns were introduced. These campaigns raised public awareness of DI and thereby reduced the secrecy surrounding the procedure. The more fundamental change was to the type of donors willing to donate. Before the removal of anonymity, donors tended to be students who were motivated primarily by money, whereas donors recruited after the change in legislation tended to be older, married men, who were motivated altruistically by a desire to assist infertile couples (Daniels and Lalos, 1995). A similar change in age, marital status and motivation of donors has been reflected in studies in New Zealand and Australia (Daniels and Lalos, 1995: p. 1873). Thus, although the predictions that removing anonymity would stop sperm donation (and so DI) have proved false, notable changes have occurred. In one sense the predictions were correct, in that the donors who donated before the passing of the law (of those anonymous donors to whom the predictors had access) did cease to donate once anonymity was removed. However, this proved to be unimportant in terms of the overall number of donors, as other donors were prepared to become non-anonymous donors.

In sum, then, the first reason for continuing anonymity is unfounded – donors will not cease to come forward. Hence only the second reason for insisting on anonymity remains, namely, that anonymity ensures that donors should have the 'correct' attitude to the procedure. Before the recent questioning of anonymity, the secrecy involved in the process of DI was taken for granted and was unquestioningly assumed to benefit all concerned (donor, parents, child and doctor). In such a framework it was in the interest of all parties to keep their involvement secret, and anonymity safeguarded secrecy for both the donor and the parents. Accordingly, the correct attitude of the donor was held to be detachment – the donor should not wish to know anything about, or have any contact with, his potential progeny (Pennings, 1997). Anonymity guarantees that the donor provides his semen – the raw material of DI – and that this is the end of his involvement; there is no hope of any future knowledge of, or contact with, any offspring resulting from his donation. This attitude is further enforced by paying the donor's 'expenses' (importantly, at least in the UK, expenses, not payment). Such reimbursement provides some reciprocity which, at least symbolically, implies an end to the encounter. In addition to providing a symbolic reciprocal act, the money which changes hands does provide motivation for some donors. Although the level of expenses is intended to be below the level of inducement, for many young men (characteristically students) the expenses are sufficient to function as inducement to donate (Daniels and Lalos, 1995; Lui et al., 1995; Pennings, 1997). Indeed, it could be argued that this perception is the one intended, as paying expenses encourages the sense of conducting a transaction, which lowers any possibility of the donor feeling any entitlement to future information or contact with any possible children. This is the traditional model in which the donor simply provides 'genetic material in order to enable others to fulfil their wish to have a child. The donor is an outsider who has no rights or responsibilities in the newly created family. The procedure ... completely severs the link between the donor and his genetic material and thus, indirectly, isolates the donor from the recipients' (Pennings, 1997: p. 1842).

Removing anonymity fundamentally alters the framework in which DI has been practised and threatens the long-established culture of secrecy. Instead of attracting donors who wish to have no contact with the offspring their sperm are used to create, donors are attracted who do not feel that anonymity is important, and therefore are willing for their donor-offspring to know who they are, and perhaps even to be contacted by them.

The conclusion which must be drawn is that those who support the continuing practice of donor anonymity do not fear that there would be no men willing to donate, but rather that these donors would be the 'wrong' type of donor. Changing the type of donor – from anonymous and financially motivated to identifiable and altruistically motivated – threatens the present model of DI. No longer would a prime concern be to keep the procedure secret and to keep the donor separate from the couple. While DI could still be used to solve childlessness, the ethos of the procedure would be very different. In particular, instead of enforcing the pretence of a 'normal' family – by which is meant the traditional (and many would argue outdated) model of father and mother and genetically related children – the change makes openness possible. Indeed, changing to identifiable donors implies disclosure to the child. For while one can inform the child of his or her donor conception, if donors are anonymous (the child would simply know she or he was conceived through an anonymous donor) one cannot give the child identifying information about the donor unless the child has first been informed of his or her status as a DI child. Thus, removing anonymity challenges the culture of secrecy, in that while anonymity is in place parents may feel that there is little point in revealing the fact of DI conception to the child as no information about the genetic father is available. However, on the removal of anonymity the reverse is the case – there is no point removing anonymity unless parents tell their children. Hence, removing anonymity can be seen as putting pressure on parents to reveal the mode of conception to their children.

Secrecy, then, in the form of donor anonymity, does not protect donors as a homogeneous class, but only a certain type of donor and thereby a certain structure of DI. Removing anonymity affects the culture of secrecy which has been at the heart of DI, and implies huge changes in the way DI is regarded by users and by society as a whole. Not only does removing anonymity put pressure on parents, but it also presumes that society will accept DI as an alternative means of family creation, in a similar manner to the way that other assisted reproductive technologies and adoption have been accepted. It could even be argued that removing anonymity introduces the presumption that there should be a relationship between donor and donor offspring, something which is anathema to the traditional concept of DI.

Secrecy and the family

The second key issue is secrecy in the family, more specifically the non-disclosure by the parents to the child. (There are other elements regarding secrecy and the family, such as between the 'parents', extended family and wider friends and acquaintances, which could be addressed, however, there is no room in this present chapter.) The practice of secrecy has been claimed to protect the family – its individuals, their relationships with each other and the family unit as a whole. An important reason which is given in defence of secrecy in the family is that it protects the family from the stigma of male infertility (Klock et al., 1994; Nachtigall et al., 1997; Lasker, 1998). Fear of admitting male infertility is cited as a key reason for non-disclosure, and this seems to be supported by the evidence, in that those who use DI to overcome male infertility are less likely to disclose to the child. For example, couples who use DI because of vasectomy, or to avoid passing on a genetic disorder, are more likely to disclose than couples in which the man is infertile (Nachtigall et al., 1997; Lasker, 1998).

Crucially, when couples use DI, unlike all other assisted reproductive technologies, there is no doubt that it is the man, and not the woman, who is infertile. For example, even though IVF (in vitro fertilization) is often used for men with low sperm counts (either naturally or after vasectomy), the focus and presumption of infertility rests with the women (Spallone, 1989). DI reveals male infertility, and so the 'cultural assumption of infertility being primarily a female problem is violated for these couples' (Lasker, 1998: p. 14). Male infertility does go some way to explain why couples do not disclose to the child, and why there is less open acceptance of DI at a wider societal level. This is linked to the wider topic of the importance of heredity and genetic relatedness; however, due to the remit of this chapter, this issue will not be discussed in detail, but should be noted as a significant topic in the debate. This chapter simply focuses upon whether secrecy is in the best interests of the child, which is the primary argument in favour of non-disclosure.

Historically, the claim that secrecy is in the best interest of the child was a strong argument in that secrecy protected the child from the stigma of illegitimacy. Illegitimacy, however, is no longer a major concern, especially when it is due to the use of assisted reproductive technologies. Thus, the claim that secrecy is in the best interests of the child must be for other reasons. The reasons that are given are: first, that not knowing about the DI conception guarantees the child stable and 'normal' family relationships, and prevents any uncertainty about identity (which could result from knowing about the DI conception); and second, that openness is damaging to the child's relationship with his or her parents, especially with his or her social father (even to the point of rejection of the non-genetic father in extreme cases). The opposing arguments for openness will in turn be presented.

First, the suggestion that keeping the mode of conception secret has a positive effect on the child by preventing any questioning about identity has recently been heavily criticized. Critics argue that knowing one's biological and genetic heritage is of fundamental importance to identity, and indeed such is the presumption behind the change in the Swedish law, and the more open practices of other countries such as Australia and New Zealand. This perception is echoed at the lay level, where there is general agreement that 'roots', in some form, are important (Edwards, 1998).

To support the hypothesis that knowing one's genetic heritage is important, an analogy has often been drawn with adoption. The ethos of adoption has changed dramatically over the last 50 years, from one of secrecy to one of openness. Those who use this analogy argue that the same thinking can be applied to the 'right' of a child to know his or her genetic parents in DI. However, although there are obvious similarities between adoption and DI – namely, at least one of the child's social parents is not the genetic parent – the analogy with adoption is frail. This is for two main reasons: first, the DI child is biologically linked to one parent (both genetically and gestationally); and second, the DI baby has not been 'given away' and therefore does not have a history of rejection to resolve. Thus, although there are similarities it would be wrong to regard this analogy as clinching the argument for openness in DI. Nonetheless, there are arguments for openness which are used in adoption that do have significance for the case for openness and thus merit exploration.

The first and most obvious parallel concerns identity – a 'right' to know one's roots, for both emotional reasons (such as discovering the kind of person one's 'father' is and knowing the reasons why he chose to donate) and for practical reasons (such as medical, in particular genetic, reasons). How far such a 'right' can be established is open to question. As noted above, those who argue for secrecy hold that if the child knew about his or her DI conception then his or her identity may be threatened. In addition, talking about a 'right' suggests that it can be granted by someone. With regard to genetic identity there are many cases where this is impossible, not only for those who have been conceived by DI but in cases of war, rape and other events which separate children from the knowledge of their genetic heritage. Thus, suggesting that knowing genetic heritage is a right, and that, without this knowledge forming a stable identity is impossible, is too dogmatic, and a view that cannot, and should not, be upheld.

This argument concerning 'roots' and identity nevertheless has considerable emotional pull, and whether one accepts it or not largely depends on one's view about the importance of genetic relatedness. In addition, there are many cases where genetic identity cannot be known, making arguments for openness that are based simply on this premise, tenuous. One could claim that knowledge of genetic parentage is desirable, but to claim it is an essential component in forming a stable identity is an exaggeration. This said, there is no doubt that keeping genetic history secret will become more difficult as the genetic revolution continues. The very nature of genetic testing is that it yields information about genetic relatives, so, by mere force of circumstance, genetic relatedness (or at least non-relatedness), and hence identity, will be revealed. Consequently, and for purely practical reasons, maintaining secrecy in DI may prove impossible. Such a scenario would force openness and thus a re-evaluation of the significance of genetic relatedness and what is meant by 'family relationships'. In sum, the argument that genetic knowledge is important for identity is not conclusive, although it may gain strength as genetic heritage becomes more important.

The second reason, which applies as much in DI as it did in adoption, is that secrecy is damaging for the family as a whole. Some may argue that in DI secrecy is not as damaging as in adoption for two reasons: first, there is less information to find out; and second, there is less chance of the secret being revealed as the only persons who need know about the procedure are the couple. However, these consequentialist arguments do not take account of the negative value connected to lying. The traditional DI assumption is that secrecy protects the family unit by ensuring that the family seems 'normal' to family, friends and society and appears the same as genetically-related families. The counter-claim, that secrecy is damaging to the family, which is used to support openness in adoption, can be applied to DI. If it proves to be the case that secrecy is damaging to the family and so to the best interests of the child, a crucial justification for maintaining secrecy will be undermined.

Two main reasons are suggested as to why secrecy is damaging to the family unit: first, that the secret will unintentionally be revealed; and second, that keeping secrets within a family is harmful in itself. The first and most obvious reason is the danger that the secret will come out, either directly, when it is told, or indirectly, in that the child growing up will form certain suspicions. Robert and Elizabeth Snowden argue that children are far more likely than their parents believe to know, or at least suspect, that they were conceived by means of DI (Snowden and Snowden, 1998). Most couples who have used DI to conceive have kept it secret from their offspring, yet they have tended to tell at least one other person. Given that these people are likely to have told one further person, it is probable that far more people know than couples are aware of, all of whom could potentially reveal the secret. Indeed, the fact that couples, who have told others, but not their offspring, often regret telling anyone can probably be attributed to fear of their secret being revealed (Nachtigall et al., 1997). Consequently, the secret is far more likely to 'get out' than the parents imagine. If this happens the chances of a breakdown in the relationship between the parents and the child, even to the extreme point where the child rejects the non-genetic father, are much greater. This reason for rejecting secrecy is relatively uncontroversial, as all accept that an accidental revelation of DI conception is clearly not in the best interests of the child. All couples accept this danger, and accordingly weigh the risk of exposure against the benefits of continued secrecy.

The second reason for rejecting secrecy is more contentious and philosophically debatable – namely, that secrecy is damaging in itself; that the simple awareness of a secret, even if it is never exposed, is harmful. Proving such a claim is difficult, not only because there is no evidence one way or the other, but also because such an absolutist position is so controversial. One possible way of approaching this issue is to consider the roughly parallel argument that lying, rather than simple non-revelation, is harmful. Making this adjustment is open to criticism, as most contributors in the field would argue that non-revelation does not equate with lying. However, in the case of DI it is possible to argue that keeping the mode of conception secret would probably necessitate lying, and even repeated lying – during the procedure (regarding time taken from work), at birth (regarding the identity of the father), in response to childhood enquiries (to the child him/herself), and so on. While it could be argued that some of these lies are less serious, such as those to an employer (which may be omissions rather than lies), lying to the child is controversial and the point at which it could be claimed that family relationships are in danger of being harmed. Moreover, it seems fair to conclude that the need for lying increases as public awareness of assisted reproductive technologies grow. While it may have been possible in the 1940s simply to lie during the procedure and when registering the birth, it is far less likely in the present climate that one will be able to avoid lying to the child. Children are increasingly likely to ask questions such as, 'Mummy, was I born like that? How was I conceived?'. Given this, and for the purposes of exploring the issue, lying rather than non-disclosure and its effect on the family and the child will now be discussed.

Asserting that lying is harmful even when never discovered is a non-consequentialist claim that lying has a negative value attached to it, namely, that a lie and a truthful statement which produce the same result are not equal. One of the clearest articulations of this type of deontological argument is found in Kant. For Kant lying is never morally justifiable, and wrong in all circumstances. Kant reaches this conclusion from two premises. First, from his formulation of the Categorical Imperative, Kant argues that the only actions which are morally justifiable are those which one would wish to be universalized: one must 'act on that maxim which can at the same time have for its object itself as a universal law of nature' (Kant, 1991, p. 99). In other words, one must judge whether one's action is moral according to whether one would wish all persons in similar situations to act in the same way, and so for the action to be the template of a moral law.

Kant is unrelenting in his condemnation of lying, shown clearly in his famous example that it is wrong to lie to a murderer about the location of his or her intended victim. In addition to the fact that one should not lie because one would be acting according to a maxim which one would not wish to universalize (namely, that it is right to lie), Kant holds that the liar is responsible for any consequences that occur as a result of the lie. For Kant these consequences are not only the direct ones (such as if the murderer finds the victim as a result of the lie) but also the wider consequences which lying has on society as a whole. According to Kant, not only do the consequences of a lie affect the individual who is lied to; the lie also harms truthfulness in general, 'For a lie always harms another; if not some other human being, then it nevertheless does harm to humanity in general' (Kant, 1994: pp. 163–4). This is because the smooth running of society depends on assuming that people deal honestly with each other; hence 'truthfulness is a duty that must be regarded as the basis of all duties founded on contract, and the laws of such duties would be rendered uncertain and useless if even the slightest exception to them were admitted' (Kant, 1994: p. 164). Such a contract argument is not unusual and has been used by many philosophers, for example, Hobbes, Hume, Warnock and even the moral projectionist J. L. Mackie, who defends 'the institution of promising' using a similar argument.

The second premise according to which Kant rejects lying is his dictum, connected to the Categorical Imperative, that one must 'act in such a way that you always treat humanity, whether in your own person or in the person of any other, never simply as a means but always at the same time as an end' (Kant, 1991: p. 91). This is a call to be a respecter of persons, which means granting other persons the conditions for them to be full moral agents, thereby facilitating their free autonomous moral action. Moral agents are guaranteed to be ends, and not means, by freely exercising their autonomy and choosing to be such. Part of allowing agents freedom and autonomy is giving them the necessary information to make reasoned decisions and so act autonomously. (This argument is elaborated by Sissela Bok (1980: p. xvii) on the subject of lying, 'Very autonomy may be at stake'.) Consequently, it is not up to individuals to decide who to lie to and who not to lie to, for 'truth is not a possession the right to which can be granted to one person but refused to another' (Kant, 1994: p. 165). Therefore, lying cannot be justified even for the most altruistic of reasons, as lying threatens the autonomy of moral agents by reducing their capacity to make rational and so autonomous decisions (see Kant, 1994). Keeping the truth from a person creates a power imbalance which results in the 'lied-to' not achieving his or her full status as a moral agent, as a possessor of freedom and reason *qua* person.

Taken together, Kant's philosophical attack on lying is robust and one of the clearest polemics against the practice. However, most people would consider Kant's position extreme, and there are few (both inside and outside philosophy) who would argue that it is wrong to lie to a murderer about the location of his or her victim. Even those who hold universalizability to be an important premise in determining morally correct actions would like to make commonly agreed exceptions which could be universalizable, and so consistent, with the Categorical Imperative and the general promotion of truthfulness. For example, with regard to lying to a murderer, the claim would be that it would not be wrong to lie, because this could be turned into a Categorical Imperative, namely, that it is always one's duty to lie to a murderer about the location of his or her intended victim. Those in favour of keeping DI secret could argue in a similar manner that all parents should lie to children conceived using DI, and genuinely wish this action to be universalized. However, while it is relatively uncontroversial to claim that lying to a murderer is correct the same cannot be said for lying to the child in the case of DI. Accordingly, even if it could be argued that instead of taking the duty not to lie as universalizable as a whole, one could universalize subsections (so that exceptions could be made), it would not be clear that lying in regard to DI would be acceptable. Lying in the case of DI is not only not necessarily in the best interests of the child, but it fails to treat the child as an autonomous moral agent. While it is not difficult to imagine an argument which would justify not treating the murderer as a moral agent (although not one which would be accepted by Kant), it would be very difficult to derive a parallel argument which justified not treating the child as an autonomous moral agent (especially when one thinks of the DI child as an adult).

Therefore, in order to justify lying one has to adopt a non-Kantian position, and most likely a non-deontological position, from which one can claim that lies are justified if the consequences are beneficial. Moreover, if the lie is in the best interests of those lied to, a lie is not only justified, but even a 'good'. From such a standpoint, 'paternalistic lies' are justified on two grounds: first, that of protection; and second, because they are in the best interests of those lied to. If these criteria are fulfilled then it is assumed that implied consent is given by the person being lied to. Implied consent can be assumed in situations where any reasonable person would wish to be lied to in the same circumstances. With regard to DI then, those who advocate secrecy claim they are justified by the consequences – a 'normal' family in which all the relations are kept intact – and because lying is in the best interest of the child, who would prefer not to know. Thus, implied consent can be assumed to be granted.

Yet even if one were to adopt this consequentialist position, and deny that there is any negative value attached to lying, it is not clear that the consequences in the case of DI do justify secrecy. To claim that lying is in the best interests of the child is doubtful, for reasons discussed above. Consequently, one cannot assume implied consent (especially when one thinks of the DI offspring as an adult rather than a child). Therefore, arguments from best interests and implied consent are flawed, leaving a basic consequentialist argument, namely, that the consequences of producing a 'normal' family justify the lies. Such a position is again questionable as it can be framed as setting the interests of the child against the interests of the family, resulting in a conflict of interests. One might want to add that for England and Wales, at least, the Children Act 1989 stipulates that the best interests of the child always come first in any decision regarding his or her upbringing (the 'welfare principle' in s.1 of the Act). There is no case law on whether best interests include knowing one's parentage, but the Act does make it plain that in a case of conflict of interests with the parents, the child's welfare comes first.

In sum, then, even if one adopts a consequentialist position and concludes that lying is not intrinsically negative, conflicts of interest still remain, and these are compounded by disagreements about what the desirable consequences are. Drawing a firm conclusion about whether secrecy in DI should be removed is an open question. It remains far from clear precisely what is in the best interests of the child in DI, and clearly there is merit in the arguments for both openness and secrecy.

Conclusion

The arguments regarding donor anonymity are ultimately concerned with the type of procedure DI should be. Those who wish to maintain anonymity wish for the culture of secrecy to continue and for donors to remain completely separate from the parents and the resulting child. Those who argue for removing anonymity are really hoping that this will result in a change to the wider practice, and that parents will reveal the fact of DI conception to their children. In practice this has not happened, and parents are still unwilling to disclose to the child even in countries which have removed donor anonymity. (Thus far only 11 per cent of parents in Sweden have informed their children of their DI conception (Gottlieb et al., 2000). However, a shift may be beginning.)

Without parental willingness to disclose to the child, making the donor identifiable is largely immaterial. Drawing firm conclusions about whether or not non-disclosure to the child is in the child's best interests is difficult. This is largely because there is very little data either way. Given this, it may be that the best, though unsatisfactory, solution is to leave decision-making entirely to the parents' discretion. Hence, for the present it seems that parents will continue to decide whether or not to tell their children, and will judge for themselves whether or not maintaining such a secret will adversely affect their families. However, if decisions about disclosure are going to be left up to parents it could be argued that all parents should be allowed to choose an identifiable donor. Without this choice they may feel that although they can disclose the child's DI status, without being able to identify the donor the child would be frustrated at the lack of further information. Conversely, parents who wish for total secrecy may wish to choose an anonymous donor, and arguably, if the choice really is to be up to the parents, this option should be available.

However said, changes in the law regarding anonymity move away from one formulation of the practice to another. By making such changes in legislation, the lawmakers are suggesting that one course of practice is preferable; in this case, that openness is better than secrecy. Indeed, what has informed the changes in the laws of certain countries is the belief that it is important for donor-offspring to have access to information concerning their genetic heritage. Moves to remove anonymity replace the presumption of secrecy with one of openness. Such a change is a major shift in the underlying ideology of DI and in the ethos surrounding the procedure. The effects of this change can already be seen in the more positive attitude the public has to DI (shown by the number of willing identifiable donors in countries which have abolished anonymity) and may eventually even bring about a change in parents' willingness to disclose to the child.

Finally, such changes in policy and all of the above arguments may simply be outstripped by increases in genetic testing and knowledge. Such practical changes, which reveal genetic non-parentage, will force openness, whether or not parents wish it and whether or not psychologists, doctors and philosophers think it is beneficial.

References

Bateman Novaes, S. (1998). The medical management of donor insemination. In *Donor Insemination: International Social Science Perspectives*, ed. K. Daniels and E. Haimes, pp. 105–30. Cambridge: Cambridge University Press.

Bok, S. (1980). *Lying: Moral Choice in Public and Private Life*. London: Quartet Books Ltd.

Daniels, K. and Haimes, E. (Eds) (1998). *Donor Insemination: International Social Science Perspectives*. Cambridge: Cambridge University Press.

Daniels, K. and Lalos, O. (1995) The Swedish insemination act and the availability of donors. *Human Reproduction* 10: 1871–4.

Edwards, J. (1998). Donor insemination and 'public opinion'. In *Donor Insemination: International Social Science Perspectives*, ed. K. Daniels and E. Haimes, pp. 151–72. Cambridge: Cambridge University Press.

Gottlieb, C., Lalos, O. and Lindblad, F. (2000). Disclosure of donor insemination to the child: the impact of the Swedish legislation on couples' attitudes. *Human Reproduction* 15: 2052–6.

Haimes, E. (1993). Do clinicians benefit from gamete donor anonymity? *Human Reproduction* 9: 1518–20.

Kant, I. (1991). *The Moral Law: Groundwork of the Metaphysic of Morals.* Translated by H.J. Paton. London: Routledge.

Kant, I. (1994). On a supposed right to lie because of philanthropic concerns. In *Ethical Philosophy,* tr. and ed. J. W Ellington 2nd edn., pp. 162–6. Cambridge: Hackett Publishing Company.

Klock, S.C., Jacob, M.C. and Maier, D. (1994). A prospective study of donor insemination recipients: secrecy privacy and disclosure. *Fertility and Sterility* **62**: 477–84.

Lasker, J.N. (1998). The users of donor insemination. In *Donor Insemination: International Social Science Perspectives,* ed. K. Daniels and E. Haimes, pp. 7–32. Cambridge: Cambridge University Press.

Lui, S.C., Weaver, S.M., Robinson, J. et al. (1995). A survey of semen donor attitudes. *Human Reproduction* **10**: 234–8.

Nachtigall, R.D. (1993). Secrecy: an unresolved issue in the practice of donor insemination. *American Journal of Obstetrics and Gynecology* **168**: 1846–51.

Nachtigall, R.D., Tschann, J.M., Quiroga, S.S., Pitcher, L. and Becker, G. (1997). Stigma, disclosure and family functioning among parents of children conceived through donor insemination. *Fertility and Sterility* **68**: 83–9.

Pennings, G. (1997). The internal coherence of donor insemination practice: attracting the right type of donor without paying. *Human Reproduction* **12**: 1842–4.

Pfeffer, N. (1993). *The Stork and the Syringe.* Cambridge: Polity Press.

Snowden, R. and Snowden, E. (1998). Families created through donor insemination. In *Donor Insemination: International Social Science Perspectives,* ed. K. Daniels and E. Haimes, pp. 33–52. Cambridge: Cambridge University Press.

Spallone, P. (1989). *Beyond Conception: The New Politics of Reproduction.* London: Routledge.

First and second trimester

Ethical and social aspects of evaluating fetal screening

Elina Hemminki

National Research and Development Centre for Health and Welfare (STAKES), Helsinki, Finland

Introduction

A current doctrine in medicine is that health care should be evidence-based, and an important tool of evidence-based medicine is health technology assessment (HTA). A typical textbook definition of HTA is that it includes studying the health, economic, social and ethical consequences of a health technology in a way that helps in deciding on its use. Health aspects include intended consequences, efficacy and effectiveness, as well as unintended consequences, adverse effects and side effects. Some commentators would also include in HTA the study of factors that influence the use of a health technology.

Specific to HTA is its aim of integrating knowledge of different aspects of a technology, in order to provide a full evaluation to help decision-makers. In practice, however, ethical and social aspects, if studied at all, have not been integrated into the HTA process. One reason for this is the difficulty of combining ethical and social aspects with other outcomes. To aggregate various factors in health, several methods have been created, including quality-adjusted life-years. To combine health and cost data, cost-effectiveness, cost benefit and other such methods have been developed. But there is no quantitative method by which to measure ethical and social consequences. Thus, they are treated as separate issues, and often added as a footnote or afterthought when an evaluation of a health technology has already been made.

The purpose of this chapter is to illustrate the importance of the integration of ethical and social consequences in HTA, using fetal screening as an example. Fetal screening is loaded with ethical and social consequences and determinants, such as views on reproduction, fetal rights, the value of disabled people, eugenic ideology, resource allocation and the structures of prenatal care. Thus, the importance of ethics and social factors may actually be easier to illustrate for fetal screening than for some other perinatal technologies – or for medical technologies in general.

When I use the words 'ethical' or 'ethics', I mean 'moral' – are we doing what is right or wrong; what is good, what is bad? By 'social' I mean consequences and aspects concerning people other than the person who is the target of a technology, as well as social structures, including health care. By 'fetal screening' I mean assessment of the quality of the fetus, i.e. an assessment to detect fetal disease, disability or a characteristic of or predisposition towards one of these, with an induced abortion as a possible consequence. This includes the testing of parents for carrier status of a genetic disease with the aim of judging the fetus's status. By 'screening', as opposed to 'testing', I mean doing a test on a general pregnant population or a segment of it defined by an unspecific risk factor, such as mother's age. I will not discuss genetic or other types of testing done because of family history or other strong risk factors, or because of a screening finding that requires confirmation.

By the term 'perinatal technologies' I mean technologies used to create human life, regulate it and improve the health of the fetus, the newborn and his or her mother. Most medical and health technologies target diseases or health. In the perinatal field many technologies deal with the regulation of life itself. Previously, medicine could only end a life already started. Now the times of solely natural creation of new human life are past, and new life can be created (or assisted), and the quality of a new human being influenced.

Consequences of fetal screening

The aim of fetal screening is to ascertain whether a fetus possesses a disease or unwanted characteristic. But in the process many other things happen; Figure 12.1 lists some of them. The knowledge of the existence of such screening may influence women's and men's images of their worthiness to have children because of their genetic makeup or other characteristics. It may also reinforce the current view of reproduction – children are not born, they are made. Fetal screening will also affect the view of pregnancy as being unreal until the quality of the fetus is guaranteed ('tentative pregnancy' as formulated by Rothman, 1987) and attachment to the fetus may be weakened. Whether it has any impact on the subsequent mother–infant relationship is unknown.

Fetal screening will influence a fetus's status – a sick fetus is not a real fetus, but something less valuable. Although it may not affect existing children with disabilities, this value judgement may in the long run create a more negative view about people with disabilities. People with disabilities, at least, sometimes interpret fetal screening as a value judgement of them. Currently it is emphasized that fetal screening is a way to give the mother/parents an opportunity to avoid having a handicapped or ill child. But this slant might easily be changed to emphasize the health of the newborn population, public health or the health level of a given society. And then we would have to face the dilemma of eugenics.

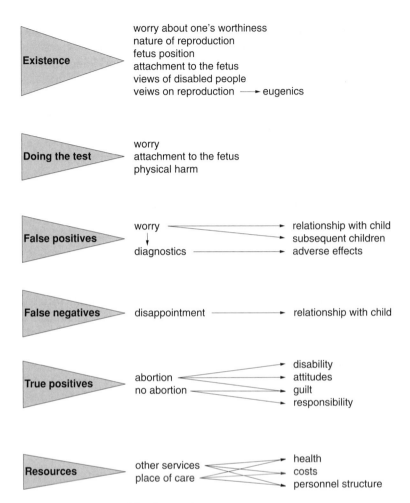

Figure 12.1. Consequences of fetal screening.

The worry and physical harm resulting from doing the screening test (Figure 12.1) varies according to the type of test. With the widely used serum test for Down's syndrome, the worry while waiting for the test result may be considerable (Santalahti, 1998). In amniocentesis (in screening by age indication) miscarriage, infection and other complications may occur. In ultrasound the initial, often uncertain diagnosis may cause worry. All these tests reinforce the concept of tentative pregnancy.

A false positive test result (Figure 12.1) means that the screening test indicates a problem or a risk for it, even though in reality the problem does not exist. Because serum tests are very unspecific (over 90 per cent of positives are false positives) and because the diagnosis, usually by amniocentesis, takes weeks, there is a great deal of well-documented stress for the pregnant woman and her partner (Santalahti et al., 1996). This worry may make the couple's lives miserable and may negatively affect the pregnancy experience, with ongoing ramifications for family relationships and subsequent pregnancies.

False negatives (when the fetus has the condition but it is not detected by the screening test) may lead to disappointment – the mother/parents falsely assume the child to be normal, and they may be totally unprepared at the birth. How this phenomenon affects their relationship with the handicapped child is unknown. They may feel guilty, or deceived by the medical profession, because they tried to avoid the birth of an affected child but failed.

In the case of true positives (when the condition is definitely confirmed from the screening test or in a diagnostic test) the option of termination, often at late gestation, has to be faced. Finding a defective fetus and aborting it avoids the birth of a disabled infant, which is the purpose and the positive side of screening. But late abortion may be psychologically difficult. Late abortions on grounds of fetal abnormality may also influence society's view of disability, fetuses and pregnancies. If the mother decides to continue the pregnancy regardless of fetal abnormalities, the parents take the responsibility. They may, both in their own eyes and that of others and society, feel that they have to bear the consequences, however difficult their lives are. This outcome was their choice; it did not merely happen to them.

There also may be mid-level consequences for health care providers. Fetal screening may have consequences for resource utilization in antenatal care. Because screening tests may require special skills and technology, they may have a notable impact on the place of antenatal care and type of personnel needed (Hemminki et al., 1999).

Special features of fetal screening

Screening is a central feature of antenatal care. Measuring of maternal blood pressure and weight, and doing various laboratory tests with the aim of identifying deviations or pathological findings are core elements. But here the purpose has been to improve the mother's or fetus's health, not to abort the fetus. It is true that abortion is not the sole purpose of fetal screening, as knowledge of a handicapped fetus may be important in planning for delivery and newborn care. In the future, fetal genetic therapy may also be an option. But for problems like Down's syndrome, neither of these factors is of any current importance. Screening is organized to offer the mother/parents the possibility of avoiding the birth of a Down's syndrome child by having an abortion.

Other special features differentiating fetal screening from other antenatal screening include its target, the involvement of other people and its relation to eugenic ideology. Usually the target of screening is an identifiable non-clinical or pre-symptomatic disease (i.e. not diagnosed by the patient or a physician) or a risk factor for a disease. In much fetal screening, achieving consensus on the concept of disease is difficult. Many say that Down's syndrome is not a disease, rather a condition or characteristic (Alderson et al., 1999). Similarly, being very short or having a genetically increased risk of ageing prematurely cannot really be defined as diseases. The borderline between screening for wanted or unwanted characteristics, e.g. fetal sex or undesirable genetic variations, can be a thin one. Which characteristics, therefore, medicine and health care systems are to define as diseases and which are not is problematic.

Fetal screening has an impact not only on the mother and her fetus, but also on the father and siblings of the child, especially in cases of genetic screening. If the fetus is found to have a genetic defect, this information is significant for people sharing the same parentage. Screening may reveal genetic information to those who did not ask for it and possibly did not want to know. Knowledge that a certain defect had led a woman to abort the fetus is especially hard for those who have the same defect. They may think that they also should have been aborted. On a societal level this question may bother handicapped people in general – if the birth of people like themselves is not wanted, they may think that they are not wanted either.

The fourth special feature of fetal screening, differentiating it from other antenatal screening procedures, is its possible relation to eugenic ideology. Eugenics was prominent in the western world early in the twentieth century, but is a source of shame today because of its connection to fascist politics and nationalistic and racist movements (Hemminki et al., 1997a). Before the technology for fetal screening was available, the reproduction of people assumed to have unwanted hereditary characteristics was regulated either through isolation in institutions, marriage prohibitions, sterilizations and other pregnancy prevention methods, or through unselective abortions if an affected woman got pregnant. In a 1997 survey, Finnish physicians were asked whether they believed that current fetal screening is based on eugenic thinking. A fifth of the physicians agreed that it was so, in whole or in part; about half said it was not; and most of the other respondents either could not say or chose the option, 'I do not know what eugenics is and cannot make a comparison' (Hemminki et al., 2000). Those physicians who agreed that fetal screening was not linked to eugenics based their opinion on the intention and voluntariness of screening, focusing on improvement of a race versus decreasing suffering among individuals.

Fetal screening is based on certain values and beliefs, such as the importance of health, the feeling that a handicapped child is worse than none at all (particularly if there is an option of having a chance to try again) and the perception that handicaps cause suffering to the child itself, the parents and/or to society. Through the organization of screening programmes and concomitant research, medicine and health care have been given the authority to define which diseases and characteristics qualify for these beliefs.

Furthermore, fetal screening assumes that fetuses are not human beings and that mothers have a full right to decide the fate of their fetuses. When a fetus has its own status – whether only when it is born or at some earlier stage – is not clearly defined. In Finland, the offical time limit between a miscarriage and birth is 22 gestation weeks, meaning that products of pregnancies spontaneously ending after 22 weeks will be recorded as children. However, induced abortion is allowed until the 24th week, and in these cases the pregnancy products are treated like fetuses.

Comparison to other perinatal interventions

Fetal screening is not the only controversial activity that occurs during the perinatal period. In the following I compare, as examples, the ethical debates on fetal screening to those on abortion, in vitro fertilization and the intensive care of preterm infants (Hemminki et al., 1997b), Table 12.1.

In fetal screening (and consequent selective abortions) ethical discussion has focused on the rights of parents to have healthy children, on the rights of disabled persons, on unintended effects of screening procedures and on the general threat of eugenics as an ideology. In discussions concerning termination of pregnancy in general, the usual ethical question is – when does life begin (e.g. Chervenak et al., 1995)? When do cells and tissues become a human being or a person? If embryos or very young fetuses are defined as human beings, all abortions are morally wrong. Only a threat to the mother's life is an argument strong enough to overcome the ethical problems of destroying an (unborn) human being. (A strict anti-abortion position would not even view the mother's life as a 'trump', since the fetus's life is of equal value.) However, because an embryo or a very young fetus is not capable of living outside the mother, it has been argued that it is not a human being in a morally relevant sense, but is part of the mother's body. This reasoning does not, however, answer the question of when does a fetus becomes a human being – at viability or at birth?

The problem is intensified by new technology which allows very premature children to survive. With the newest intensive care technology, younger and younger infants spontaneously born too early can be kept alive. Concern has been raised over the fact that many of the infants kept alive exhibit disabilities, some of which are serious. Although the balance between additional surviving healthy infants and additional disabled infants saved is highly positive, with far more healthy than disabled survivors, the absolute numbers of children with disabilities may have increased as a result of neonatal intensive care (Hagberg et al., 1993).

Table 12.1. Ethics discussions on some perinatal activities

	Fetal screening[1]	Abortions[2]	Neonatal intensive care	In vitro fertilization
Start of life	−	+	..	−
Saving fetuses/infants	P↓	+	P↑	−
Right to have children	..	..	..	+
Preventing disability	P↑	..	−	−
Preventing death	−	P↓	P↑	..
Rights of disabled	+	..	−	−
Eugenics	+	..	−	+

Key: +, commonly; −, not commonly discussed, should be; .. not relevant;
P↓ purpose to decrease; P↑ purpose to increase.
[1]Including selective abortions.
[2]Abortions because a child in general is not wanted.

Regarding in vitro fertilization (IVF), ethical discussions have concerned the right to have one's own children, the right to parenthood (if donated cells are used), restrictions on who can be a mother (e.g. marital status, age) and the ample possibilities for eugenic practices. IVF pregnancies, however, also result in much higher proportions of preterm and small infants, who have a higher risk of disability.

Thus, for these four common perinatal activities, different ethical aspects have been highlighted (Table 12.1). This is surprising, since the ethical issues actually overlap. For example, although selective termination of pregnancy after screening is sometimes only possible after the twentieth week of gestation, little of the ethical literature on screening has concerned the start of life and its ending, issues so central in the abortion discussion. This is especially problematic for selective abortions between 22 and 24 weeks. In many countries the official statistical limit for abortion and birth is 22 weeks of gestation, and newborns born spontaneously at that age often receive treatment to keep them alive, sometimes even successfully.

A second incongruity is this. In fetal screening, fetuses with disabilities are actively targeted, but IVF results in a higher rate of preterm pregnancies and neonatal intensive care in survival of preterm infants. Surviving preterm infants have more disabilities than other infants, yet the debate about disability is almost entirely absent from the literature on IVF.

Finally, when fetuses are screened using chorionic villus biopsy or amniocentesis, some pregnancies with healthy fetuses will be unintentionally terminated as a result of such screening itself. This contradicts the ethos of efforts toward trying to save very premature babies. In multiple IVF pregnancies, the practice has emerged of terminating some of the fetuses to reduce the number of infants to be born and thus the risk of prematurity (see Chapter 16). However, the terminated fetuses are not per se more sick than those left intact.

Integration of ethics and social consequences into health technology assessment

From the health technology assessment perspective there are two issues for ethics: first, how to make ethical thinking consistent over the range of different interventions; and secondly how to integrate ethics into other aspects of HTA. As I have argued in the preceding section, there is a great deal of inconsistency in what ethical factors are thought crucial in different interventions. Perhaps this is explained by the general marginality of ethics in medicine until comparatively recently, by increasing specialization in health care provision, by each intervention's unique history and rationale, and by the different main purposes of the activities (Hemminki et al., 1997b). It is unlikely that any one ethical principle can regulate the whole of medical practice. But it would be useful to think of common principles that apply to different interventions, to classify the interventions by the ethical principle on which they are based and to acknowledge the ethical principles with which they are in conflict.

The marginality of ethics in HTA is a more difficult problem to resolve. Often medical ethics figures only as an afterthought, brought up when the technology is already in use. Ethical aspects are not easily quantifiable, compared with other aspects (effectiveness, adverse effects and costs). Ethics, unlike costs, has a low status in HTA, and ethicists are not typically core people in the field.

Many reasons for the marginalization of ethics in HTA can be offered. The first is specialization – on the one hand, ethics has been left to ethicists, who are not typically core people in HTA, and on the other hand, ethics is not included in the education of people who promote and do HTA. Secondly, ethical questions are difficult to define and operationalize. It would require a lot of theoretical and methodological thinking and research to be able to compare, for example health and ethical consequences jointly in the way one currently compares health and economic consequences. Furthermore, individualistic thinking emphasizes autonomous choices as the answer to various ethical problems, forgetting the societal perspective of consequences and control. The myth of the objectivity of research is strong among health and economic researchers, and they may find the explicit value requirements of ethics difficult. Ethical consequences are often likely to be negative for the dissemination of a technique. It is easier to find examples of techniques that are effective but ethically unacceptable, than to find an example of an ineffective technique which for ethical reasons should be used. Producers of technology are influential in HTA – they finance and do much of the HTA, and they are not eager to promote evaluations which are likely to bring up negative sides of their products.

In HTA, social aspects/consequences are neglected even more than ethical aspects – rarely are they added even as an afterthought. Probably many of the reasons I have listed above for the neglect of ethical aspects apply also for social aspects, but to varying degrees. Specialization certainly applies, but ethical questions are difficult to define and operationalize. Individualistic thinking is likely to be very important. Even though public health people think in terms of groups and societies, the units of measurement are usually on an individual level, which are then summed up to form a group effect. It is not common in HTA to think about what kind of spill-over effects a health technology has outside its group of target individuals.

What can be done?

The current state of affairs where the value of a health technology is judged only on the basis of some of its consequences, and the use of the technology is promoted on the basis of such deficient information (in addition to commercial and other interests), is not satisfactory. The first step is to acknowledge this problem. If the limited and narrow nature of current research were defined as an important problem, interest in finding solutions might be raised.

A feasible point for introducing ethics and social aspects into HTA could be to bring these points into research via resource allocation. Before a new technology is developed, a societal and professional ethical and social discussion should occur – do we want this kind of technology? It may be argued that this is a naive and unrealistic approach. Before research is done, one cannot predict which of its fruits will and can be used. Other counter-arguments include the claim that such considerations result in censorship and harm all innovative basic research, and the possibility that someone somewhere will do such research anyhow. It is possible that ethical and social pre-evaluation in basic research is unrealistic, but such steps could be taken prior to product development. Further, active research support for and dissemination of ethical and social aspects of health technology is likely to be helpful. When we have the technology ready, arrangements similar to those currently in place for drugs could be introduced – drugs are not allowed to be marketed before assessment.

Currently the typical order in evaluating a therapy is first to study its efficacy (and short-term adverse effects). Then, using the costs of the therapy and calculated benefits, an implicit or explicit estimate of cost-effectiveness or cost utility is made to decide about utilization. In case of technologies that are ethically or socially potentially controversial, the order of evaluation could be different. An initial ethical and social evaluation would be done, then an initial cost-evaluation (i.e. can the system afford it if it were effective for planned indications?) would be followed by an evaluation of efficacy and effectiveness – but only in affirmative cases.

The outcomes to be used in HTA should be many-sided, and qualitative techniques to combine different kinds of data should be developed. Currently HTA evaluations try to give an overall estimate of the health value of a technology, in isolation from the social situation and people. This is relatively artificial even in regard to health effects, and when social and ethical dimensions are introduced, the need to inspect a technology within a context becomes very evident and necessary.

Commercial and professional pressures are strong factors influencing the dissemination of health technology. Most new technologies are produced by profit-making companies, or their products are needed in producing the technology, and commercial pressures are clear. But professionals may also have profit motives – their own income may be influenced by the use of a technology, and above all, their professional image and esteem, both personally and as a disciplinary group, may depend on it. Because evaluations currently are narrowly done and the crucial ethical and social elements are usually not there, the strong commercial and professional pressures are likely to lead to unnecessary, premature or too widespread use of health technology. Currently the use of technology runs ahead of proper evaluation. More conservative adoption of health technology, including regulation of technology introduction and marketing, would be welcomed. Acknowledging ethical and social consequences may help to achieve this.

References

Alderson, P., Goodey, C. and Appleby, J. (1999). The ethical implications of antenatal screening for Down's syndrome. *Bulletin of Medical Ethics* **147**: 13–17.

Chervenak, F.A., McCullough, L.B. and Campbell, S. (1995). Is third trimester abortion justified? *British Journal of Obstetrics and Gynaecology* **102**: 434–5.

Hagberg, B., Hagberg, G. and Olow, I (1993). The changing panorama of cerebral palsy in Sweden. VI. Prevalence and origin during the birth year period 1983–1986. *Acta Paediatrica* **82**: 387–93.

Hemminki, E., Rasimus, A. and Forssas, E. (1997*a*). Sterilizations in Finland: from eugenics to contraception. *Social Science and Medicine* **45**: 1875–84.

Hemminki, E., Santalahti, P. and Louhiala, P. (1997*b*). Ethical conflicts in regulating the start of life. *Perspectives in Biology and Medicine* **40**: 586–91.

Hemminki, E., Santalahti, P. and Toiviainen, H. (1999). Impact of prenatal screening on maternity services – Finnish physicians' opinions. *Acta Obstetrica et Gynecologica Scandinavica* **78**: 93–7.

Hemminki, E., Toiviainen, H. and Santalahti, P. (2000). Finnish physicians' opinions on prenatal screening. *British Journal of Obstetrics and Gynaecology* **107**: 655–62.

Rothman, B.K. (1987). *The Tentative Pregnancy: Prenatal Diagnosis and the Future of Motherhood.* New York: Penguin Books.

Santalahti, P. (1998). *Prenatal Screening in Finland – Availability and Women's Decision-Making and Experiences.* National Research and Development Centre for Welfare and Health Research Report 94. Helsinki: STAKES.

Santalahti, P., Latikka, A.-M., Ryynänen, M. and Hemminki, E. (1996). Women's experiences of prenatal serum screening. *Birth* **23**: 101–7.

13

Prenatal counselling and images of disability

Priscilla Alderson

Institute of Education, London, UK

Prenatal counselling and associated tests have become routine parts of prenatal care in many countries (Reid, 1990). The main intentions are to offer women the choice about whether to continue with a pregnancy when a fetus is impaired, and to contribute to reducing the incidence of disability with its attendant distresses and costs (HTA, 1998). This chapter reviews contrasting views about prenatal counselling, its advantages and disadvantages. Medical and counselling images of disability are compared with the views of adults who have conditions that are tested for prenatally. The evidence poses questions for bioethical reflection about the nature of disability (is it mainly physical impairment or social restrictions?) and about the possible impact of prenatal screening and counselling on maternal–fetal relationships. These questions include not only personal, mother–child relationships, but also the way that parenting generally, like pregnancy, may be becoming tentative and provisional, instead of the unconditional acceptance of the child as 'a gift of God' common in traditional rhetoric, at least, if not in practice.

Prenatal counselling

Prenatal testing and counselling have expanded since prenatal diagnosis of Down's syndrome, thalassaemia and sickle cell anaemia began through amniocentesis in the late 1960s. Chorionic villus sampling (cvs), another diagnostic test which also draws fetal material from within the maternal abdomen, has since been developed. There are now two further and less invasive methods: examination of serum from maternal blood tests; or, from about 12–15 weeks gestation, nuchal translucency (swelling in the fetal neck) by ultrasound scanning. Both these tests can indicate higher risks of the fetus having a chromosomal disorder or spina bifida (Wald et al., 1992), and increasingly serum screening and ultrasound scanning are routinely offered in wealthier countries. In Britain, in areas where there are many members of ethnic minority groups affected by sickle cell anaemia or thalassaemia, universal prenatal screening for these conditions has been implemented or proposed. The monogenetic condition most likely to affect Caucasians –

cystic fibrosis – is not yet routinely screened for, but, as with other mono-genetic conditions, prenatal tests are often offered to families known to be affected. The tests may be preceded or followed by counselling, which ranges from giving medical results to detailed discussion about the nature and meaning of the tests, the results and the possible choices they offer (Green and Statham, 1996; Marteau et al., 1988).

There is a crucial difference in knowledge of the condition being tested for between people with an affected close relative who have personal experience and who opt-in to have prenatal tests, and the 'healthy' unaffected majority of pregnant women who are routinely screened unless they opt-out. The latter group is likely to need much more counselling before being able to make an informed choice about whether to have a test. Yet because personal opt-in testing involves far fewer people and tends to be done by clinical geneticists, whereas mass screening involves far more people and is done by generalist prenatal staff, the latter group usually receive less counselling (Clarke, 1994, 1997).

Prenatal counselling can begin before conception, when people in a 'high risk' group or family are tested for their carrier status of single gene condi-tions. The same tests during pregnancy indicate, if both parents are carriers, that the fetus could be a carrier or have the full condition. So a positive result leads on to decisions about whether or not to have the more invasive definitive tests of amniocentesis or cvs, and whether or not to continue with the pregnancy.

Advantages of prenatal counselling

Advocates of universal prenatal screening and counselling say that the servi-ces offer every woman information and opportunities to choose. Preconcep-tual tests for carrier status may influence decisions about choosing a partner and becoming a parent. With fetal tests, parents may be more accepting of an impaired child if they are able to prepare emotionally before the birth, and are also able to feel that they chose to have the child rather than feeling imposed upon. Termination of affected pregnancies obviates the emotional, practical and financial costs of supporting disabled children, and also pre-vents the suffering which the child and family would otherwise endure. 'Therapeutic termination' is usually cited as the 'effective remedy' which validates screening programmes (HTA, 1998). Decades of preconceptual and prenatal screening in Cyprus have contained the costs of treating thalas-saemia, which would otherwise have overwhelmed the national budget (Modell and Kuliev, 1993).

Fetal tests and prenatal selection now enable women from families with a known severe genetic disorder to have healthy children, whereas previously they could only choose between either the risk of having an impaired child or else remaining childless. Efficient screening programmes involve the kinds of scientific and statistical knowledge which raise standards in evidence-based health services (Thornton, 1994) and also raise standards and the status of the nursing, midwifery and counselling professions (Sigmon et al., 1997).

The prenatal literature, confirmed by our research observations (see Acknowledgements), tends to emphasize the burdens of having an impaired child. For example, Professor Lilford calculates a net gain to society of screening 100 000 pregnancies, involving 3000 amniocenteses (2960 with negative results) incurring the inadvertent miscarriage of 30 unaffected fetuses, in order to reduce the incidence of Down's syndrome from 100 to 60 live births (Painton, 1997). He considers the costs are justified by the severity of Down's syndrome. There is frequent mention of 'risk', 'handicap', 'mental retardation', 'bad/faulty/dangerous gene', 'problem', 'trouble' and 'suffering' (see review by, for example, Shakespeare, 1999). Pathology tends to be stressed, rather than the unpredictable range from very mild to very severe. For example, a paper in a leading medical peer-reviewed journal begins, 'Spina bifida occurs in one of 2,000 births and leads to life-long and devastating physical disabilities including paraplegia, hydrocephalus, incontinence, sexual dysfunction, skeletal deformities and mental impairment' (Scott et al., 1998). 'Including' could imply that all cases with spina bifida have these and other defects, although the accurate meaning would be 'may include'; some people with spina bifida have none of these problems. However, by implication, the greater the costs of disability, then the greater the benefits of prenatal prevention.

Universal screening and counselling are guided by principles of respect for prospective parents' autonomy, the justice of fair distribution and cost containment, and the beneficence of preventing suffering and promoting scientific public health and other health services, as well as by reasoned utilitarian values (Bromham, Dalton and Jackson, 1990; Ettorre, 1999). The intention is to promote healthier and happier maternal–fetal and subsequent mother–child relationships.

Disadvantages of prenatal counselling

Concerns about prenatal testing and counselling range from the effects on individuals to broader social effects. Screening of large populations raises unnecessary anxiety among the vast majority of women whose pregnancies are 'normal', although many have to go through anxious waiting for ominous screening results to be clarified (Green, Statham and Snowdon, 1994). Frequently, women are screened without their full knowledge or consent (Green, 1994; Marteau, 1995). Prenatal counselling services tend to be under-resourced and fall below recommended standards, so despite their best efforts staff seldom have enough time to counsel well (Clarke, 1994; Smith, Shaw and Marteau, 1994). The diagnostic fetal tests are risky. Amniocentesis and cvs each incur a one per cent risk of miscarriage, and some clinics warn that autopsies after termination find on average that one fetus in every 200 is 'normal' after a false positive result. False positive and false negative results are further complicated when risks and reassurance are misunderstood, and are reduced to statistical terms, which confuse many women – and also many prenatal counsellors (Sadler, 1997; HTA, 1998). Pregnancy is being transformed from a healthy 'natural' experience into a pathological 'tentative' state in which women are increasingly bound by medical opinion, invasive surveillance and 'manufactured uncertainty' (Rothman, 1994, 1998). Despite being intended to prevent suffering, termination of pregnancy for fetal abnormality can cause intense distress and regret (Green and Statham, 1996; Santalahti, 1998).

New reproductive technologies align with other current trends, such as risk management, consumerism and economic pressures (Beck 1992; Winkler, 1998) to encourage women to expect to have a 'perfect' baby, closer to a consumer commodity than a valued person with ordinary human failings. Some analysts see these trends as undermining the status and value of children (O'Neill, 1994; Brazier, 1996), others criticize them as 'feto-centric' (Rothman, 1996: p. 26). Either way, there is a growing tendency to set the interests and rights of mother and fetus in opposition, as illustrated by Bromham et al. (1990). This conflict has been critically analysed by Callahan and Knight (1992) who show how, in cases of enforced Caesareans in the US, fetal distress has tended to be linked to maternal disadvantage. Better living standards and health care could benefit both mother and fetus, preventing occasions for conflicts of interests. Women who escaped from having enforced surgery tended to give birth normally, so questioning the medical expertise on which fetal rights arguments are based.

While women's lives are complicated by pregnancy, many women welcome pregnancy as personally fulfilling and status-enhancing – as demonstrated by the demand for infertility services. Yet during recent decades, universal prenatal screening has encouraged a tendency towards treating every pregnancy, however greatly desired, as provisional, creating a culture of 'Do you really want it? Take it or leave it.' The technologies contribute towards accentuating conflicts between maternal and fetal interests through their ability to scan and screen the fetus as a separate identity, and their emphasis on 'abnormality'. Decisions about 'therapeutic' abortion are treated as medically informed technical choices about 'handicap' rather than as moral decisions that profoundly affect human relationships, identity and obligations, and the meaning of parenthood as an unconditional or else a provisional relationship.

Further concerns include the following questions. Are women truly informed and respected, or are the choices they are asked to make illusory, overly constrained by economic and social pressures, or unwanted burdens for women who would prefer not to know or to choose? Economically, could the considerable funds and resources devoted to prenatal screening be used more effectively to prevent and treat disease and disability, which are far more commonly acquired than innate? (Oliver, 1996). How scientific can prenatal counselling be, given high rates of false positive and false negative results of initial screening, and the inability to assess how severely affected a fetus is, with the unknown impact of the potential child's future lifestyle? Although opt-in individual testing at the request of women who have affected relatives with a genetic condition is beneficial, there is a strong case for showing that mass prenatal screening causes more harm than good (Clarke, 1997).

Disabled people's perspectives

The pros and cons listed so far can all be based on mainstream medical and moral assumptions: that health and independent personal fulfilment are the highest goods; that it is therefore right to prevent and avoid illness and disability, to the extent of preventing disabled lives; that such lives inevitably will be costly, dependent lives of suffering; and that it is kind and responsible to the potential person and to the family, especially the mother, to relieve them of these burdens.

Yet these assumptions raise questions. What do disabled people think about the images of disability publicized by the screening services, and their effects on human relationships? Is life with the screened-for conditions inevitably so seriously impaired, dependent, sad and unproductive? What do people who live with these conditions think about the value and quality of their life and about prenatal screening? How do they feel when close relatives consider having an abortion of a fetus with their condition? The next two sections consider these questions, beginning with the activists' views.

Radical views of disabled people

Disability activists contrast the term 'people with a disability or handicap' with that of 'disabled people' (Oliver, 1996; Asch, 1999, 2000). They argue that the former phrase emphasizes a deficit in the person, and the latter term denotes how they are disabled more by an uncaring society than by any impairment or learning difficulty (Goodey, 1991; Ward and Simons, 1998) they may have. Oliver, a professor who uses a wheelchair, argues that his mobility is limited by the poor design of local buses rather than by his physical state. Disability activists claim equal civil rights, access and opportunities with everyone else, and they oppose the discriminatory language of 'special need'. They criticize the medicalization of disability, saying that they wish to be treated by doctors when they are ill or injured or have a condition which can be cured or palliated, but not otherwise. Many disabilities are not susceptible to any medical treatment and, according to the activists, in cases when doctors cannot do good they can do harm, both to the individual and more generally, by pathologizing disabilities. With other critical researchers, they challenge geneticization (Lippman, 1991), its eugenic tendencies (Paul, 1992) and its fatalistic reductionism to genetic influences and away from social influences and human agency (Rose, 1995). Language blurs thought in general policies and individual practices. As Steinberg (1997: p. 117) notes, talk of 'an "offending gene" implicitly bespeaks an "offensive person"'.

Shakespeare (1999) reviews openly eugenic and influential medical comments about screening services. Yet he asks whether both medical and activist images of disability are not 'losing the plot'. Perhaps they are equally extreme, one exaggerating pathologies, the other over-denying them, and neither attending to the lived realities of people's daily lives which, Lippman (1994) urges, should be examined carefully. Issues include women making responsible prenatal decisions, the goodwill of the staff who work with them, and the diverse and expert but little-known views of disabled people. Shakespeare tries to steer a middle course between the polarities of denial of the limitations of very severe disability, on the one hand, or else fearful pity and dread about very severe disability, on the other. Interviews to be described later consider how disabled people work between these polarities in their everyday realities.

Attempts to analyse maternal–fetal relations and prenatal decisions are trapped in another powerfully dismissive demarcation: pro-life versus pro-choice. All discussion is too easily assigned to one side or the other, with superficial approval or rejection. Yet decisions about a greatly desired though impaired pregnancy illuminate the complications in right-to-life arguments versus women's actual right to choose freely when they want neither available option – neither a severely impaired child nor an abortion.

Disabled and other feminists discuss this middle ground (Degener, 1990; Morris, 1991; Asch, 1999, 2000). Crow (1996: p. 208) says they should acknowledge that impairment, instead of being 'irrelevant, neutral and sometimes positive', really is a 'quandary' of 'contradictions and complexities'. Ramazanoglu (1989) argues that feminist research is a matter of examining and holding together contradictions instead of futile attempts to ignore or resolve them superficially, and this links to concepts of 'maternal holding on' watching and waiting (Ruddick, 1990) in contrast to 'masculinist' decisive rapid intervention which prenatal counselling tends to facilitate.

The next section reviews a few of the responses of disabled people during our research interviews.

Research with disabled people

During a European project (see Acknowledgements) researchers investigated the views on prenatal screening of physicians, midwives, pregnant women, the general public, experts and reports in the mass media and professional journals. A small study also obtained the views of adults who have a condition which is screened or tested for prenatally. In the UK, we interviewed 40 people, 10 each with cystic fibrosis (CF), sickle cell anaemia or thalassaemia and five each with Down's syndrome or spina bifida.

Two aspects of the interviews provided information relevant to prenatal screening. The first, through general questions about their family and friends, education and work, problems, enjoyments and aims, built up a picture of interviewees' views on the quality and value, and the possible suffering and costly dependence of their lives. The second aspect was to ask interviewees directly for their views about being or becoming parents themselves and about prenatal screening choices. Did they agree with the assumption underlying screening policies that it is reasonable and perhaps preferable to prevent lives such as theirs?

Before reviewing some of the replies, a note about research method is necessary. As reviews of Medline and other website data-sets show, the medical literature on these conditions is mainly drawn from medical records and research about associated pathology, and from quantitative psychological surveys of anxiety, depression, intelligence and quality of life. The research relies on standardized questionnaires that measure levels of difficulty. Researchers use a slightly impersonal 'objective' manner in order to be fair and to elicit comparable replies from everyone. They focus on disability, asking questions such as 'How does your illness affect your daily life?' rather than considering other possible factors.

In contrast, we used qualitative methods, a less formal interview style, and open questions asking for detailed replies; we looked for variety instead of measuring common factors. We contacted small groups of people through informal networks in order, we hoped, to avoid seeming perhaps intimidatingly professional, and to stress that we saw them as persons rather than patients. For terms such as 'patient', 'disease' and 'suffering', we substituted the more neutral ones of 'person', 'condition' and 'experience'. With each potentially negative question about problems or difficulties, we also asked a positive one about rewards and successes. Everyone was sent a leaflet before they agreed to take part about the topics we would raise, and about their rights: to consent or refuse; to withdraw or withhold information; and to maintain confidentiality. We were worried at first about whether we should risk asking questions that might be painfully probing, but we were soon reassured by the responses; almost everyone talked calmly and frankly as if they were used to discussing issues such as screening for their condition.

Table 13.1. The 50 interviewees

Conditions	Thalassaemia	Cystic fibrosis	Sickle cell	Spina bifida	Down's syndrome
Interviewees	10	10	10	5	5
Men	5	2	6	1	4
Women	5	8	4	4	1
Age range	26–39	17–30	21–33	18–33	20–43
Median age	33	24	29	26	30
Mainstream school	10	9.5	9	4.5	2?
Special school	–	0.5	–	0.5	?
Done college/courses	6	4	8	3	5
University	4	5(7)	2	1	–
Live with: parents	6	3	4	3	2
friend(s)	–	4	1	–	2
partner	1	2	2	0.5	0.5
Have children	1	1	3	1	–
Live on own	3	1	3	1.5	5
Have done paid work	10	9	7	4	3
Now do paid work	9	4	5	4	–
Student	–	2	1	2	2

Most taped interviews lasted about an hour; towards the end we said that, although we would like to use all the detail which interviewees had supplied in our reports, we would have to select and summarize their comments for published papers. We asked interviewees to help us to complete summary sheets, noting their key responses to each main topic in a few sentences. This worked very well, as the previous discussion had helped to order and clarify their views, and the sheets gave them some editorial control over how we would use their views.

In contrast to mainstream medical and psychological traditions, our approach, methods and language yield different and, we would argue, more realistic insights into the daily lives of people with serious congenital conditions. Table 13.1 summarizes the background detail of the numbers of men and women interviewed, their ages, education, employment and households. Cohabitation was higher than shown in the Table because some had formerly lived with partners. Table 13.1 shows that most interviewees contribute, now or in the past, by doing paid work instead of incurring the 'lifetime costs of care' which are used in some calculations to show that prenatal screening is cost-effective (Wald, 1992). All the interviewees are literate and numerate –

two groups are highly educated, five people with CF had been to university and two more planned to go there. The groups also did a great deal of voluntary work. Among the people with Down's syndrome, for example, one helped to run a youth club, one taught on courses about empowerment, assertion and safer sex for people with learning difficulties and was an artist, and two were actors who shared in creating plays about disability and genetics. All the interviewees related a wide range of activities that they enjoyed doing.

This is not to claim that these interviewees are representative. Too little social research has been conducted to discover what a representative group with, say, sickle cell anaemia would be like. Qualitative research such as this study cannot produce measurable, generalizable findings about the abilities and experiences of these five groups of people. Yet the study can challenge general assumptions, by showing how these interviewees did not fit the negative images propounded in the prenatal medical literature. To give a flavour of the interviews, the next sections will describe a few of them.

Examples from the interviews

To give an example of the informality, my first interview about cystic fibrosis (CF) was with Tim, aged 23 (names have been changed). I was worried when he showed me into the family living room where his sister and girlfriend were already sitting, as I expected that their presence would inhibit him. I avoid the standard research practice of asking families to regroup to allow for a private interview, partly because their decisions and family dynamics are such useful data and partly because I would assert a potentially inhibiting power balance. The point of meeting at their home or other place of their choice is to respect their status – they are the experts who are helping me. Tim could have arranged a private meeting if he had wanted to. During the interview he spoke about his shorter life expectancy, and when the young women objected he said that they always avoided the subject, but he wanted to talk about it with them. I was pleased that he seemed to use the interview for his own purposes, and their presence was a spur to talk rather than a constraint. Tim worked as a retail manager, and used his days off to attend hospital. Like other interviewees he tried to make his employment record at least as good as that of his colleagues, to prevent his condition being used as an excuse to dismiss him. In common with other people his age, Tim longed to earn enough to live with his girlfriend and leave his parents' home. Like many of the interviewees, when asked about his hopes and aims, Tim spoke freely about being a partner and becoming a parent, spontaneously raising these issues and relieving me of the worry that I might upset or embarrass him by introducing them.

Some of the people with CF had successful careers. Jane was delighted to return to work and to caring fully for her family after her recent heart transplant, but others were frustrated at not being able to find suitable work. They found it hard to live on benefits in cold damp homes, unsuitable for their lungs. Life expectancy for many people with CF is now over 40, but they felt that out-dated images of the sickly child who dies young are still too prominent and deter employers from accepting them.

To illustrate the range of people, the most disabled person with CF was Jenny aged 24, who wished that she could use her English degree to be a journalist. Having returned to live with her parents, she would 'like to be able to do things more spontaneously, have more energy, spend less time with my parents and have more self-identity, be stronger and more confident'. She sang and composed, and like several others enjoyed clubbing but found the smoky atmosphere a problem. Her boyfriend helped her to do her daily chest physiotherapy. Jenny said that she would love to be married and have children but felt that no one would want to take on the responsibility of caring for her and that she was not strong enough to have a child. She was unusual among the group in speaking of her pessimism and depression, but like all of them she distinguished between problems attributable to CF and problems attributable to other factors such as lack of transport and suitable employment. Asked what she might say to a woman who has been told that the baby she is expecting has CF, Jenny replied, 'I would say have the child because I would much rather be alive than not, and nowadays treatment is good. Twenty years ago maybe I would have said no. A baby now with CF has much better chances than I have'. Jenny's family did not talk much about her shorter life expectancy. 'I'm glad of that and I don't dwell on death and illness. I just get on with doing what I want to do'.

In contrast, Rob, aged 26, regrets being told 'practically since I was born that I might die soon. It has stopped me from making plans and getting on with my life, like going to university or doing things which might be boring for a few years but lead on to something better'. When asked what he found helpful in his life, Rob talked, like several others, about being independent and inter-dependent rather than dependent. Asked what he might want to change about himself, again like some of the others Rob replied, 'I'm happy with my character, I'm very happy with what's happening in my life at the moment', and he was more keen to talk about how to change society. 'I'd rip it up and start again, the materialism and back-biting and callousness. If that was sorted out, the smaller issues of tolerance and intolerance would drop into place'.

Everyone spoke in many different ways about discrimination and intolerance of disability being the main social problems they would change. For example, one man with Down's syndrome described being pushed and shoved in the street by his neighbours, and another was fed up with being treated by new work colleagues as if he were stupid, though he added, 'They learn in the end, and then they realize that are the ones who look silly'.

The 10 people with thalassaemia and 10 with sickle cell anaemia experienced the hidden disability of chronic illness like the CF group. Sometimes they have crises which require hospital treatment. They too described a range of rewarding and frustrating experiences, enthusiasms and problems. Their conditions did not appear to dominate their lives in most cases, and much time was spent talking about the many things they had in common with their 'ordinary' peers: work or unemployment, income, housing, relationships, leisure activities and ambitions.

The five people with spina bifida showed the lack of correlation between physical disability and social fulfilment. Angela, who became upset during the interview and cried though she said she wanted to continue talking, was the least physically disabled one. In her mid-30s, she worked in a shop, where few of her colleagues knew she had any disability. She was actively involved with church and other groups, but said she wished that she had more friends and a boyfriend. The other more disabled people with spina bifida included a young single mother who was also a college student, and Richard and Vivian who both used wheelchairs. Richard was a keep fit enthusiast who worked at a sports centre and planned to go to Australia to see the paralympics. He enjoyed going to city clubs with friends, and could haul himself in his chair up and down stairs, so he used underground trains despite officials trying to stop him. He said that when he joined mainstream secondary school, the wheelchair users were all taught mobility and coping with stairs and pavement kerbs, which helped him to become very fit. He said, 'I see myself as able-bodied as anyone else'.

Vivian's spine was too severely curved for surgical correction to be possible. We sat on the floor in her flat and she constantly shifted her weight to relieve her pain. She worked in journalism and also gave expert advice about access to public buildings. She passionately believed in and worked for disabled people's rights. Much of Vivian's income went on her transport costs and domestic help. Like Richard she had a very busy social life 'I'm a great one for socializing. You do feel low and in pain and angry with people and it is important to have friends and to go out for a drink', and she talked enthusiastically about her many interests. Vivian was planning to have a baby and she talked of her mixed feelings about taking folic acid to reduce the risk of the baby having spina bifida, yet 'being proud that I have spina bifida' because it had given her such experience, knowledge and opportunities she would not otherwise have had.

The 40 respondents' views on prenatal screening ranged from believing that it was very useful through to unhappiness that it was offered to anyone. Those with thalassaemia, sickle cell anaemia and CF were more likely to favour screening, provided it was accurately informed regarding their condition, which they tended to doubt was the case. They also tended to say that they would respect any decision made by prospective parents after being properly informed, whether to continue or end a pregnancy affected by their condition, though they hoped the pregnancy would continue and some had mixed feelings. One woman with CF said, 'CF doesn't do any good, but people with CF do. I'm angry that people assume abortion is advisable for CF or Down's but I respect the right of each person to choose in their own case. I'm not sure that many can make informed decisions... It's difficult, it's expensive and wasteful to test everyone, and if these scary policies come about, what kind of world would it be? Would anyone have babies?'

Many spoke eloquently about the dangers and hurt to them of discrimination, and the crucial importance of respect for every type of person. These views perhaps led them to be non-judgemental of other people, including the prenatal decisions they make. However, the people with Down's syndrome or spina bifida, conditions which are most routinely screened for, tended to be more unhappy about screening. For example, two men with Down's syndrome, who had been talking intently about their acting, suddenly looked very sad when asked about screening, and said they did not want to talk about it, as if the subject was too painful. They knew about screening, having created plays relating to it.

Discussion

The research could be criticized for being too homogeneous about widely diverse conditions. However, the interviewees had far more similarities than differences, including the ways they reflected on their lives, and their belief that they suffered from the general stigma of disability more than from their actual condition. Perhaps these interviewees are unusually healthy and capable for people with their conditions. Yet even so, there are probably many other people like them, living as actively as they do with their condition. This raises questions about why the prenatal literature, policy makers and counsellors make so little mention of the potential range of each condition from mild to severe, of the increasingly effective treatments which Jenny mentioned, and of the possibility that some therapeutic abortions may prevent potentially rewarding lives. A further complication for prenatal predictions is the mismatch, shown particularly by the people with spina bifida, between the degree of severity of physical disability and the way people value and enjoy their lives.

The implications of the interviews for prenatal counselling and maternal–fetal relations

The overall impression given by the interviewees was of very interesting, thoughtful and pleasant people. Most of them appeared to value and enjoy their lives, sometimes despite pain and serious illness, as much as any average group of 40 young adults might say they do. One man with sickle cell anaemia was in such pain that his interview took place over three separate visits, but this was because he was so keen to take part. Their friends appeared to value them, and so did their families, with one exception as might be expected in any group of 40 adults (her mother had died and her father had remarried). Most interviewees had far more in common with their 'ordinary' peers than differences, and none showed any clear reason why their life would have been better prevented.

One woman with CF commented, 'I feel up today because I'm talking to you, and I'll feel down on another day'. Yet she also spoke frankly about her problems and fears, as well as about things she enjoyed. Even allowing for the artificial nature of the research interview, and the way our methods partly shape the evidence, as is inevitable in every type of research, the interviewees provide compelling evidence for questioning the assumptions on which prenatal policies and counselling are based – that it is reasonable to prevent such lives. The interviewees challenge the view that it is kinder to terminate any affected pregnancy, however mildly the fetus might be affected, because life is so awful for the severest cases.

Repeatedly, interviewees spoke of the crucial importance to them of being involved in mainstream society – schools and colleges, homes and jobs, clubs and pubs and friendships. They tended to find exclusion, rejection and prejudice more painful and disabling than the direct effects of their condition. Some saw rejection as a linked, indirect effect of their condition, but then another more impaired person would talk of overcoming a similar difficulty. They tended to stress their need to see beyond their condition as a personal predicament, and to press for greater inclusion by challenging negative attitudes in society, and by showing how they could be involved. They were grateful to parents who encouraged them to be strong and who, as one woman with Down's syndrome said of her mother, were ready to 'fight for my rights [even through] the High Court, the High Court of Justice!'

Several interviewees were concerned that prenatal counselling could be seen as official medical endorsement of prejudice against them, condoning the restrictions they most wanted to see removed from education, employ- ment and their neighbourhoods. Some of them helped to train medical students, and they criticized inaccurate medical images of disability, such as the sickly child advertisements that raise funds for medical research. Our research aim was to listen to and report seldom-heard voices, and here are some comments made by people with spina bifida.

- 'We're disabled by attitudes and lack of access', said Vivian.
- Angela said that 'parents should accept their child on any terms'.
- On prenatal screening, Vivian commented, 'You can't decide for people who haven't had their lives yet ... and I'd rather be alive than dead. I'm really proud of having spina bifida, it's not like AIDS or cancer [which her mother had died of] ... It's made me make a real effort to do lots of things and to take risks... I don't need to be cured and I don't want to be anybody else... You can't just get rid of people and go back to the Nazis'.
- Christel felt that she had become more mature than her friends through becoming a mother, 'Having a baby wisens you up'.
- Richard believed, 'If you're old enough to decide you want a child, you should be old enough to handle the child, no matter what disability or ability... If [a child] is going to have parents that care for it, then I don't think that it should need screening... I think the counselling is partly driven by ignorance'. If spina bifida is diagnosed prenatally, 'I would say, "keep the baby, try and make the most of it because there are ways round things"'.

Richard was referring to a theme that ran through the interviews – of adaptation, ingenuity and a resilience that grows through accepting and surmounting difficulties. This is in contrast to prenatal screening policies which propose efforts to prevent and avoid difficulties, as if human beings cannot or should not have to experience them, and as if disability is not inevitable for most human beings, at least at the beginning and end of life. The interviewees quoted earlier suggest that this approach is unrealistic, because ordinary people's lives so often involve problems – such as with relationships, loss, frustrating limitations or poverty. Fearful avoidance of disability, rather than promoting ways to support disabled people's lives, is liable to diminish people rather than freeing them into new achievement and confidence.

The interviewees also worried about future trends. These are vividly highlighted by the consultation document on pre-implantation genetic diagnosis, PGD (HFEA, 2000; King, 2000), which is considered in the final part of this chapter. PGD involves genetic testing of embryos at about the eight-cell stage, after in vitro fertilization (IVF) and before selected embryos are implanted into a uterus. The Human Fertilisation and Embryo Authority asks which criteria should be used to decide when PGD may be appropriate, such as expectancy of a very short life, a life of very poor quality or one of great suffering. The difficulty in these criteria is the current limitations in predicting how severe an impairment might be or might become, how much it may be ameliorated by social or medical support, and how the affected person and family may experience similar difficulties either as hardship and suffering or as part of a worthwhile rewarding life. Some parents value their child's very short life far more than no life at all (Delight and Goodall, 1990). Quality of life fluctuates greatly for many people, and suffering is especially hard to gauge in people with severe mental impairments and those who appear to be unaware and unable to relate, which are further proposed criteria for using PGD. Unawareness may include unawareness of suffering, which would obviate the criterion of suffering, and uncertainty again prevails over the diagnosis and prognosis of unawareness. Children who have been dismissed as 'vegetables' are perceived by others to experience profound feelings, such as by the researcher who commented, 'Cabbages do not cry' (Oswin, 1971).

Apart from difficulties in deciding when to resort to PGD, there are broader concerns that PGD adds to the medical and state-funded prenatal screening technologies, in appearing to endorse discrimination against impaired people as unwanted burdens who are better excluded from society. The argument that prenatal selection is different from ending such lives after birth, and affects attitudes towards impaired fetuses only, is unconvincing. The interviewees show that some disabled people feel threatened and disadvantaged by the prejudices which are, perhaps inadvertently, promoted through prenatal screening. The emphasis on particular impairments when selecting an embryo or fetus as worth preserving suggests that any policy difference between preserving an embryo or a person with, say, thalassaemia is not one of principle but of practicality. Abortion is permissible and euthanasia is not, and people with thalassaemia are able to assert that their life is worthwhile. Babies and young children are in a vulnerable position between fetus and 'independent viable person'. Rather than justifying the view that parents' attitudes will be unaffected by screening and PGD programmes, perhaps it should be the responsibility of those who wish to introduce the programmes to guarantee that attitudes are not being affected. Social exclusion, school exclusion and family exclusion (in numbers of teenagers living on the streets) are increasing rapidly, as are expectations that children should conform to ever more specific milestones, school tests and behaviour standards with an unjust 'zero-tolerance' which does not allow for contingencies and disadvantages. Prenatal programmes are not responsible for these changes, but they are part of them, and are powerful medical and official indirect endorsements of them.

Another theme of injustice is when public rejection, expressed through national prenatal programmes, is made to appear to be a matter of private grief and responsibility, as when each individual woman faces the 'choice' of termination of pregnancy, a choice constrained by social and economic circumstances. Disabled activists refuse to accept this way of reducing the political to the personal, in individuals' 'triumph or tragedy stories' (Oliver, 1996). Yet pregnant women seldom question the way prenatal health professionals tell these stories, and describe certain impediments as incompatible with a reasonable lifestyle. For this reason, some commentators urge that PGD and similar services should only be offered to affected families who specifically request such tests, and not to the general population. They are concerned that technological imperatives, free-market economics and medico-legal defensiveness will ensure that PGD soon develops into a mass service, as IVF comes to be performed more easily and safely. Tests which screen 'negatively' for one or a few specific impairments are soon likely to become multi-package tests to screen simultaneously for numerous impairments, and then tests to select 'positively' for growing numbers of preferred features such as intelligence or height. 'Non-directive' counselling of pregnant women about whether to keep a fetus differs from simply informing pre-pregnant women about which fetus they might prefer to acquire. The same questions can appear to be far less connected with morality or the responsibility of mother to child. Gradually, technology reframes and distances moral choices and the most intimate relationships. When the embryo and fetus, and implicitly the baby and child, are presented to women by health professionals as a means of fulfilling adults' dreams of perfection, rather than as ordinarily imperfect mortals to love as ends in themselves, then maternal–child as well as maternal–fetal relationships are likely to become ever more tentative and conditional.

Acknowledgements

This chapter draws on sociological research funded by the European Commission, Prenatal Screening in Europe Project no. 11 BMH4-CT96-0740, 1996–1999; by the Finnish Academy, 1998–1999; and by the Wellcome Bioethics Programme, 1999–2001, Cross Currents in Genetics Towards the Millennium. I am grateful to everyone who took part in the research, and to my co-researchers, although I am responsible for any shortcomings and opinions in this chapter.

References

Asch, A. (1999). Prenatal diagnosis and selective abortion: a challenge to policy and practice. *American Journal of Public Health* **89**: 1649–57.

Asch, A. (2000). Why I haven't changed my mind about prenatal diagnosis: reflections and refinements. In *Prenatal Testing and Disability Rights*, ed. E. Parens and A. Asch. Washington: Georgetown University Press.

Beck, U. (1992). *The Risk Society: Towards a New Modernity*. London: Sage.

Brazier, M. (1996). Embryos, property and people. *Contemporary Reviews in Obstetrics and Gynaecology* **8**: 50–3.

Bromham, D., Dalton, M. and Jackson, J. (Eds) (1990). *Philosophical Ethics in Reproductive Medicine*. Manchester: Manchester University Press.

Callahan, J. and Knight, J. (1992). Women, fetuses, medicine and the law. In *Feminist*

Perspectives in Medical Ethics, ed. H. Holmes and L. Purdy, pp. 224–39. Indianapolis: Indiana University Press.

Clarke, A. (1994). *Introduction to Genetic Counselling: Practice and Principles*. London; Routledge.

Clarke, A. (1997). Prenatal genetic screening: paradigms and perspectives. In *Genetics, Society and Clinical Practice*, ed. P. Harper and A. Clarke, pp. 119–40. Oxford: Bios.

Crow, L. (1996). Including all our lives: reviewing the social model of disability. In *Encounters with Strangers: Feminism and Disability*, ed. J. Morris. London: The Women's Press.

Degener, L. (1990). Female self-determination between feminist claims and "voluntary" eugenics, between "rights" and ethics. *Issues in Reproductive and Genetics Engineering* **3**: 87–99.

Delight, E. and Goodall, J. (1990). Love and loss: conversations with parents of babies with spina bifida managed without surgery. *Developmental Medicine and Child Neurology* **32**(8, Suppl. 61): 1–58.

Ettorre, E. (1999). Experts as storytellers in reproductive genetics: exploring key issues. In *The Sociology of the New Genetics*, ed. P. Conrad and J. Gabe, pp. 539–59. Oxford: Blackwell Sociology of Health and Illness Monograph.

Goodey, C. (1991). *Living in The Real World: Families Speak About Down's Syndrome*. London: The Twenty One Press.

Green, J. (1994). Serum screening for Down's syndrome: experiences of obstetricians in England and Wales. *British Medical Journal* **309**: 769–72.

Green, J., Statham, H. and Snowdon, C. (1994). *Pregnancy: A Testing Time. Report of the Cambridge Prenatal Screening Study*. Cambridge: Centre of Family Research.

Green, J. and Statham, H. (1996). Testing pregnancy. In *The Troubled Helix*, ed. T. Marteau and M. Richards, pp. 140–63. Cambridge: Cambridge University Press.

HFEA (Human Fertilisation and Embryology Authority) (2000). *Consultative Document on Pre-Implantation Genetic Diagnosis*. London: HFEA.

HTA (Health Technology Assessment) (1998*). Antenatal Screening for Down's Syndrome*, vol. 2, no. 1. Southampton: HTA.

King, D. (2000). *Response to the HFEA Consultative Document on Pre-Implantation Genetic Diagnosis*. London: CAGHE.

Lippman, A. (1991). Prenatal testing and screening. *American Journal of Law and Medicine* **17**: 15–50.

Lippman, A. (1994). Prenatal testing and screening: constructing needs and reinforcing inequalities. In *Introduction to Genetic Counselling: Practice and Principles*, ed. A. Clarke, pp. 142–86. London: Routledge.

Marteau, T. (1995). Towards informed decisions about prenatal testing: a review. *Prenatal Diagnosis* **15**: 1215–26.

Marteau, T., Johnson, M., Plenicar, M., Shaw, R. and Slack, J. (1988). Development of a self-administered questionnaire to measure women's knowledge of prenatal screening and diagnostic tests. *Journal of Psychosomatic Research* **32**: 403–8.

Modell, B. and Kuliev, A. (1993). A scientific basis for cost-benefit analysis of genetic services. *Trends in Genetics* **9**: 46–52.

Morris, J. (1991). *Pride Against Prejudice*. London: The Women's Press.

Oliver, M. (1996). *Understanding Disability: From Theory to Practice*. Basingstoke: Macmillan.

O'Neill, J. (1994). *The Missing Child in Liberal Theory.* Newfoundland: University of Newfoundland Press.

Oswin, M. (1971). *The Empty Hours.* Harmondsworth: Penguin.

Painton, D. (Ed.) (1997). *Antenatal Screening and Abortion for Fetal Abnormality: Medical and Ethical Issues.* London: Birth Control Trust.

Paul, D. (1992). Eugenic anxieties, social realities and political choices. *Social Research* **59**: 663–83.

Ramazanoglu, C. (1989). *Feminism and the Contradictions of Oppression.* London: Routledge.

Reid, M. (1990). Prenatal diagnosis and screening. In *The Politics of Maternity Care*, ed. J. Garcia, R. Kilpatrick and M. Richards, pp. 300–24. Oxford: Clarendon Press.

Rose, S. (1995). The rise of neurogenetic determinism. *Nature* **373**: 380–82.

Rothman, B.K. (1994). *The Tentative Pregnancy: Amniocentesis and the Sexual Politics of Motherhood.* London: Pandora.

Rothman, B. K. (1996). Medical sociology confronts the human genome. *Medical Sociology News* **22**: 23–35.

Rothman, B.K. (1998). *Genetic Maps and Human Imagination.* New York: W.W. Norton.

Ruddick, S. (1990). *Maternal Thinking: Towards a Politics of Peace.* London: The Women's Press.

Sadler, M. (1997). Serum screening for Down's syndrome: how much do health professionals know? *British Journal of Obstetrics and Gynaecology* **104**: 176–9.

Santalahti, P. (1998). *Prenatal Screening in Finland – Availability and Women's Decision-Making and Experiences.* National Research and Development Centre for Welfare and Health Research Report No. 94. Helsinki: STAKES.

Scott, N., Adzick, L., Sutton, L., Crombleholme, T. and Flake, A. (1998). Successful fetal surgery for spina bifida. *Lancet* **352**: 1675–6.

Shakespeare, T. (1999). Losing the plot? Medical and activist discourses of contemporary genetics and disability. *Sociology of Health and Illness* **21**: 669–88.

Sigmon, H., Grady, P. and Amende, L. (1997). The National Institute of Nursing explores opportunities in genetics research. *Nursing Outlook* **45**: 215–19.

Smith, D., Shaw, R. and Marteau, T. (1994). Informed consent to undergo serum screening for Down's Syndrome: the gap between policy and practice. *British Medical Journal* **309**: 776.

Steinberg, D. (1997). *Bodies in Glass: Genetics, Eugenics and Embryo Ethics.* Manchester: Manchester University Press.

Thornton, J. (1994). Genetics, information and choice. In *Consent and the New Reproductive Technologies*, ed. P. Alderson, pp. 35–51. London: Institute of Education.

Wald, N., Kennard, A., Densem, J., Cuckle, H., Chard, T. and Butler, L. (1992). Antenatal maternal serum screening for Down's syndrome. *British Medical Journal* **305**: 391–3.

Ward, L. and Simons, K. (1998). Practising partnership: involving people with intellectual disabilities in research. *British Journal of Learning Disabilities* **26**: 128–31.

Winkler, M. (1998). The devices and desires of our own hearts. In *Enhancing Human Traits: Ethical and Social Implications*, ed. E. Parens, pp. 238–50. Washington DC: Georgetown University Press.

14

Models of motherhood in the abortion debate: self-sacrifice versus self-defence

Eileen McDonagh

Department of Political Science, Northeastern University, Boston, USA

The power of problem definition

Many political commentators argue that problem definition is the most important component of the policy formation process. Problem definition is crucial because it defines how we first identify public issues, which in turn influences how we define appropriate solutions. Over time, the initial way a problem is defined then crystallizes policy debates, producing what can then become a very rigid framework, all but impossible to expand or modify (Rochefort and Cobb, 1994: vii, pp. 4).

The abortion issue, particularly in the US, is a classic example of the power of problem definition for determining not only policy outcomes for American women, but also the crystallization of policy debates. Constitutionally, in the course of nearly 30 years of Supreme Court reasoning, abortion rights have become rigidly defined as a problem of decisional autonomy, that is, as a problem of privacy and choice. Politically, during that same time period, the problem of abortion has been defined by pro-life activists (as we would expect), but also by pro-choice advocates (as we might not expect) on the basis of a very traditional model of motherhood, one invoking cultural and ethical depictions of women as maternal, self-sacrificing nurturers.

The combination of defining the problem of abortion rights constitutionally in terms of the privacy of choice and politically in terms of a traditional view of motherhood has produced a rigid, serious policy consequence – namely, failure to obtain access to abortion services for women in the form of public funding of abortions. Correction of this policy consequence requires a redefinition of the problem of abortion rights from both constitutional and political perspectives, which entails, as part of that redefinition, a transformation of the traditional model of motherhood to include nontraditional elements. To understand more clearly what is involved in this transformative process, let us review the current status of how a traditional model of motherhood underlies the current way the problem of abortion is defined.

Problem definition: constitutionalism and politics

In the United States, the Due Process Clause of the Fourteenth Amendment of the Constitution prohibits the state from depriving 'any person of life, liberty, or property without due process of law'. This Due Process right of privacy has been interpreted by the Supreme Court to mean that a state may not interfere with a person's choice about whom to marry, how to educate and raise one's children, or the choice to use contraceptives. When the Supreme Court established the constitutional right to an abortion in *Roe* v *Wade* in 1973, it did so by ruling that the Due Process right to privacy was 'broad enough to encompass a woman's decision whether or not to terminate her pregnancy' without interference from the state. This decision was a breakthrough for women's rights because it immediately struck down numerous state laws that had severely limited procurement of an abortion (Ginsburg, 1985; Klarman, 1996).

However, in *Roe*, the Court also established that the fetus is a separate entity from the woman. The Court reasoned that because a pregnant woman 'carries [potential life] within her', she 'cannot be isolated in her privacy' and her 'privacy is no longer sole'. As the Court put it, because a pregnant woman carries a fetus, 'any right of privacy she possesses must be measured accordingly'. As the Court stated in *Roe*, 'the right of personal privacy includes the abortion decision, but ... this right is not unqualified and must be considered against important state interests in regulation. [including] the state interests as to protection of ... prenatal life'. Thus, in *Roe*, the Court established that it is constitutional for the state to protect the fetus from the moment of conception and that a pregnant woman's right of privacy to make a choice to terminate pregnancy can be limited by, or balanced against, the state's interest in protecting the fetus as a separate entity from the consequences of that choice. Prior to viability, although the state may not prohibit an abortion per se, the state may protect the fetus by requiring restrictive regulations, such as 24-hour waiting periods and informed consent decrees, and by prohibiting the distribution of any information about abortion in publicly funded family planning clinics. These policies are constitutional even in the case of an indigent woman suffering from a medically abnormal pregnancy that could cripple her for life. What is more, law scholars concur that the Due Process foundation for abortion rights, as interpreted by the Court, means that it would be constitutional for a state to prohibit the use of public resources to assist a woman in obtaining an abortion, even if her pregnancy is subsequent to rape or incest, and even if her pregnancy threatens her with death.

After the stage subsequent to viability, the state in promoting its interest in the potentiality of human life may not only prohibit state assistance in obtaining an abortion, but may also prohibit a woman from choosing an abortion, 'except where it is necessary . . . for the preservation of the life or health of the mother'. Thus, although *Roe* has proved resilient in the ensuing decades for retaining the constitutional right to choose an abortion, defining the problem of abortion rights in terms of privacy has proved completely inadequate for establishing a constitutional right to state assistance for obtaining one. This is consistent – the Due Process right of privacy to be free of government interference when making choices about one's own life or reproductive options does not usually include a constitutional right to government assistance in exercising one's choice. Hence, the constitutional right to choose to use contraceptives, as established in 1965 in *Griswold*, does not include the constitutional right to government funding to purchase contraceptives. Similarly, the constitutional right to choose whom to marry does not include a constitutional right to government funding of one's wedding. Nor does the constitutional right to choose what to read include the constitutional right to government funding to purchase books of one's choice.

Thus, the constitutional problem with using privacy and the Due Process Clause for defining abortion rights is that a Due Process depiction of the abortion issue reinforces the Court's disconnection between the constitutional right to an abortion and abortion funding. Since the right to make a choice without government interference – such as the right to choose an abortion or whom to marry – does not include the right to government assistance in exercising that choice, there is little, if any, constitutional leverage to apply to the abortion access issue.

When we turn to the political arena, we run into a similar dead-end to procuring access to an abortion, as a result of the problem definition of abortion. The journalist William Saleten has followed the abortion debate for some years. Based on his experience, he draws attention to the conservative political message developed not only by pro-life activists, but also by the pro-choice community over the last decade. Starting at least in the mid-80s, around the time of the *Thornburgh* decision, pro-choice activists became so fearful that the right to an abortion would be overturned in court that they began to develop powerful conservative strategies with which to reach out to the American public.

The conservative message, as Saleten analyses it, was premised on conveying a persuasive view of abortion rights that would be suitable for the mass media and for electoral campaigns. As a consequence of this political goal, general issues about women's rights were relegated to the sidelines of the message. In their stead, issues were stressed that were easy for the mass public to affirm, such as the encroachment of big government. As a result, the right to an abortion came to be politically framed as the right to get the government out of your life; that is, the government should have nothing to do with your right to have an abortion. This idea takes the form of bumper stickers, such as 'Get the state out of my uterus!' However clever such bumper stickers might be, the problem with access to abortion in general and abortion funding in particular is that the goal is to get the government into women's lives in the form of providing abortion services. Thus, rather than getting the state out of a woman's uterus, access to public funds, public facilities, and public personnel for abortion services involves getting the state into a woman's uterus, so to speak. The pro-choice strategy of politically defining the abortion message to be getting the government out of women's lives, therefore, is counterproductive as a claim for public funding of abortion services.

The traditional model of motherhood and abortion rights

Underlying the problem definition of abortion rights is a traditional view of motherhood – one that rests upon a relational view of women, defined in terms of an ethic of care, inclusive of a nurturing, if not a sacrificial, relationship between mother and fetus. Relying on the traditional model of motherhood to define the problem of abortion, however, does not give us the necessary arguments to justify public funding of abortions. To gain for women state assistance in procuring abortion services, therefore, requires a redefinition of the problem of abortion, one that draws upon a model of motherhood that incorporates non-traditional elements into the way women are envisioned when seeking an abortion. Expanding the traditional model of motherhood that currently underlies the definition of abortion rights in the US to include a non-traditional model of motherhood holds the promise of securing not only the constitutional right to an abortion, but also the constitutional right to abortion funding.

To reframe the abortion debate to make it possible to secure a constitutional right to abortion funding, we must reconsider the central ethical and legal issue that haunts abortion policies – what justifies killing the fetus? When we look more closely at the way pro-choice advocates answer that question when explaining why they support abortion rights or why they themselves procured an abortion, we find that their justification for abortion rights, far from carrying a non-traditional message about women's rights, relies upon and reinforces some of the most traditional components of motherhood by invoking the principles of 'lifeboat' ethics.

The traditional model of motherhood depicts women in a nurturing relationship with the fetus and with others in need of care. The key to this relationship is that there is no inherent conflict between any of the parties. What creates difficulties for those in the relationship is an external context defined by a scarcity of resources. In order to fulfill her role as nurturer, a woman is forced to choose how to provide the greatest good for the greatest number; to do so, she must make a calculation of whom or what to sacrifice. Presumably, she would gladly sacrifice herself, if this would be most beneficial to all concerned, which, in the case of an abortion, could include the decision to continue a pregnancy. However, when using the traditional model of motherhood to justify the non-traditional goal of obtaining an abortion, it turns out that the pro-choice utility calculation can indicate that the best way to help the most people is to sacrifice the fetus by aborting it.

From a political vantage point, this is a strategic way to 'have your cake and eat it too', since such a justification leaves in place traditional cultural assumptions about women as care-givers, even while expanding the non-traditional options open to women in the form of the right to an abortion as an instrument of care-giving not to the fetus, of course, but to others. We can see a good example of the use of a traditional model of motherhood as a means to achieve the non-traditional goal of abortion rights in the way Kate Michelman, long-term President of the National Abortion Rights Action Leagues (NARAL), justifies her own abortion. Michelman is a master-politician, one who has been in the limelight for decades, representing pro-choice positions. What is significant about Kate Michelman, therefore, is that when she tells her story about why she obtained an abortion, that story reveals a premise that the best way to present the abortion issue is to embed it within a traditional model of motherhood. To put it another way, Michelman's justification for abortion exemplifies the political power of obtaining non-traditional goals for women by infusing those goals with the most traditional imagery associated with women.

Kate Michelman explains how she became acutely aware in 1977 about the need for women to have the right to obtain an abortion. In her words:

I was a thirty-year-old mother of three, pregnant with my fourth child, when my husband left me for another woman. I had hoped to have six children, but I had no car, couldn't get credit, and no longer had a husband to provide for me and my children. I could not feed the three children I already had, much less support an additional child. At that moment I understood the kinds of choices women have to make and how they affect the very fabric of a woman's life. I decided to get an abortion. (in Tribe, 1990: p. 134.)

What is most significant about this very strategic, political story is that Kate Michelman embeds the right to an abortion in a very traditional model of motherhood. Michelman's story employs a traditional view of a woman whose identity is defined in terms of her childbearing goals, child care responsibilities and economic dependency on a husband. The key to this story is to discern what justifies the non-traditional act of killing the fetus. The answer is that Michelman defines motherhood traditionally as a nurturing set of relationships in which there is a scarcity of resources. She lacks a husband, a car, credit and the economic resources to feed and care for an additional child. Something has to be sacrificed if any are to survive. The killing of the fetus by means of an abortion, therefore, is justified as a sacrifice necessary for the survival, if not the good, of the greater whole. The fetus must be sacrificed by the mother in order for the mother to be able to continue the nurturing of the other children already born. Thus, rather than the mother nurturing the fourth child, the fourth child, the fetus, must be sacrificed.

Lifeboat ethics and justification for killing

Michelman's story not only illustrates a traditional view of motherhood in the context of obtaining a non-traditional goal for women – abortion rights – it also corresponds to a specific ethical model that justifies killing – lifeboat ethics. The Model Penal Code (Philadelphia: American Law Institute), prepared and published by the highly respected American Law Institute, analyses the lifeboat model in terms of a justified choice of evils. The context of the lifeboat model involves a situation in which the homicidal actions of an individual that ordinarily would be criminal are nevertheless defensible because these acts are the only way to save other lives. As stated in the Code, 'conduct that results in taking life may promote the very value [life] sought to be protected by the law of homicide' in the first place. The example provided by the Model Penal Code is:

[Suppose someone] makes a breach in a dike, knowing that this will inundate a farm, but taking the only course available to save a whole town. If he is charged with homicide of the inhabitants of the farm house, he can rightly point out that the object of the law of homicide is to save life, and that by his conduct he has effected a net saving of innocent lives. The life of every individual must be taken in such a case to be of equal value and the numerical preponderance in the lives saved compared to those sacrificed surely should establish legal justification.

In other words, the lifeboat model justifies killing when the sacrifice of one life is necessary to secure the lives of a greater number. As Dame Mary Warnock asserts, when faced with a choice of two people dying, or one person dying at the expense of another, the decision is easy – though it is the lesser of two evils, the latter is preferable to the former. As the journalist Polly Toynbee (2000) notes, the ethicist Professor Bernard Williams offers these hypotheticals in support of the view that it is preferable to sacrifice the lives of a few if necessary to save the lives of many. For example, if ice cave explorers find themselves trapped and the only way to escape is to kill one of their members so that the rest may live, then it is ethical to do so because this is a situation that is 'an unavoidable emergency . . . [that is] of no one's contriving'. Similarly, if a rail trolley is speeding toward a man pinned to the tracks, it is imperative to change onto another track to avoid killing him; however, if the other track in question had five men pinned to it, then it would be preferable, and thus permissible, to stay on the original track in order to save the five men at the expense of one.

Of course, real-life examples involving more than hypotheticals are excruciating in their complexity. A recent example in the UK concerned the decision whether to separate conjoined twins, Mary and Jodie (false names used to protect their identity), who were joined at the lower abdomen and who shared one set of lungs and heart. Their separation absolutely entailed the death of one, but failure to separate most likely would have entailed the death of both within six months, due to the strain of supporting two lives on only one set of heart and lungs. As the journalist Steven Morris (2000) observes, ethicists approach this problem in two ways. Utilitarians believe it is more ethical to 'save one life even at the cost of another'. However, absolutists (Morris, 2000) take a different stance, asserting that 'it can never be right to sacrifice a life... [As] [t]he Archbishop of Westminister Cormac Murphy-O'Connor, said: "There is a fundamental moral principle at stake no one may commit a wrong action that good may come of it" '.

The law of some nations, however, does allow for the separation of conjoined twins, even when the operation necessarily entails the loss of life of one of them. In 1993, for example, doctors at the Children's Hospital of Philadelphia, USA, made the difficult decision to separate conjoined twins, knowing full well that this would mean the death of one of them. However, doctors believed that both twins would die unless this operation was conducted, so with the permission of the parents of the twins, they separated them; one died as a result of the operation, and the other one lived for ten months after the operation. According to Mr. Justice Johnson, however, who gave the initial High Court judgment in the case of the conjoined twins born in the UK, 'The court would never authorise a step to actively terminate a life, even to relieve misery, [but would authorise] treatment to be withdrawn, even if this leads to death'. (The Court of Appeal permitted the operation to proceed, but overruled Johnson's reasoning insofar as it relied on this implicit parallel between the healthy twin as a 'life-support' device and a ventilator, which can lawfully be withdrawn.)

In the US, although the lifeboat model has its complications, it nevertheless underlies pro-choice arguments that seek to justify why a woman has a right to kill the fetus. This justification legally and culturally maps onto a traditional model of motherhood, because the nurturing aspect of the woman seeking an abortion is not the issue. Initially, the presumption is that everyone in the lifeboat is in harmony with everyone else. As Michelman puts it, she was a 30-year-old mother of three, pregnant with her fourth child, planning to have a total of six children, who had assumed the economic support of a husband. The initial situation is one of traditional, harmonious, family life. More broadly, we can characterize this type of justification as a sacrifice model having four main components:

(1) It applies to a situation where there is a group – more than one person –

in a closed system, context, or environment, such as a lifeboat, having no access to outside resources.

(2) In the closed system there are not enough resources to go around to take care of everyone; hence, someone or something in the group must be sacrificed for the sake of the greater whole.

(3) There is no necessary adversarial relationship between any of the entities in the closed system. Thus, the lifeboat model can be an environment of harmony and love, but it is also a tragic one because there are not enough resources for everyone to survive. Thus, in order for the greater number to survive, there has to be some sort of sacrifice that will make it possible for more rather than fewer to continue their existence. In the context of the abortion debate, the entity that is sacrificed is the fetus.

(4) Perhaps most importantly, the lifeboat model of sacrifice is consistent with a traditional image of women whose primary concern is a relational one, based on how to meet the needs of others. Hence, one of the most strategically powerful characteristics of the lifeboat model as a justification for abortion rights is that it involves no role change for women. Women who choose an abortion do so in order to be good mothers to children already born or ones who will be born at a later time. Abortion becomes a means of providing for, or taking care of, others. The problem is defined simply in terms of being a mother with too many to care for, and without adequate resources. The only solution is to sacrifice one entity, the fetus, in order to be able to nurture others. Such a sacrifice affirms rather than challenges maternal norms and roles for women.

The problem with the sacrifice model

The problem with the sacrifice model of motherhood, however, is that it cannot be used to argue for the need for abortion funding. In a normal lifeboat scenario, no one calls upon the state to help toss someone overboard. Rather, the hope is that the state will provide the resources necessary to avert the lifeboat crisis altogether. That is, the lifeboat model implies that if the state arrives in the form of outside assistance, then everyone in the lifeboat can survive. If the state could provide a conjoined twin with a needed heart and lungs, for example, that would obviate the question of sacrificing the life of one twin for the sake of the other; such a solution, obviously, is infinitely preferable to deciding the ethical and legal issues implied in killing the one twin who lacks those vital organs in order to save the other twin who has them. Similarly, if the state could arrive in time to save all ice cave explorers, thereby obliterating the need to sacrifice the life of one in order to save the lives of the others, that would solve the ethical and legal complications of the sacrifice model; there would be no longer a justification for killing one of the ice cave explorers because there would no longer be a context lacking resources for all.

So, too, in all lifeboat contexts. If by a miracle, or by state action, the lifeboat context can be eliminated and there can be enough resources to provide for all in the lifeboat, then the rationale for sacrificing a member of the group disappears, and with that disappearance, the language of justification for the killing of anyone or anything no longer applies. This is because the key principle in a lifeboat context is that there is no initial or inherent conflict among the parties, only a contextual lack of resources.

Abortion and the traditional model of motherhood

The use by pro-choice advocates of the sacrificial, lifeboat model for abortion rights, therefore, is a double-edged sword. On the one hand, its strength is that it can justify abortion in a context of scarcity that employs a model of motherhood involving no role change for women. Women can be depicted as justified in seeking an abortion, without ever raising the issue of a conflict between the mother and the fetus. A woman seeks an abortion, as Kate Michelman presents it, because she lacks the resources to be a good mother at that particular time in her life. She does not have the time, money or educational requisites, so the fetus is sacrificed in order that she and others for whom she is responsible can survive. Use of a traditional model of motherhood to justify the right to an abortion is a crucial source of political power. It allows pro-choice advocates to meet pro-life advocates on the same footing, by arguing that pro-choice women are dedicated to being good mothers, and that obtaining an abortion is a necessary means a woman must sometimes use in order to be a good mother. Invoking traditional role norms for women in the context of justifying the right to an abortion has been an effective use of traditional roles to gain non-traditional goals.

On the other hand, there has been a serious flaw in the formula that links traditional roles for women with the right to an abortion. Most significant is that such a justification contains no principle that can be used to claim the right to state assistance in providing an abortion, that is, killing the fetus. In contrast, the lifeboat model argues just the opposite; the purpose of state assistance is to provide resources so that it is not necessary for anyone or anything to be sacrificed in a lifeboat scenario; the state's job is to solve the problem of scarce resources so that all may survive. In this respect, the lifeboat model provides a better argument for funding childbirth than it does for funding an abortion.

Thus, to find a solution to the problem of access to abortion, including abortion funding, we must turn to a different model of motherhood, one that employs non-traditional roles for women and one that activates the other major justification for killing – self-defence.

The non-traditional model of motherhood and abortion rights

The non-traditional model of motherhood

The key issue in redefining the problem of abortion is to recognize that medically and legally pregnancy is a condition in a woman's body 'resulting from the presence of the fetus'. What is more, pregnancy is a condition that massively alters and transforms a woman's body and liberty. Specific hormones and proteins in a woman's body, for example, are elevated to hundreds of times their base level, thereby indicating that a fertilized ovum is present and affecting her body. While most of the changes resulting from the fetus's effects on a woman's body subside about a month after birth, a 'few minor alterations persist throughout life'. In a medically normal pregnancy: some hormones in a woman's body rise to 400 times their base level; a new organ, the placenta, grows in her body; all of her blood is rerouted to be available to the growing fetus; her blood plasma and cardiac volume increase 40 per cent; and her heart rate increases 15 per cent. These are just a few of the massive changes that ordinarily result from the fetus's effects.

From choice to consent

In *Roe*, the Court established that the fetus was a separate entity from the woman and that it was constitutional for the state to protect the fetus. With this in mind, the key issue in redefining abortion rights is to recognize that it follows that a woman not only has a right to choose what to do with her own body, but also a right to consent to the transformations of her body and her liberty resulting from the fetus as a separate, state-protected entity. If we accept that the fetus is indeed a separate entity, a move which pro-choice advocates have more typically resisted, we can actually derive a novel pro-choice argument. The traditional common-law position, still the dominant one in English law, is that the fetus has no separate legal personality: 'until born alive, a foetus is not a legal person' (Montgomery, 1997: p. 401). In American constitutional law, the Supreme Court has refused to rule on whether the fetus is a person, stating only that even if the fetus were a person, it would not be included in the protections of the Constitution because the Fourteenth Amendment refers to 'born' persons. Thus, at the moment, in the United States the fetus lacks a legal, personhood status. Yet it is constitutional for the state to protect the fetus, which means that the fetus is in a category with other entities that are not legally people but are nevertheless under state protection, such as endangered wildlife species.

What the consent argument does is to hoist anti-abortion campaigners with their own petard by focusing not merely on what the fetus 'is', but on what the fetus 'does'. Whether the fetus is or is not a person, what it 'does' is to seriously harm a woman, if she does not consent to the condition of pregnancy. This is because one way in which the law of medical negligence defines harm is in terms of absence of consent. If a physician, for example, performs life-saving surgery without consent, that physician legally is deemed to have harmed the patient, even if the surgery saved the patient's life. In the case of pregnancy, if a woman consents to the effects of the fetus, we have an example of the symbiotic ideal of mother and child that cultures so often idealize. However, given the quality and quantity of the transformations of a woman's body and liberty resulting from a fetus, if a woman does not consent to pregnancy, even a medically normal pregnancy constitutes serious harm.

We can see why a medically normal pregnancy constitutes harm, if it is non-consensual, by considering what would happen if a born person were to affect another born person's body in even a fraction of the ways a fetus affects a woman's body. The magnitude of the injuries would be easy to recognize, if a born person injected into another's body, without consent, hormones 400 times their normal level, or someone, without consent, took over the blood system of another to meet her or his own personal use, or someone, without consent, grew a new organ in that person's body. Without consent, such effects of one born person upon the body of another born person would be instantly recognizable as massive bodily injury, entailing a legal charge of battery or assault.

Self-defence

Legally and culturally, the lifeboat context is one of two major situations in which killing is justified. The other major justification for killing another living thing, including a person, is self-defence. The law recognizes and affirms the right of people to use deadly force to defend themselves against even the threat of certain types of harm, much less actual harm. From a review of state-level self-defence statutes, it is apparent that there are three major types of harm which justify the right of a person to use deadly force in self-defence: harm that threatens a person with death; serious bodily injury; or a severe loss of liberty.

The threat of death involves an irreversible injury of existential proportions – the ending of one's life. Clearly, in this most extreme of all types of injury, legal norms support the right of people to defend themselves with deadly force against even the threat of such an injury. However, the second type of harm recognized as justifying the use of deadly force in one's self-defence is when the threat of injury reaches a quantitative level that the law considers it to be serious bodily injury. Legal norms try to assess 'how much injury is sufficient' to warrant that label, and courts and legal norms sometimes define the requisite quantity in terms of how much tissue damage is involved, how the use of body organs or parts is impaired, or how much time it takes for the victim to recover. The Model Penal Code defines a serious bodily injury as an injury 'which creates a substantial risk of death or which causes serious, permanent disfigurement, or protracted loss or impairment of the function of any bodily member or organ', where protracted means as much as four weeks.

The third category of harm refers to one's liberty. These are injuries where the key issue is a person's consent to interact with another person. Injuries that justify the use of deadly force in self-defence include rape, kidnapping and slavery. In all three cases, it is not that the action is necessarily wrong; rather, it is that the action occurs without consent. Sexual intercourse with consent is not a crime; without consent, it is rape. Travelling with somebody is not a crime, unless one person is coercing the other against her or his will, then it is kidnapping. Similarly, agreeing to work for someone is employment. To be forced and coerced to work by somebody is involuntary servitude or slavery.

States across the USA affirm the right to use deadly force in self-defence when a person is threatened with death, serious injury or a severe intrusion of liberty. Forty-two states, for example, have passed statutes explicitly affirming people's right to use deadly force when another private party threatens them with a sufficient quantity of bodily injury, referred to variously as 'serious bodily harm', 'serious physical injury', 'great bodily harm', 'great personal injury', 'imperil of bodily harm', 'grievous bodily harm', or as in the case of Michigan, 'brutality'. Thirty-six states explicitly affirm a person's right to use deadly force in self-defence when threatened with forcible rape, even when that rape is not aggravated by physical injuries in addition to the rape itself. Thirty-five states legislatively recognize people's right to use deadly force in self-defence against kidnapping. Only one of these states, Indiana, stipulates that the kidnapping must occur with the use or threat of force; kidnapping alone is sufficient in the other states. Twenty-seven states specifically affirm the right to use deadly force when threatened with slavery, either by explicit reference to their own state constitutions or to the federal Constitution. In addition, some states affirm the right to use deadly force in self-defence when threatened with assault, robbery, arson, burglary and any other forcible felony. Similarly, the Model Penal Code states that deadly force in self-protection is justified when a person believes that 'such force is necessary for the purpose of protecting [herself or] himself against the use of unlawful force by such other person ... [such as] against death, serious bodily injury, kidnapping or sexual intercourse compelled by force or threat'.

In US law, therefore, self-defence is an affirmative right, meaning that juries must be instructed that these injuries justify the use of deadly force in self-defence. In a Texas case, for example, a woman shot and killed a man in self-defence as he tried to rape her. An Appellate Court ruled that she had a right to instruct the jury about her justified use of deadly force in self-defence, to the effect that:

You [the jury] are further instructed on the law of self-defense that a person is justified in using deadly force against another to prevent the other's imminent commission of aggravated kidnapping, murder, rape, aggravated rape, robbery, or aggravated robbery. (Goldway, 1978.)

Similarly, the Supreme Court of Michigan concluded that a lower court had erred when it refused to instruct the jury that 'force, including deadly force, may be used to repel an imminent forcible sexual penetration'. The Supreme Court of Connecticut reached a similar conclusion when it ruled that a trial court should have instructed the jury that the 'defendant could use deadly force if necessary to repel sexual assault involving forced penetration as well as serious bodily harm or death'.

Courts view the right to self-defence as grounded upon the most basic tenets of natural law, and although 'society may prescribe rules of caution and prudence to be observed by persons before exercising the right', society may not 'completely abrogate' the right of self-defence. Some commentators argue that the federal Constitution 'precludes criminalizing and punishing an act done in self-defense ... [because] since the sixteenth century, a homicide resulting from an act done in self-defense was justifiable and not unlawful'. For this reason, we should classify the right of self-defence as a right 'so rooted in the tradition and conscience of our people as to be ranked as fundamental' and given the protection of the Due Process Clause of the Fourteenth Amendment.

Self-defence with deadly force, therefore, 'justifies the actor's conduct; it does not simply excuse it'. Self-defence reflects our cultural understanding, as translated into law, that when one party aggresses sufficiently upon another, it is preferable to free the non-aggressor of the aggressor's intrusion than it is to preserve the life of the aggressor. For this reason, 'a person who properly acts in self-defence engages in socially approved conduct'.

Self-defence and abortion rights

The self-defence model applied to abortion rights is older than *Roe* v *Wade* itself. It dates back to a 1971 article by the moral philosopher Judith Jarvis Thomson. Thomson asks us to imagine a situation in which we wake-up one morning to find ourselves attached to a famous violinist. If we break that attachment, the violinist dies. The question posed is whether we have a moral obligation to stay attached to the violinist, or whether we are morally justified in breaking the attachment, even if that means the violinist's death. Thomson argues that the demands made upon us to remain attached to the violinist exceed that required of morally responsible people. Hence, it is morally permissible to detach ourselves from the violinist, even if that action necessarily results in the violinist's death. The analogy with abortion is that even if the fetus is dependent upon the woman for its survival, the types of demands it makes upon a woman exceed what any moral person need make. Thus, a pregnant woman is justified in being a bad Samaritan by refusing to accede to the fetus's dependency needs, even if it entails killing the fetus to separate her from it.

From self-sacrifice to self-defence

We can build upon Thomson's claim that a woman has a right to be a bad Samaritan by developing a constitutional right to abortion based on self-defence. The positive value of such an endeavour is that it provides a new claim for not only the right to an abortion, but also the right to abortion funding. The negative aspect is that it entails a role change for women, one that metaphorically substitutes a battlefield model of motherhood for the lifeboat model of motherhood. Is this necessarily a bad thing? From a constitutional perspective, the answer is clearly 'no', since a self-defence model of motherhood opens the door to a constitutional right to abortion funding.

In our society, however, the presumption is that the state acts to defend people against harm. The private right of self-defence, therefore, is meant to be a means of last resort when the state is not available to assist in one's self-defence. Ideally, the state acts to defend people's bodies and liberty from harm resulting from other entities. The power of redefining abortion rights in terms of self-defence, therefore, is that it provides a way to establish an affirmative claim that the state must act to protect women's bodies and liberties from non-consensual effects resulting from the fetus.

What the fetus does

We can contrast the lifeboat model and the self-defence model of state action in this way. As we discussed, people in a lifeboat, suffering from scarce resources, may conclude that the only solution to secure the survival of the greater whole is to sacrifice someone in the lifeboat by killing them. If the state were to arrive in the form of a rescue ship, however, the sacrifice would no longer be necessary, and the state would not act to assist in such a sacrifice. On the other hand, if the state arrived to find one person in the lifeboat assaulting another, the state would be expected to act to stop the harm resulting to the victim. It is what the fetus *does* to a woman, therefore, not what it *is*, which is the decisive principle that establishes not only a woman's right to terminate pregnancy by means of an abortion, but also her right to state assistance.

Contingent equal protection

It is important to note that the Supreme Court has established that the Constitution does not guarantee a person a substantive Due Process right to assistance from the state to protect a person from harm. However, the Equal Protection Clause of the Constitution does require the state to treat people who are similarly situated in a similar way. The key question, therefore, is with whom is a woman similarly situated when she seeks an abortion? According to the traditional model of motherhood, she is similarly situated to a person in a lifeboat lacking resources necessary for all to survive. According to the non-traditional model of motherhood, however, she is situated in a non-consensual relationship with another entity, the fetus, which is seriously harming her. We do not know, according to American constitutional precepts, whether the fetus is a person or not. However, we do know that the fetus is under state protection. Thus, there are two possibilities:

(1) The woman is suffering harm resulting from the fetus, which is a non-human, yet state-protected entity, such as wildlife that causes harm.

(2) The woman is suffering harm resulting from the fetus, which is a human being. In the first instance, the state does protect people from harm resulting from state-protected wildlife, such as grizzly bears and wolves, even when the victims are negligent by entering restricted park areas where there is great danger of such harm from wildlife. Thus, state protection of wildlife does not negate state assistance to people suffering harm resulting from that wildlife. Hence, if a woman suffering a non-consensual pregnancy is legally viewed as similarly situated to a victim of harm resulting from a state-protected, non-human entity, such as wildlife, equal protection precedents mandate that the state must provide a pregnant woman with assistance to protect her from that harm, that is, with assistance to procure an abortion as the necessary means for stopping the harm resulting from the fetus.

In the second instance, if the fetus is viewed as a person, the claim for state assistance in protecting a woman from harm resulting from the fetus is also evident. The state routinely protects victims of harm resulting from other people, and the same would apply to the fetus. Of course, even if the fetus were a person, it would have no conscious intentions or control of its behaviour. Yet the state stops mentally incompetent people, which may include those on drugs, the mentally ill, or persons with learning difficulties, from harming others. The Equal Protection Clause, thus, would mandate that the state also must stop the fetus from harming a woman.

Thus, whether or not the fetus is in the category of a person or of a state-protected non-person, when the fetus harms a woman in a non-consensual pregnancy, it situates her with other victims of harm. Since the state does assist people whose bodily integrity and liberty are harmed by other entities, the state is obligated to protect a woman whose bodily integrity and liberty is being harmed by a fetus. To do otherwise violates the Equal Protection Clause of the Fourteenth Amendment, not on grounds of sex discrimination, but rather on the grounds that the state is not protecting a woman's fundamental right to bodily integrity and liberty in a similar way the state protects others.

Abortion as role change

Despite pro-choice advocates' use of a traditional model of motherhood to define abortion rights, the termination of a pregnancy by destroying a fetus at some level challenges assumptions about nurturing role norms associated with women (Gelb and Palley, 1987). As the law scholar Robin West (1988) observes, 'American feminism is primarily strategic'. Hence, it is understandable that pro-choice advocates, for strategic, political reasons, wish to minimize the challenge of that role dissonance by framing the abortion decision in terms of women's traditional identities as mothers. In such representations of the abortion decision, a woman chooses an abortion in order to be a good mother, either to the children she has already borne in the past or to the children she intends to bear in the future. The particular fetus that is aborted at most is a 'problem' or poses a 'dilemma' to the woman – but it is not in conflict with her. In fact, currently most pro-choice advocates eschew depicting the abortion decision in terms that even mildly suggest an adversarial relationship between a woman and a fetus.

There is much to value, of course, in locating the abortion decision within the framework of women's traditional roles, and such a portrayal of the abortion decision as part and parcel of women's traditional role norms has been enormously effective in gaining public and political support for abortion rights. Such portrayals, however, have not been effective in gaining constitutional support for a woman's right to government assistance in obtaining an abortion. It is for this reason, therefore, that it is necessary and time to redefine the problem of abortion rights, even if this redefinition requires expanding traditional role norms for women to include non-traditional ones. We must find new depictions of the fetus and the pregnant woman, depictions that can secure for women not only the right to an abortion, but access to one as facilitated by public assistance. A consent to pregnancy approach does just that. The consent model meets the standards in the law for using deadly force in self-defence to stop that harm. Thus, all pregnancies – not just medically abnormal ones – not only are harmful, if a woman does not consent to pregnancy, but all non-consensual pregnancies meet legal standards for the use of deadly force in self-defence to stop them.

Roles and goals

As we know from the work of policy analysts, such as Joyce Gelb and Marian Palley (1987), the problem of definition has been at the core of the feminist agenda throughout its history, and particularly in its activist phase during the 1970s. How a problem is defined is crucial, and of particular importance is whether the problem involves merely role equity or role change for women. Problems defined in terms of role change for women pose much greater obstacles than those that do not.

Hence, one of the most strategically powerful characteristics of the lifeboat model as a justification for abortion rights is that it involves no role change for women. Women who choose an abortion do so in order to be good mothers to children already born or ones that will be born at a later time. Abortion becomes a means for providing for, caring for, or taking care of, others. The problem is defined simply in terms of being a mother with too many to care for, and without adequate resources. The only solution is to sacrifice one entity, the fetus, in order to be able to nurture others. Such a sacrifice affirms motherhood rather than challenges maternal norms and roles for women. In this way, the traditional ethic of sacrifice, which some pro-choice advocates currently invoke to justify the right to an abortion, is powerful because it taps into a traditional model of motherhood. By so doing, it exemplifies a potent formula used more than once by feminists seeking non-traditional goals – namely, the linkage of a non-traditional goal with a traditional model of motherhood. It was this formula that accounted for the success of feminists in the US in the early decades of the twentieth century who sought to obtain a constitutional guarantee of women's right to vote. In the Progressive era, mainstream woman's suffrage leaders did not challenge traditional role norms identifying women as maternal nurturers whose lives were dedicated to helping others. On the contrary, they used the traditional depiction of women as mothers and self-sacrificial caretakers to argue for why society would improve if women were entitled to vote.

Thus, although the goal of the right to vote involved non-traditional behaviour for women, premising entry into the public realm, an equal exercise of the suffrage with men, nevertheless the means used to achieve that goal invoked traditional depictions of women's greater moral and ethical commitment to the care of others. What is significant about women's enfranchisement in the early twentieth century in the US is that it was decidedly not based on equality arguments about the sameness of men and women, but rather upon difference arguments based on the dissimilarity of men and women, even though from a political perspective. Ironically, the utility of the traditional model of motherhood was its ability to obtain a non-traditional goal for women – voting rights.

However, it is also correct to note that achieving the right to vote, while necessary, was scarcely sufficient for implementing a broader agenda of women's rights. Thus, it required a feminist social movement in the 1960s and 1970s to challenge women's inequality in marriage, employment, education, sexual experience and psychological well-being. And it was in this follow-up social movement stage of completing the policy agenda for women's rights that the traditional model of motherhood was also challenged. Betty Friedan's *The Feminine Mystique* (1965) is notable not only because it was a best-seller, but also because it was a direct attack on the traditional model of motherhood that depicted women's lives and identities through the eyes of those for whom they cared, for whom they exercised an ethic of care. In Friedan's forceful view, such traditional norms robbed women of a sense of self, so that they suffered from the 'problem that had no name'.

Understanding the discontinuity created in the early twentieth century by using a traditional model of motherhood to achieve the non-traditional goal of woman's suffrage can inform today's efforts to obtain access to abortion funding. While in the short-term a traditional model of motherhood may gain an important legal and political right for women, such as the right to vote in the early twentieth century or the right to an abortion in the latter part of the twentieth century, in the long-term, changing women's options in society eventually challenges the very traditional basis used to garner new options in the first place. The historical as well as theoretical resistance to dismantling traditional views of women, yet the necessity to do so to complete the rights agenda, becomes an enduring motif in American law and politics. In the case of abortion rights, therefore, we must confront the task of expanding ethical norms appropriate for women to include the norm of self-defence as a justification for the right to obtain an abortion. Only by so doing can we complete the agenda, in order to obtain both a constitutional and a political guarantee of access to abortion services.

References

Friedan, B. (1965) *The Feminine Mystique*. Harmondsworth: Penguin.

Gelb, J. and Palley, M.L. (1987). *Women and Public Policies*, 2nd edn. Princeton, NJ: Princeton University Press.

Ginsburg, R.B. (1985). Some thoughts on autonomy and equality in relation to *Roe* v. *Wade*. *North Carolina Law Review* **63**: 375–86.

Goldway, C. (1978). The constitutionally of affirmative defenses. *Columbia Law Review* **78**: 655–78.

Klarman, M.J. (1996). Rethinking the civil rights and civil liberties revolutions. *Virginia Law Review* **82**: 1–67.

Montgomery, J. (1997). *Health Care Law*. Oxford: Oxford University Press.

Morris, S. (2000). Twins must have fatal surgery. *Guardian Unlimited Archive* Aug. 26. www.guardianunlimited.co.uk/archive/article/0,4273,4055528,00.html

Rochefort, D.A. and Cobb, R.W. (1994). *The Politics of Problem Definition: Shaping the Policy Agenda.* Lawrence, Kansas: University of Kansas Press.

Thomson, J.J. (1971). A defense of abortion. *Philosophy and Public Affairs* 1: 47–66.

Tribe, L. (1990). *Abortions: Clash of Absolutes.* New York: W.W. Norton.

Toynbee, P. (2000). Two into one. *Guardian Unlimited Archive.* Sept. 8. www.guardianunlimited.co.uk/archive/article/0,4273,4060914,00.html

West, R. (1988). Jurisprudence and gender. *University of Chicago Law Review* **55**(1): 1–72.

15

Who owns embryonic and fetal tissue?

Donna L. Dickenson

Centre for the Study of Global Ethics, University of Birmingham, UK

Background: why does ownership of embryonic and fetal tissue matter?

Until very recently the question of who owns embryonic or fetal tissue was of limited commercial importance, although there were applications of aborted fetal tissue in the treatment of Parkinson's disease, diabetes mellitus and other conditions. With a few exceptions the use of embryonic tissue was, so to speak, a non-issue (Boer, 1994), although the use of ovarian fetal tissue was specifically forbidden by Parliament.

By mid-1999, however, commercial exploitation of stem cells had been termed the most controversial ethical issue in biomedicine (Capron, 1999). The threshold event occurred in November 1998, when two separate teams of US scientists claimed that they had managed to isolate human embryonic and fetal cells and grow them indefinitely under laboratory conditions. These pluripotent and/or totipotent cells are effectively the parent cells for all bodily tissues, with an unlimited capacity to divide and the theoretical potential to become any body tissue. (Some authors equate pluripotent and totipotent cells, but others distinguish between totipotent cells, at the 2–4 cell stage, which are capable of giving rise to every cell line in the body and to an entire human individual, and pluripotent cells, which are derived from the blastocyst at a slightly later stage of development, when the outer and internal cells have already become differentiated.) Provided that the subsequent differentiation of embryonic stem cells can be controlled, it may conceivably be possible to use embryonic and fetal tissue to produce bone marrow, blood and brain tissue for transplant – eventually perhaps, any bodily tissue or organ, although this possibility is some years distant. For example, healthy cultured cardiac cells could be injected into damaged heart muscle following myocardial infarct. (In mice, heart muscle cells have been derived from embryonic stem cells injected into, and successfully integrated with, the heart muscle of adult animals.) Neurological stem cell transplants might be particularly promising because the risk of rejection is moderated by the brain's unique immunological status (Nuffield Council, 2000: p. 4). As one of the scientific teams stated,

We could make universal donors. More specific cells could become transplant therapies for diabetes, spinal cord injury, neurodegenerative disorders like Parkinson's
disease, muscular dystrophies, arteriosclerosis and wound healing.

The use of stem cells would also streamline pharmaceutical testing; new drugs
could be tested for safety and efficacy on cultured stem cells before being
tested in humans. Thus pharmaceutical and biotechnology firms are hugely
interested in the use of such cultured cells and in the development of tissue
banks of both undifferentiated and specialized cells and tissues. Six to eight
pluripotent cell lines have already been developed, in the US and Singapore,
although some estimates (as of July 2001) cite up to 30 worldwide (Phillips,
2001). Eventually the need for embryo 'donations' should lessen as the self-
replicating stem-cell lines grow in size. But does this mean that the ethical
issues will disappear? Hardly. The enormous commercial value of these cell
lines, which will increase with their size, raises profound issues of justice and
exploitation, particularly issues of property rights.

Both the US teams were funded by the Geron Corporation, an American
biotechnology company which is now seeking a patent on the technologies.
At the time of writing, late in 2000, the UK's Roslin Institute, which produced
the Dolly cloning technique, was reported to be exploring collaboration with
the Wisconsin researchers, with a view towards deriving cells from adult
patients that could be cloned using isolated embryonic stem cells. The aim is
to develop cell therapy rather than manufacturing tissues and organs, with
the advantage of avoiding immunological rejection problems. By a remarkable coincidence, the Geron Corporation also has a major interest in the
commercial arm of the Roslin Institute. The globalization of stem cell
research and application is already upon us. It will almost certainly mush-
room into an international trade in embryonic stem cells. German research
groups already are using embryonic stem cells imported from other 'less
moral' countries such as Denmark, Finland, Spain, Sweden and the UK, since
the German Embryo Protection Act of 1990 prohibits any retrieval of cells
from embryos, under criminal penalties (Lunshof, 2000).

One of the US teams, based at the University of Wisconsin, produced their
cells from blastocysts developed in vitro as part of infertility treatment. The
second team, from Johns Hopkins, used what they called primordial germ
cells, which would eventually have become gametes. Interest has mainly
focused on embryonic stem cells (ES cells) rather than embryonic germ cells
(EG cells), where attempts to derive adult cells in mice have led to abnormalities. Use of ES cells has also been assumed to be less ethically debatable,
because it does not require abortion, or because pre-embryos are thought to
have a lesser moral status than fetuses. I think it is far from obvious, however,
that use of ES cells is ethically trouble-free; that is because I shall focus not on
the status of the fetus/embryo, but on the rights of the mother.

The Wisconsin method uses embryos grown in vitro, developed through fertilization of the mother's ova with the father's sperm – primarily 'spare' embryos which are not to be implanted. (It would also be possible to create embryos from gametes 'harvested' expressly for this purpose.) Stem cells are derived from the inner cell mass of the blastocysts; the outer cellular layer, which would normally develop into the placenta, is dissolved. Since the blastocysts are used before implantation, the mother's 'sweat equity' is reduced, but she has still undergone the labour of stimulation with fertility drugs (superovulation) and extraction of ova – painful and moderately risky procedures.

The Johns Hopkins method of using primordial gamete cells relies on aborted fetal tissue, into which the mother has put the labour of early pregnancy. John Gearhart's team at Johns Hopkins derived stem cells from primordial germ (gonadal) cells of fetuses aborted five to nine weeks after fertilization. Oddly, although using aborted fetuses might appear to be the more ethically and legally controversial of the two methods, the Hopkins technique does not contravene federal restrictions, whereas limitations have been imposed on the use of the Wisconsin method. The ethically significant difference seems to be that life is not deliberately created in the Hopkins case, as by the admixture of gametes to form early-stage embryos, and the fetus is dead before research starts, even if the cells are still alive. In the Wisconsin method, the embryo is effectively killed by removal of the outer layer of the blastocyst (Capron, 1999).

Although the two techniques raise separate moral and legal questions, commentators have united in approaching both of them almost solely through focusing on the moral status of the embryo or fetus. So far as the mother (and sometimes father) are concerned, the only legal and ethical issues are usually held to concern the quality of consent to further uses of the embryonic and fetal tissue. For example, the Nuffield Council on Bioethics group (2000: p. 1) concluded that 'the removal and cultivation of cells from a donated embryo does not indicate lack of respect for the embryo'. UK Parliamentary debate before the Human Fertilisation and Embryology (HFE) Act of 1990 had culminated in agreement that embryo research is morally acceptable if confined to the period before development of the primitive streak, and if no embryo on which research has been performed is re-implanted in a uterus. Since a donated embryo from IVF (in vitro fertiliz-ation) procedures is normally 'surplus' to requirements, and will not be implanted in a uterus, the Nuffield Council committee concluded that there were no moral objections to use of such embryos to create a stem cell line, provided that parental consent was obtained to this further use. The alterna-tive is to allow the embryo to perish; the embryo has no future life, and thus it is not being robbed of any entitlement to life. Although the embryo does not benefit, it loses nothing, whereas other future persons may benefit from therapeutic research using embryonic stem cell lines (Nuffield Council, 2000: paragraph 22).

This is a straightforward utilitarian line, which appears to consider that the only deontological arguments that might be deployed concern the fetus. But even if we concede that the embryo or fetus has no rights which could give rise to duties to refrain from stem cell development, that says nothing whatsoever about the rights of the parents, and particularly about the rights of the woman. The remainder of this chapter will concentrate on the risks of exploitation of pregnant women, and conversely on the arguments in favour of their possessing a property right in stem cells derived from their embryos or fetuses, in addition to the procedural right to give or withhold consent to the further use of those tissues. This new focus is particularly urgent if the UK does implement the Nuffield Council recommendation to allow research involving human embryos for purposes of developing tissue from embryonic stem cells, amending existing legislation (Schedule 2 of the HFE Act). At present there is no plan to create ES cells deliberately for this purpose, provided that sufficient cells can be obtained from donated surplus IVF embryos. However, even this comparatively modest proposal raises difficulties about possible exploitation of vulnerable couples undergoing IVF, and particularly about the claim-rights of women.

These rights can be viewed in a Lockean fashion, as derived from the labour which women put into the processes of superovulation and egg extraction (for ES cells) or early pregnancy and abortion (for EG cells). Alternatively, a Marxist feminist interpretation would emphasize the added value which women put into the 'raw material' of gametes. If the Marxist interpretation is preferred, one would focus interest on women's alienation from their reproductive labour, and on the exploitative transfer of rights in the products of that labour to private commercial companies. For the purposes of this discussion, either the liberal or the Marxist model is valid. However, most of my discussion will be more Lockean than Marxist.

Property, persons, pregnancy and progeny

It is important to emphasize that Locke does not say we own our bodies; only God does. What we do own is our labour, which is the expression of our moral agency or personhood; this is what Locke is referring to when he declares that 'Every man hath a property in his own person' (Waldron, 1988; Dickenson, 1997). To extrapolate this argument to organs and tissue, no other parts of the body are owned, because we do not put labour into creating our own bodies. Only the products of pregnancy can be viewed as rightfully belonging to the pregnant woman, because she puts labour into them. On a straightforwardly Lockean account, women should have a presumptive property right in the products of pregnancy.

In the *Moore* case it was arguable that even if Moore lacked a right in his

T-cells, the hospital and researchers did as well, resulting in a stand-off (Gold, 1996). What we have here is an excellent example of the old maxim, 'Hard cases make bad law'. The *Moore* case exhibited such egregious abuses of the patient's informed consent that the legal judgment turned almost entirely on those abuses. (Not only was Moore never told that his original splenectomy had yielded T-cells with remarkable immune powers, developed into a \$3 billion cell line; he was asked to keep returning to donate all manner of other bodily products on the pretext of further therapy and check-ups.) The wider issue of development rights in Moore's cell lines was decided in a manner that arguably breaches previous legal precedents (Gold, 1996), by awarding all such rights to the researchers and the hospital board of regents. It may be that the patient does not own the tissue, but does that necessarily mean that the researcher or hospital does? If we wish to avoid commodification of tissue by allowing the patient tradeable rights, why are we so willing to allow commodification by allowing them to the researchers?

The assumption in the case of ES and EG cells, however, must be that the woman has a presumptive right in these cells, outweighing the rights of the clinic and researchers. Possibly some such inchoate recognition of pregnant women's property rights in fetal and embryonic tissue actually lies behind the provisions in both the Polkinghorne report and the report of the US National Bioethics Advisory Committee (NBAC) prohibiting women from directing the uses to which such tissue should be put (Polkinghorne Committee, 1989; NBAC, 1999). Yet whereas women's exercise of rights in the tissue derived from their pregnancies is closely scrutinized, we can predict that if somatic cell transfer ever becomes a possibility, donors will be able to specify the use to which that tissue will be put. If there were similar rules for embryos to the Polkinghorne rules forbidding directed donation for aborted fetal cells (to family members or other named individuals), the commercial appeal of the somatic cell technique would vanish, since the main use is to be transplantation of autologous cells or tissues grown from stem cell lines derived from embryos cloned from patient's own DNA (Capron, 1999: p. 27).

In the case of both ES and EG cells, of course, the father has also made a genetic contribution, but, I would argue, not a donation of his labour. It is obscene in more than one sense to compare masturbation to produce sperm with superovulation and egg extraction. To argue for the father's ownership of either blastocysts grown in vitro or embryos, then, one would have to assert that his right derives from his ownership of his sperm or genes, but I have already argued that we do not actually own parts of our body, including gametes and genes. The 1990 HFE Act supports this interpretation insofar as it pays gamete donors expenses; the Authority and the clinics it licenses are not purchasing gametes, but recompensing donors for loss of time and travel expenses. I have argued elsewhere that abuses have occurred under the Act (Dickenson, 1997), not least the clinics' practices that have effectively left women paying to donate gametes, but the principle in the Act is clear. In the US, common law has sometimes supported the notion of the father's genetic ownership of the fetus, as in the *Baby M* case. Here a commercial 'surrogate' mother was required to hand the baby over to the contracting couple, but on legal reasoning which actually invalidated the notion of contract at the same time as upholding the particular contract. In the judge's words, the father 'cannot purchase that which is already his', by virtue of his genetic input (*In the Matter of Baby M*, 1987). This case represents the unpleasant extreme of allowing ownership by virtue of genetic property in the body. Nor is it clear why the gestational mother, who was also the genetic mother, was not seen to 'own' the baby, on this reasoning. It is not a model I wish to follow.

Far from affording the pregnant woman rights in the embryonic and fetal tissue that she has laboured to create, most current policy documents concentrate on making sure that she freely gives up any such rights, through giving a clear and separate consent to use of the tissue for research and therapeutic purposes. This exhortation in the name of the 'gift relationship' (Titmuss, 1997) is the strategy suggested separately by the NBAC Report (1999) in the US, and by the Medical Research Council working party and the Nuffield Council commission in the UK. The advisory report from the Geron corporation ethics group (Lebacqz et al., 1999) is slightly franker in advising that women donating embryonic or fetal tissue should be told about market value, but one suspects that this proviso is inserted merely to stave off *Moore*-type legal actions. Given the vulnerability of IVF patients, and their typical gratitude towards the clinicians for giving them any chance of a child, there is plenty of room for exploitation. As Lori Knowles puts its, there is a 'tension between the altruism individuals are supposed to exhibit by donating their tissue for research and the current patent system, which encourages companies to stake lucrative property claims in that research' (Knowles, 1999: p. 38).

'In law, a tangible thing is either a person or property, and if it is one it cannot be the other' (Knowles, 1999: p. 39). In the US and UK, although palpably not in Germany, it is widely agreed that the blastocyst is not a person. Therefore it must be property, as the Geron Corporation is happy to agree; but it does not follow from this that the property necessarily belongs solely to the Geron Corporation or its equivalents. In the *Moore* case it was argued that granting any form of property rights to the tissue donor, Moore, would impede the free flow of scientific research – but so, of course, do patents on cell-lines and genes by biotechnology companies. The issue of *whose* property, for *whose* benefit, needs a wider airing than it has so far received in the stem cells debate. As Knowles (1999: p. 40) cogently states:

Fears about a market in human body parts and about commodifying human reproduction have prompted many to suggest that couples should not sell their embryos. The same arguments are used to argue that donors should not share in the profits resulting from research on their embryos. In property law, however, restrictions on sales are prompted by the nature of the property itself, not by the status of the person claiming a commercial interest. Therefore, if it is wrong to commercialise embryos because of their nature, then it is wrong for everyone. It is simply inconsistent to argue that couples should act altruistically because commercialising embryos is wrong, while permitting corporations and scientists to profit financially from cells derived by destroying those embryos.

Models of ownership for embryonic and fetal tissue

What are the models to follow in the stem cell debate? We could adopt one of at least three possible approaches to ownership of embryonic and fetal tissue.

Status quo

In this model we would uphold the law's primary concentration on obtaining consent from the donor of the tissue, rather than conferring property rights on her. This is the basis of guidelines from the American College of Medical Genetics, which establish that patients must be asked for consent before research is done on tissue samples (American College of Medical Genetics, 1995). It was also roughly the approach of the UK Polkinghorne Committee (1989), although the scope of profitability and commercial application of tissue has moved on enormously since then. Given, however, that 'informed consent is no part of English law' (*Sidaway*, 1985) this is unlikely to provide satisfactory protection for women. The very favourable public image of IVF is another problem: there is not going to be much pressure on IVF clinics to justify what they do with blastocysts obtained as part of infertility treatment. Couples may be pressured to agree that 'spare' blastocysts can be used for commercial purposes, perhaps in exchange for reduced cost of treatment cycles.

This first model continues to maintain what has become a fiction in actuality, if a fact in law: that tissue extracted after procedures is no longer of any interest to anyone. Yet between 1976 and 1993 Merieux UK collected 360 tons of placental tissue annually from UK hospitals for sale to French drug companies (Nelkin and Andrews, 1998). Almost certainly, none of the mothers was asked for consent to this use of the placenta grown in her body, and expelled as the final stage of her labour in childbirth. In Canada, a similar practice was reversed after a Sicilian woman asked for the placenta, in order to carry out the custom of eating it; only then did the extent of the scandal become known (J.-L. Baudouin, pers. comm., 1999).

Similar issues arise in relation to umbilical cord tissue. In 1988, a French team under Dr Elaine Gluckman developed a process for turning umbilical cord blood into a substitute for bone marrow in transplantation. The team originally envisaged communal, non-profit banks of umbilical cord blood, but the process was quickly taken over by private firms, who marketed their own reprocessed blood back to the mothers as a form of insurance, to be stored for their babies (Sugarman et al., 1997). Likewise, a method of cryo-processing stem cells from neonates was patented by the US-based Biocyte Corporation in 1991, assuring the firm rights over therapeutic services in both the US and Europe.

In the face of full-scale commercialization elsewhere of life forms, following the 1980 US decision in *Diamond* v *Chakrabarty* and the 1998 decision by the European Parliament to support patenting of life in order to maintain competitiveness with the US, we need better protection than the common law has previously afforded us. The amount of original input necessary to obtain a patent is minimal – for example, a patent on a diagnostic test for Down's syndrome was given to a researcher who merely established a correlation between a particular hormone level and the syndrome, not the test itself. Researchers have been given patents on particular gene sequences without even having established their function. Not much labour has been 'mixed' with the natural substance in these cases.

What restrictions have the biotechnology companies so far imposed upon their researchers? The Geron Ethics Advisory Board code (Lebacqz et al., 1999: p. 31) specifies that 'the blastocyst must be treated with the respect appropriate to early embryonic human tissue'. This means 'ensuring that it is used with care only in research that incorporates substantive values such as reduction of human suffering' (Lebacqz et al., 1999: p. 33). But as Knowles points out, this is a very low threshold, met by almost all medical research. In any case, Geron had already obtained and begun stem cell research on embryos before appointing an ethics board to draw up guidelines, implying that these guidelines were purely an afterthought (Tauer, 1999).

There are straws in the legal wind, however, of which the UK *Kelly* decision (*R.* v *Kelly*, 1998) on theft of body parts could be one (an argument which I shall develop further in the third option). Other jurisdictions also offer alternative legal models, for example, France, where human tissue cannot legally be bought or sold, although limited use of embryonic tissue is allowed (in contradistinction to the apparently ethically correct but commercially wide-open situation in Germany.). This leads us on to the second option.

Strict regulation of commercialization

So far, this second approach has not manifested itself much in practice in the US or the UK, and it is likely to face even greater obstacles as commercial interests gather further momentum. To some considerable extent, however, the UK already regulates assisted reproduction, through the statutory regulatory body established by the HFE Act 1990. In vitro research on human embryos is illegal without a licence from the Human Fertilisation and Embryology Authority (HFEA), for both the project and the premises in which it operates. The uses of fetal tissue (relevant to EG cells) are regulated by guidelines set down by the Polkinghorne Committee (1989), aimed at maintaining a strict divide between the decision to undergo an abortion and the decision to allow further uses of aborted tissue. The Polkinghorne review also concluded that research ethics committee approval must be sought for 'all proposals for work with fetuses or fetal tissue, whether alive or dead, and whether classed as research or therapy, because of the high level of public concern'. In the wake of the Bristol inquiry and the Alder Hey hospital scandal over the retention of dead children's organs, the public is no doubt still concerned. But there are no statutory provisions in the UK governing the uses which can be made of aborted fetal tissue; as with the *Moore* judgment, the focus is solely on the correctness of the procedure, not on the uses made afterwards of the 'tissue' removed.

No research can be authorized on embryos older than 14 days, but that provision would still allow the method developed by the Wisconsin team, using blastocysts, under license from the HFEA. None the less, there are mounting commercial pressures, by which I include pressures from the leading IVF clinics, to repeal the 14-day rule and to end regulation altogether. These pressures were manifest in the deliberations of the Chief Medical Officer's expert advisory group on therapeutic human cloning, where IVF specialists argued that schedule 2 of the HFE Act already permitted stem cell line development – even though the techniques described in this chapter, and the cloning technologies which give them commercial importance, were completely unknown at the time the Act was passed in 1990. This argument was successfully resisted by the legal expert on the committee, but pressure will continue to mount for altering schedule 2 – particularly now that the Nuffield Council on Bioethics has recommended doing so. Likewise, the HFEA and the Human Genetics Advisory Commission have recommended that the Secretary of State should add two further purposes to the primarily reproductive diagnostic ones now mentioned in schedule 2: 'developing methods of therapy for mitochondrial diseases' and 'developing methods of therapy for diseased or damaged tissues of organs' (HGAC/HFEA, 1998). This latter proviso, very broadly couched indeed, would effectively give *carte blanche* to the IVF clinics for commercial exploitation of stem cell lines. The arguments for therapeutic benefit of stem cell commercialization seem to be in the ascendant in the UK at the moment, which does not augur particularly well for strict regulation.

In the US, the NBAC has approved stem cell research if done with close oversight, as long as embryos used as sources of stem cells would otherwise have been discarded. Federally funded research is now permitted on stem cells themselves, so long as the work of deriving cells from embryos is done with private money – getting around a ban which has existed since 1996 on embryo research. This seems an unattractive variant of regulation, however, leaving the biotechnology companies to garner federal funding for further development of the cell lines which they have already produced themselves (Cahill, 1999).

Some commentators (e.g. Gold, 1996; Knowles, 1999) have proposed that commercial researchers and firms should be permitted to 'commodify' stem cells and other bodily tissues, but only under the condition that they return a share of the profits to the National Health Service or the wider political community. In this model, donation would remain altruistic, but firms should be obliged to make cell lines widely available and to price the products derived from them at an affordable level – under pain of penalties from a patented biotechnology products review board. As a pragmatic solution, this proposal is attractive, but I want to propose something different.

Vesting control over all tissue in the mother, and treating alienation of it from her as theft

A feminist model sensitive to women's alienation from their reproductive labour might want to take a more radical tack than regulating commercial interests. I have already hinted that the recent decision in *Kelly* might be construed favourably to women, provided we make two assumptions:

(1) embryonic or fetal tissue is akin to parts of a corpse (even though it has never been a living person) and putting labour into bodily parts of a non-living body conveys some sort of property right;

(2) the labour which the woman puts into superovulation and egg harvesting (in the case of blastocysts and other forms of human embryo) and into pregnancy and childbirth (in the case of umbilical cord blood and placental tissue) gives her a right over the tissue.

This need not be a fully-fledged property claim, and given the legal and philosophical incoherence of the concept of property in the body, it probably should not be. It need only be as great as the scope delineated in *Kelly* – enough to protect the tissue from being appropriated by others, under penalty of the Theft Act. In his influential model, *A Theory of Property*, Stephen Munzer argues that 'persons do not own their bodies, but they do have limited property rights in them' (Munzer, 1990: p. 41). These he views as primarily powers (to transfer, waive and exclude others from the use of one's body parts) rather than as claim-rights (to possess, use, manage and receive income) (Munzer, 1990: p. 22; following Honore, 1961).

Even with these two assumptions, there are still problems. Vesting control over tissue in the mother may not be sufficient to protect the woman from exploitation by commercial interests. Those interests surpass any in surrogacy, where it is difficult enough to distinguish between allowing women to contract as equals and opening them to exploitation. Arguably, thinking of the mother as having any kind of property interest in fetal tissue or the tissue by-products of pregnancy is also false to the uniqueness of the relationship between the woman and the developing fetus (Mahowald, 1994).

None the less, the great advantage of this model is that it recognizes what women do and endure in infertility treatment, pregnancy and childbirth. It gives them a property in the labour of their persons and the products of that labour. This is not the same as owning a baby, which is not what we are talking about in the case of embryonic stem and germ cells. It is difficult to believe that placental tissue could have been 'harvested' without anyone's noticing that the mother might have something to say about it. Yet the ignoring of women's labour is pervasive throughout the discussion of rights over fetal and embryonic tissue (Mahowald, 1994). This third model makes sure that women's labour gets noticed.

If the second model is unlikely to succeed, however, why should the third have any chance at all? One reason is that it foregrounds the need to assign an owner to the tissue, that is, the bankruptcy of the traditional doctrine of *res nullius* in the face of commercial interests that want to make very sure that the *res* is definitely not *nullius*. Whereas regulation, in the second model, accepts that commercial interests or academic researchers own the tissue, but must bow to a certain degree of societal control over their actions, the more radical model actually affords a better chance of litigation establishing that their ownership is not free and clear. If all the women whose placentas were 'harvested' had to be compensated or indeed acknowledged, that would be quite a disincentive.

Near where I live, a motorway was planned to cut through an area where rare butterflies abounded, 'Alice's Meadow'. Hundreds of local people each bought a one-metre square of the meadow, and all their claims had to be adjudicated before eminent domain could be given. The motorway went elsewhere. It's a thought, isn't it?

Acknowledgement

Grateful acknowledgement is made to Donald Bruce of the Church of Scotland project on ownership of life-forms and to Tom Murray of the Hastings Center. An earlier version of this paper was presented at the First Reproductive Ethics workshop of the TEMPE project (Teaching Ethics: Materials for Practitioner Education), Cork, June 2000, with funding from the European Commission (DG-XII) under the Fifth Framework programme.

References

American College of Medical Genetics (1995). Guidelines. *American Journal of Human Genetics* **57**: 1499–500.

Boer, G. (1994). Ethical guidelines for the use of human embryonic tissue. *Journal of Neurology* **242**: 1–13.

Cahill, L.A. (1999). The new biotech world order. *Hastings Center Report* **29**: 45–8.

Capron, A. (1999). Good intentions. *Hastings Center Report* **29**: 26–7.

Diamond v. *Chakrabarty* (1980). 447 U.S. 303.

Dickenson, D. (1997). *Property, Women and Politics: Subjects or Objects?* Cambridge: Polity Press.

Gold, E.R. (1996). *Body Parts: Property Rights and Ownership of Human Biological Materials.* Georgetown: Georgetown University Press.

HGAC (Human Genetics Advisory Commission) and HFEA (Human Fertilisation and Embryology Authority) (1998). *Cloning Issues in Reproduction, Science and Medicine.* London: Department of Trade and Industry.

Honore, A.M. (1961) Ownership. In *Oxford Essays in Jurisprudence*, Series 1, ed. A.G. Guest, pp. 107–47. Oxford: Clarendon Press.

In the Matter of Baby M, 217 N.J. Supr. 313 (1987), affirmed in part and reversed in part, 109 N.J. 396 (1988).

Knowles, L.P. (1999). Property, progeny and patents. *Hastings Center Report* **29**: 38–40.

Lebacqz, K., Mendiola, M., Peters, T., Young, E. and Zoloth-Dorfman, L. (1999). Research with human embryonic stem cells: ethical considerations. *Hastings Center Report* **29**: 31–6.

Lunshof, J. (2000). Burning issues in genetics: Germany. *Workshop on Ethics and Genetics, European Commission TEMPE Framework 5 programme, Maastricht,* 9 June.

Mahowald, M. (1994). As if there were fetuses without women: a remedial essay. In *Reproduction, Ethics and the Law: Feminist Perspectives*, ed. J.C. Callahan, pp. 199–218. Bloomington: Indiana University Press.

Moore v *Board of Regents of the University of California* [1990]. 271 Cal Rptr 146, Cal. Sup. Ct.

Munzer, S. (1990). *A Theory of Property.* Cambridge: Cambridge University Press.

NBAC (US National Bioethics Advisory Commission) (1999). *Ethical Issues in Human Stem Cell Research*, vol. 1. Maryland: NBAC.

Nelkin, D. and Andrews, L. (1998). *Homo economicus*: commercialization of body tissue in the age of biotechnology. *Hastings Center Report* **28**: 30–9.

Nuffield Council on Bioethics (2000). *Stem Cell Therapy: The Ethical Issues, A Discussion Paper.* London: Nuffield Council on Bioethics.

Phillips, S. (2001). Business versus the Bible. *The Times Higher*, 27 July: p. 17.

Polkinghorne Committee (1989). *Review of the Guidance on the Research Uses of Fetuses and Fetal Material.* London: HMSO.

R. v *Kelly* [1998]. 3 All ER 741.

Sugarman, K., Kaalund, V., Kodish, E. et al. (1997). Ethical issues in umbilical cord blood banking. *Journal of the American Medical Association* **278**: 938–43.

Sidaway v *Bethlem RHG* [1985]. 1 All ER 643.

Tauer, C.A. (1999). Private ethics boards and public debate. *Hastings Center Report* **29**: 43–5.

Titmuss, R. (1997). *The Gift Relationship: From Human Blood to Social Policy.* 2nd edn. New York: New Press.

Waldron, J. (1988). *The Right to Private Property.* Oxford: Clarendon Press.

16

The fewer the better? Ethical issues in multiple gestation

Mary B. Mahowald

Department of Obstetrics and Gynecology, University of Chicago School of Medicine, USA

Until the last part of the twentieth century, Hellin's Law governed the predictability of multiple births – the natural occurrence of twins in the general population is 1/100, and the frequency of each higher multiple is determinable by multiplying the denominator by 100, so that the frequency of triplets is 1/10 000, the frequency of quadruplets is 1/1 000 000, and so on. Since the advent of fertility drugs in the 1960s and in vitro fertilization (IVF) in the 1970s, the incidence of multiple gestations has increased markedly. By the late 1980s, the rate of multiple births had more than tripled; it appears to be rising still (Hammon, 1998: p. 338).

With each higher order of multiples, risks to both fetus and pregnant woman escalate. For women, the risks include anaemia, preterm labour, hypertension, thrombophlebitis, preterm delivery and haemorrhage. Tocolytic therapy to avoid preterm delivery introduces further risks. For fetuses or potential children, the risks include intrauterine growth retardation, malpresentation, cord accidents and the usual sequelae of preterm delivery, such as respiratory distress, intracranial haemorrhage and cerebral palsy (Hammon, 1998: p. 339).

Conflicts between the interests of pregnant women and their fetuses are not new; attempts to induce abortion and to rescue fetuses have occurred through most of human history. Although medical advances have considerably reduced the mortality and morbidity risks of childbearing for most women and their offspring, that same technology has introduced methods by which people who would not otherwise reproduce can have biologically related children. These methods are mixed blessings when the pregnancies they facilitate exacerbate the risks of gestation for women and their fetuses. They are also mixed blessings when, while providing a means to desired motherhood for some, they occasion pressures on others to undergo risks they would not otherwise encounter.

In what follows I describe different methods of fetal termination in multiple gestation, and critique the terminology used in discussing these methods. The perspective I bring to this analysis is a version of feminism which demands that differences be identified and evaluated for the extent to which they are associated with inequality (Mahowald, 2000: chapter 4). To illustrate a range of morally relevant variables, I sketch a number of cases, both real and concocted, examining these from my egalitarian feminist standpoint. I conclude that, while greater efforts are needed to reduce the incidence of multiple gestation, fetal termination with pregnancy preservation is justified in certain circumstances.

Methods of fetal or embryo termination in multiple gestation

According to one of its foremost practitioners, 'Most cases of multiple pregnancy are iatrogenic and avoidable by more diligent use of fertility drugs and better patient management' (Evans et al., 1997: p. 771). Although iatrogenic practice has not been reported in the well-publicized cases of the McCaughey septuplets and the Chukwu octuplets, we do know that these gestations were initiated through use of fertility drugs, that at least one newborn died and others suffered lasting impairment, and that the women involved faced severe health risks with long-term adverse consequences (Associated Press, 1998; Tribune News Services, 1999). We also know that the high multiplicity of these gestations could probably have been avoided, even after the administration of infertility drugs, if ultrasound monitoring indicated maturation of multiple follicle cells (Manier, 1998: p. 1). At that point, clinicians might have declined to administer a second drug that would trigger the release of eggs. Alternatively or additionally, the patient might have agreed to refrain from intercourse until her next cycle, when the risk of multiple gestation would be reduced by modifying her drug dosage.

Obviously, prevention of multiple gestation is desirable and can probably be accomplished in most cases. As already acknowledged, however, the possibility of high multiples occurs in nature, albeit rarely, and the mortality and morbidity of these gestations for women and some of their fetuses can only effectively be reduced by terminating other fetuses. In other words, the criterion on which to base the medical prognosis for women and their potential children in multiple gestations is 'the fewer the better'. How, then, does one reduce many gestating fetuses or embryos to fewer?

An apparent, relatively easy answer occurs in the context of in vitro fertilization, when higher order multiples can be avoided by declining to transfer more than three or four embryos after fertilization, storing or disposing of extra ones in some other way. In fact, this is the usual practice of reproductive endocrinologists, who tend to consider higher order multiples a failure rather than a success. The recommendation to transfer only three or four is thought to strike a balance between the risk of multiples and the risk of not achieving a pregnancy at all. This approach does not adequately answer the question raised, however, because multiple gestations are still possible, regardless of whether fertilization occurs in vitro or in vivo. Moreover, the disposition of untransferred embryos poses additional questions, which I have addressed elsewhere (Mahowald, 2000: chapter 12).

Current techniques by which to limit the number of embryos or fetuses in a multiple pregnancy involve either direct termination or removal of in vivo embryos. The removal procedures are performed through transcervical suctioning at 8 to 11 weeks' gestation or through transvaginal aspiration usually at six to seven weeks' gestation. Unfortunately, the transcervical technique is associated with a high (50 per cent) incidence of total pregnancy loss, and the transvaginal technique precludes rudimentary detection of anomalies such as nuchal folds (suggestive of Down's syndrome). Transvaginal aspiration also precludes the possibility of spontaneous loss of embryos, which could make further termination unnecessary. (Some practitioners of transvaginal aspiration wait until about 10 weeks so as to allow for spontaneous loss, but the approach is more difficult and risky at that point.) In the light of these limitations, the most common method of terminating some of the embryos or fetuses in a multiple gestation is direct termination at 9 to 12 weeks through transabdominal needle insertion of potassium chloride into the fetal thorax; the goal of this procedure, to 'achieve cardiac standstill', is later confirmed (or otherwise) by ultrasound (Evans et al., 1997: p. 772). If cardiac function has not ceased, the procedure may be repeated.

As in the preceding paragraph, the terms fetus and embryo are used interchangeably in discussions of this issue because the distinction between embryos and fetuses is not cleanly definable by duration of gestation. Some authors (e.g. Grobstein, 1995) use the term 'pre-embryo' for the embryo that has not yet implanted in the uterus. I find this term misleading because it suggests, inaccurately, that the genetic material essential to development has not yet been assembled in the newly fertilized organism (cf. Mahowald, 1995b).

Eight weeks of gestation is often stipulated as the threshold between embryonic and fetal development, but this is a broad generalization. Cardiac function begins weeks earlier and lung function or kidney function much later. In general, embryonic development starts at fertilization and continues until all components of the basic organ system are initiated; fetal development consists mainly of their elaboration. Depending on the duration of a multiple gestation, then, procedures for reducing the multiple may involve embryos or fetuses. Because common parlance often uses the term fetus to describe the developing organism from fertilization to birth, I will hereafter also do that.

More on terminology

The language used to name procedures to reduce the number of developing fetuses in an established gestation is controversial in its own right. Among the terms utilized are selective birth, selective abortion, selective reduction, fetal reduction and multifetal pregnancy reduction (Berkowitz et al., 1996). Others that could be utilized are partial abortion or partial feticide. The term 'selective birth' has been used for cases of multiple gestation in which a specific fetus had been identified as anomalous and targeted for termination. (Targeting could occur for other reasons, such as sex selection.)

Prenatal detection of the anomaly is not possible until weeks, sometimes months, after detection of the number of gestating fetuses. Ultrasound guided cardiac injection of the targeted fetus is then the means through which termination is accomplished. Obviously and perhaps misleadingly, the term 'selective birth' focuses on the fetuses that are not targeted. 'Selective abortion' would more accurately describe the procedure, but only if abortion is defined as termination of the fetus rather than termination of pregnancy.

'Selective reduction' is accurate if specific fetuses are targeted and if the pregnancy itself is not thought to be 'reduced'. But women, after all, are neither more nor less pregnant, regardless of the number of fetuses they are carrying. What is reduced, therefore, is the *number* of gestating fetuses. In situations in which *selective* reduction of fetuses occurs, the actual procedure is direct termination of the targeted fetus or fetuses. In these cases, 'selective termination' would be a more accurate representation of what is intended and done. If abortion is defined as termination of the fetus rather than termination of a non-viable pregnancy, 'selective abortion' would be accurate when specific fetuses are targeted and 'partial abortion' would be accurate in other cases as well. (Clinical texts usually define abortion as termination of a non-viable pregnancy; popular understandings tend to identify it with termination of fetuses. Cf. Mahowald, 1982.) If abortion is defined as termination of a (non-viable) pregnancy, terminating one fetus while maintaining the pregnancy through another (or others) is not equivalent to abortion.

Years ago I used the term 'fetal reduction' to describe interventions to reduce the number of developing fetuses in multiple gestations (Mahowald, 1993: pp. 87–90). I now consider the term 'reduction' misleading or ambiguous. It is misleading because it obscures the fact that the procedure in most cases entails direct killing of at least one fetus, and in other cases makes it impossible for some fetuses to survive, which to many is morally equivalent to killing. It is ambiguous because 'reduction' is not equivalent to 'termination'. Although 'termination' is the more honest description, a fair and adequate definition of the procedure needs to include the aim of maintaining the pregnancy by preserving some fetuses.

'Multifetal pregnancy reduction' is the term most commonly used by those who perform the procedure (e.g. Berkowitz et al., 1996: p. 1265; Rorty and Pinkerton, 1996: p. 55; Evans et al., 1997: p. 771). It is also the vocabulary preferred by the American College of Obstetricians and Gynecologists. This terminology, however, raises some of the same problems cited above – pregnancy is not reducible, and even if it were, the term 'reduction' mischaracterizes the intervention. To be adequate, a definition of the procedure would indicate that it involves terminating fetuses while preserving pregnancy. Awkward but accurate definitions could therefore be any of the following: fetal termination with pregnancy preservation; fetal termination and preservation in multiple gestation; reducing the number of fetuses in multiple gestation; abortion with pregnancy preservation; and partial abortion. As already suggested, the last two definitions are only accurate if abortion is defined as termination of the fetus rather than termination of pregnancy. Hereafter, I will use the first definition, which I consider simplest, clear and accurate – fetal termination with pregnancy preservation, which I will shorten to FTPP.

Egalitarian feminism and FTPP cases

An egalitarian version of feminism gives priority to equality, broadly construed, as an ethical consideration. Individual liberty may therefore be subordinated to other goods in order to render the different capabilities of individuals as equal as possible – for example, in Amartya Sen's notion of equality of capability (Sen, 1995). But what are the capabilities to be considered with regard to FTPP and to whom do they belong?

Different capabilities belong to different individuals whose interests may be promoted or impeded through FTPP. Although fetuses are not legally persons, and their personhood is morally debatable, they are in fact living, human and genetically distinct from the women in whom they develop. Many human fetuses have the capability of becoming persons both legally and morally. In high order multiple gestations, however, that capability is so greatly and unalterably reduced (without intervention) that the scenario is morally different from, say, a twin gestation, where the capability of both fetuses becoming legal and moral persons is high. The following cases illustrate this morally relevant difference along with other variables that influence the capabilities of individuals. Consideration of these variables is crucial to ethical decisions about whether FTPP should be requested or performed. Case 2a is one in which I was personally involved; case 3a is the well-publicized case of the McCaughey septuplets. Although the other cases are fictitious, all of the features enumerated have occurred in real cases.

- Case 1a: Normal twins – during her second prenatal visit, a 36-year-old mother of five children, aged 2 to 12 years, is told that she has a twin gestation. She tells her doctor that she thinks she can handle a single newborn but not two at once. 'I simply don't have time for twins', she says. Having heard about FTPP, she asks whether this is an option for her. The alternative of adoption is suggested but rejected. The woman has the financial resources to cover the costs of FTPP.

- Case 1b: Same case as 1a except that one fetus has Down's syndrome.
- Case 1c: Same case as 1a except that one fetus has trisomy 13.
- Case 1d: Same case as 1a except that the woman cannot pay for FTPP.
- Case 2a: Infertility drug + twin gestation – an affluent childless woman undergoing infertility treatment for two years becomes pregnant after taking Perganol. She has been told that this drug might cause multiple gestation. At eight weeks' gestation, ultrasound confirms the presence in utero of two fetuses, both of which appear healthy. One week later, the woman asks her physician to reduce the number of fetuses to one. Although the patient is informed that this procedure involves risk of losing the other fetus also, she persists in her request for FTPP, indicating that if this cannot be done, she will seek abortion of both fetuses, and 'try again' for another pregnancy.
- Case 2b: Same case as 2a except that the twins are known to be a male and a female, and the woman asks the physician to target the female fetus.
- Case 2c: Same case as 2a except that the woman asks the physician to target the male fetus.
- Case 2d: Same case as 2a except that the woman has a triplet gestation and wants to have a singleton.
- Case 2e: Same case as 2a except that the physician has never performed FTPP.
- Case 3a: Infertility treatment and high-order multiples – after having a daughter with the assistance of a fertility drug (Metrodin), Bobbi McCaughey asks her doctor for similar assistance to have a second child. Six weeks later, ultrasound shows that she is carrying septuplets. Doctors present the option of FTPP as a means by which to optimize the chance of a live healthy birth of at least one child. The option is rejected on grounds that it is morally equivalent to abortion.
- Case 3b: Same as 3a except that fertilization occurs in vitro, allowing transfer of fewer embryos.
- Case 4: Quadruplet gestation after IVF or natural fertilization.

From an egalitarian feminist standpoint, the variables in the above cases need to be identified because they are sometimes associated with inequality or unjust discrimination. The variable of ability to pay, for example, expands the options of some women while restricting those of others; it may thus exemplify classism. Targeting disabled fetuses or fetuses of a specific sex suggests unequal regard for one individual or group as opposed to another; it may thus exemplify ableism or sexism. In high-order multiple gestations, however, consideration of FTPP is mainly based on the desire of most pregnant women to have a healthy child. Most women not only desire this goal but pursue it at some cost to themselves, for example, by refraining from practices they might otherwise enjoy, such as alcohol consumption or smoking. In addition, many potential parents hope to have children who are bright, attractive, and athletically or artistically gifted; such hopes or desires are hardly to be equated with discrimination towards those who are not so endowed. The efforts of most pregnant women to promote the health or welfare of their intended offspring are beneficent or non-maleficent, and in some cases altruistic, rather than discriminatory.

Cases 1a–d and 2a–e are similar in that they involve relatively minor medical risks to the women and their fetuses. However, the rationale for FTPP in Cases 1a–d may be tied to the woman's responsibilities to children already born, whereas the rationale in Case 2a is apparently tied solely to the woman's wish to have one child rather than two. Some infertile women are especially anxious about their ability to be the 'perfect mother' they aspire to be, and this anxiety may be exacerbated when the woman has conceived twins. The physician's sensitivity to such anxiety is morally appropriate, but does not imply that termination of the fetus is morally justified or that the physician is morally obliged to accede to the request. Libertarian feminists would support the woman's request in all of the cases described except perhaps Case 1d; they might even maintain that clinicians are obliged to comply with such requests. Whether egalitarian feminists would support FTPP in any of these cases depends not only on the woman's wishes and welfare but also on variables such as responsibility for children already born. Egalitarian feminism might therefore support FTPP in Case 1a but not in Case 2a, unless the moral status of the fetus is either denied or considered less compelling than respect for the autonomy of the pregnant woman.

From an egalitarian feminist standpoint, the variables introduced in Cases 1b and 1c suggest the relevance of considerations of beneficence towards the potential child. FTPP that targets a fetus with trisomy 13 may be defended on grounds that this condition is usually fatal within the first year of life; given the probable necessity of burdensome treatment that outweighs its expected benefit to the potential child, FTPP may be viewed as fetal euthanasia. FTPP that targets a fetus with trisomy 21 or Down's syndrome cannot be described as fetal euthanasia unless conditions other than mental retardation support a similar rationale. Most individuals with Down's syndrome live a life that is relatively happy; accordingly, prevention of their birth cannot be justified on grounds of beneficence towards them. Still, the increased burden of care and its impact on other family members, coupled with the woman's desire to avoid these burdens by targeted FTPP, may override an obligation of beneficence towards the fetus or potential child. This position is weakly supportable by those who attribute some moral status to the fetus; it is obviously better supported by those who deny that status.

Egalitarian feminists support access to health care regardless of ability to pay; this makes Case 1a morally comparable to Case 1d – FTPP should be offered or not offered in both situations. For libertarian feminists, however, the two situations are not comparable, and denial of FTPP for the woman who cannot pay for it is justifiable if its provision would necessitate the restriction of other women's liberty, e.g. through their having to subsidize their poorer counterparts. Unfortunately, medical centres that provide reproductive assistance generally operate according to the libertarian model; only those who can pay out of pocket or through their insurers obtain treatment.

In all of the cases described, libertarians might be stymied by the need to respect the autonomy of clinicians as well as patients. In case 2a, for example, the physician who was asked to perform FTPP was reluctant to do so. After observing the twin gestation on ultrasound, he considered himself successful in helping her to achieve a desired pregnancy. When she did not agree that this was good news, he was not only disappointed but somewhat angry. The physician recognized, however, that the moral content of the request was equivalent to requests with which he had complied in the past – that he help some women to continue their pregnancies and help others to terminate them. He acknowledged that he did not in general find abortion morally objectionable.

Although the physician did not mention it at the time, I later learned of a variable that undoubtedly contributed to his reluctance – he had never performed FTPP (cf. Case 2e). In his hands, therefore, there was probably greater risk of losing both fetuses and of harming the pregnant woman than in a more experienced physician's hands. From both libertarian and egalitarian feminist standpoints, the pregnant woman deserved to know this if in fact the physician was willing to comply with her request. Instead, he bypassed that disclosure when he referred the woman to a medical centre in which FTPP had been done successfully, telling her that his reason for doing so was his moral discomfort about performing it. Quite apart from moral reticence, the physician's lack of experience provided adequate grounds for referral elsewhere. The appropriateness of the decision was demonstrated one year later when he performed FTPP for the first time, and all three fetuses of a triplet gestation were lost.

FTPP that targets either male or female fetuses, as in Cases 2b and 2c, is hardly justifiable on grounds of beneficence towards the fetus or potential child. From an egalitarian feminist standpoint, Case 2b (targeting the healthy female fetus) is more problematic than Case 2c (targeting the healthy male fetus) because FTPP is much more likely to be sexist in its rationale and societal impact when females rather than males are targeted. In contrast to both of these cases, Case 2d describes an increased risk for the pregnant woman and three fetuses, making considerations of beneficence more significant than in twin gestation (while less significant than in high order multiple gestations). Still, considerations of beneficence may not support FTTP in triplet gestations because it does not improve the odds of taking home a healthy baby (Berkowitz, 1996; Souter and Goodwin, 1998). Although maternal risk may be reduced through FTTP, it also exacts a high emotional toll, particularly for those who have undergone the rigours of infertility treatment in order to become pregnant in the first place. Unlike women who choose FTTP for higher order multiples, those with twin or triplet gestations are unable to base their decisions 'on the understanding that they are saving some of the children by sacrificing others' (Souter and Goodwin, 1998: p. 69).

In Cases 3a, 3b and 4, the rationale for requesting FTPP is to save lives rather than to lose them. Most clinicians agree that the relatively good outcome in the McCaughey case is not one that can reasonably be expected to recur. It has been alleged by some that proper management of Bobbi McCaughey's treatment would have avoided the risks of a septuplet pregnancy. The means of saving lives (direct killing) is morally problematic, but not intervening seems morally tantamount to allowing patients to die when they can be saved. If the only way of having any fetuses survive is to remove or terminate some of them, the moral reasons for doing so are surely more compelling than in other cases. In fact, it seems more pro-life to reduce the number of fetuses in such a situation than to permit the continuation of a pregnancy in which all of the fetuses would otherwise be expected to die. A libertarian feminist standpoint would support FTPP in this case on the same grounds as it supports it in the other cases, respect for the pregnant woman's autonomy. An egalitarian feminist standpoint would also support FTPP but on additional grounds, namely, the moral imperative to save lives that can be saved. (Different feminist standpoints are supported by feminist standpoint theory, which I have described and defended in Mahowald, 1995a.)

Within the context of that imperative, targeting some fetuses rather than others for removal or termination is egalitarian in that the criterion for selection is blind to the different characteristics of the fetuses themselves. The operator selects those that may most easily be reached so as to minimize the risks of the intervention for others and for the pregnant woman.

Case 3b differs from 3a (the McCaughey case) only in the manner in which pregnancy was initiated. Most cases of multiple gestation occur through infertility drugs rather than through IVF. With IVF in the US, the recommended number of embryos transferred is three or four; this maximizes the woman's chance of giving birth to a healthy infant while minimizing the risk of high order multiple gestation. To reduce risks for both women and fetuses, clinicians are obligated to follow this recommendation. Even when it is followed, however, a quadruplet pregnancy can result, as described in

Case 4, and this obviously increases concerns about mortality and morbidity.

Prior to advances in reproductive and perinatal technology, the septuplet and octuplet births that have been reported could not have occurred; these were not 'natural' multiple gestations but gestations induced by ovulation stimulation. Because of the demands of confidentiality, suspicions that the cases were mismanaged from a medical point of view cannot be confirmed. Family physicians and generalist obstetrician-gynaecologists who lack specialized training in infertility treatment can and do prescribe infertility drugs without utilizing techniques that would minimize the risk of high-order multiples. Whether administered by generalists or specialists, however, infertility treatment has become a profitable business that egalitarian feminists are loathe to support because it increases the gap between those who can afford it and those who cannot.

Regarding Case 4, the difference between a naturally induced quadruplet gestation and one triggered by fertility drugs is relevant because of the possibility of avoidance in the latter cases. Multiple births induced by infertility treatment are generally suspect on feminist grounds because of the probability that gender stereotypes influenced the decision to pursue treatment in the first place. While egalitarian feminists concur in this suspicion, we also critique the relative unavailability of reproductive assistance to poor infertile women who seek such assistance without being driven to do so through gender stereotypes. To the extent that women autonomously choose infertility treatment, they are responsible for the associated risks of multiple gestation about which they have a right to be fully informed. From an egalitarian feminist standpoint, a woman's fulfillment of that responsibility means taking account of the impact of her decision not only on herself and her potential children but also on the wider society, which is hardly likely to benefit by high order multiples.

Given the impact of gender stereotypes, the risk of multiple gestation to women and to potential children, concerns about overpopulation and responsibilities to children already born, some feminists maintain that fertility drugs should be outlawed. As one feminist put it, 'Only when women are willing and able to define themselves in terms larger than "mom" will they come to accept that they are just fine exactly the way they are – childless – and that there is a natural rhythm to the planet which may not include their having children, and that the concept of "mother" can be broadened to include the whole world' ('Zoe', 1999). This broadened concept is not only applicable to women regardless of whether they have children; it is also applicable to men. To the extent that both sexes become mothers in this sense, society in general will implement the nurturant or care-based ethic that Sara Ruddick characterizes as a feminist politics of peace (Ruddick, 1989).

An egalitarian version of feminism calls for individuals to take account of the broader societal context by opposing injustice towards any non-dominant group. Because the capabilities of women and their potential children may be further reduced through multiple gestation, FTPP may be defended in high multiple gestations as a means through which to promote their equality with those who are dominant. In twin and triplet gestations, whether it promotes the equality of women or children remains questionable.

In high-order multiple gestations, the pregnant woman's right to FTPP is supportable solely on grounds of the risk to her of sustaining the pregnancy. Reports of septuplet and octuplet pregnancies provide ample evidence of how severe these risks can be. For example, Nkem Chukwu, who conceived octuplets, was hospitalized for three months and fed intravenously during much of her hospitalization. In the final two and a half weeks of her gestation, she lay almost upside down to relieve pressure on her abdomen, suffering nosebleeds as a result. Following delivery, she required additional surgery to stop internal bleeding (Associated Press, 1998). Even if no fetuses were expected to survive, risk to the mother would justify the procedure, as it does in cases of late abortion for maternal health reasons. The expectation that mortality and morbidity risks will be decreased through FTPP strengthens the argument, but this can be countered by pointing to the fetuses that are terminated rather than those that may be saved.

Although egalitarian feminists do not regard potential persons as equal in value to actual persons, many acknowledge responsibility for potential children as morally relevant to decisions about FTPP. This acknowledgment is based on a sense of responsibility to those already born and the impact of decisions on them; it may also stem from a sense of responsibility for potential children. In other words, responsibilities for potential persons are not as great as responsibilities to actual persons, but they still have moral weight.

From an egalitarian feminist standpoint, even if the fetus has moral status or standing, FTPP is morally justifiable so long as (1) its moral status is deemed less compelling than the pregnant woman's autonomy, or (2) the decision is not based on the desire to avoid the birth of a child or children with disabilities (Silvers et al., 1998). Those who view the moral status of the fetus in gradualist terms are unlikely to impute greater value to it than to women's autonomy as early in gestation as FTPP is usually performed. Even later, however, the decision may, and often is, based on the desire to insure the live birth of at least one child rather than the desire to avoid the birth of one or more who are disabled. In other words, survival and avoidance of morbidity are separable goals. Some individuals and couples simply want to maximize their chance of having a living child, whether able or disabled.

Moreover, FTPP to avoid the birth of a child or children with disabilities does not itself imply disvaluing either fetuses or persons with disabilities. Such decisions may instead be based on the inability of the woman or couple or the inability of society to provide adequate care for the potential child or children. Because the same rationale is applicable to gestations of singletons, both able and disabled, it surely does not constitute discrimination against those who are disabled. Rather, it describes the forced option that some women face in the context of tragically limited supports for potential children. It is possible, therefore, to affirm equal respect for the disabled while undertaking FTPP so long as the mere fact of the disability does not determine the choice. Not the disabilities themselves but their inevitably and overwhelmingly burdensome consequences to the children as well as the women who raise them are the grounds for interventions.

A final argument in defence of FTPP in cases of high-order multiple gestations is based on an analogy with the right of born persons, whether able or disabled, to decline life-saving or life-sustaining treatment. If competent, informed adults have a legal and moral right to die by refusing such treatment, and if there are circumstances in which such refusals on behalf of others are viewed as reasonable by most people, it hardly seems just to prevent cessation of treatment in comparable circumstances for those who are incompetent, such as children or fetuses. Or, to put it differently, if we are morally bound to respect the right to die as well as the right to live in other humans, why should fetuses not be accorded similar respect? Abortions typically entail imposition rather than refusal of treatment, but FTPP is more like refusal than imposition of treatment, at least in situations of high order multiples, because sustaining such pregnancies without FTPP requires even more medical technology than FTPP itself. The technology required to continue high-order multiple gestations also entails greater risk, discomfort and cost to the pregnant woman. Beyond her right to FTPP for the sake of her own health, then, FTPP in effect is the means by which she may decline the medical technology that would otherwise be required to sustain a pregnancy associated with severe fetal morbidity. She thus acts on behalf of the fetuses that are terminated as well as those whose chance of survival is thereby enhanced.

Conclusion

When multiple gestation occurs, whether naturally or through reproductive interventions, women should have the legal option of undergoing FTPP just as they have the option of abortion in singleton pregnancies. In neither case, however, should ability to pay be the criterion by which some women are refused and others offered the procedure. Again as with abortion, physicians should not be legally obliged to perform FTPP if they are morally opposed to it, so long as they refer the woman elsewhere. For women themselves, the moral parameters of FTPP decisions include many relevant variables. In my delineation of real and concocted cases, I have illustrated some of these – the burdens and benefits of maintaining versus reducing the number of fetuses, the goals of FTPP in particular cases, whether fetuses are targeted for reasons involving social prejudice, and responsibilities to already born children as well as potential children. In general, I conclude that FTPP in high order multiple gestations is morally justifiable in order to save lives and reduce severe morbidity for the pregnant woman as well as surviving fetuses. This rationale is adequate even if fetuses are imputed to have moral standing, so long as women give their full, informed consent to the procedure.

In cases involving twins and triplets, FTPP is not comparably justifiable because it does not increase the likelihood of having a healthy baby to take home. (Data on FTPP in twin and triplet gestations show outcomes no better than the outcomes in twin and triplet gestations when FTPP is not performed; see Souter and Goodwin, 1998. If these data were proved wrong, my view would change.)

None the less, reducing triplets to twins probably results in lower costs and fewer days in the hospital, along with a decrease in the moderate morbidities associated with prolonged hospitalizations and preterm delivery. (I have developed this argument more fully in Silvers et al., 1998.) While FTPP in triplet gestations is defensible as a means of avoiding those burdens, efforts to avoid them introduce concerns about discrimination against those who are disabled. From an egalitarian feminist standpoint, such decisions can and should stem from different criteria, such as responsibilities to other persons and lack of societal support of care for those who are disabled. From that same standpoint, FTPP is hardly defensible in twin gestations unless fetuses have no moral standing or their standing is subordinated to the autonomy of the pregnant woman. In other words, other factors being equal, the case for FTPP in high order multiple gestations is compelling, the case for FTPP in triplet gestations is less compelling, and the case for FTPP in twin gestations is the least compelling.

In sum, nature's paradigm is a wise dictum for potential practitioners of FTPP – humans were designed to have one baby at a time. Although the successes and excesses of the infertility industry have apparently supplanted Hellin's Law, 'the fewer the better' remains an applicable guideline for infertility specialists as well as for women.

References

Associated Press (1998). Work just begun for octuplet mom. *New York Times*, 31 December, http://www.nytimes.com/aponline/a/AP-Octuplets.html

Berkowitz, R. (1996). From twin to singleton. *British Medical Journal* 313: 373–4.

Berkowitz, R.L., Lynch, L., Stone, L. et al. (1996). The current status of multifetal pregnancy reduction. *American Journal of Obstetrics and Gynecology* 174: 1265–6.

Evans, M.I., Littman, L., Richer, R. et al. (1997). Selective reduction for multifetal pregnancy: early opinions revisited. *Journal of Reproductive Medicine* **42**: 771.

Grobstein, C. (1995). Human development from fertilisation to birth. In *Encyclopedia of Bioethics*, ed. W.T. Reich, pp. 847–51. New York: Macmillan.

Hammon, K.R. (1998). Multifetal pregnancy reduction. *Journal of Obstetric, Gynecologic and Neonatal Nursing* **27**: 338.

Mahowald, M.B. (1982). Concepts of abortion and their relevance to the abortion debate. *Southern Journal of Philosophy* **20**: 195–207.

Mahowald, M.B. (1993). *Women and Children in Health Care.* New York: Oxford University Press.

Mahowald, M.B. (1995a). On treatment of myopia: feminism, standpoint theory and bioethics. In *Feminism and Bioethics: Beyond Reproduction*, ed. S. Wolf, pp. 95–115. New York: Oxford University Press.

Mahowald, M.B. (1995b). The fetus: philosophical and ethical issues. In *Encyclopedia of Bioethics*, ed. W.T. Reich, pp. 851–6. New York: Macmillan.

Mahowald, M.B. (2000). *Genes, Women, Equality.* New York: Oxford University Press.

Manier, J. (1998). Risky, costly, multiple births not inevitable. *Chicago Tribune*, 23 December: p. 1.

Rorty, M.V. and Pinkerton, J.A.V. (1996). Elective fetal reduction: the ultimate elective surgery. *Journal of Contemporary Health Law and Policy* **13**: 55.

Ruddick, S. (1989). *Maternal Thinking: Towards a Politics of Peace.* New York: Ballantine Books.

Sen, A. (1995). *Inequality Reexamined.* Cambridge, MA: Harvard University Press.

Silvers, A., Wasserman, D. and Mahowald, M.B. (1998). *Disability, Difference, Discrimination: Perspectives on Justice in Bioethics and Public Policy.* New York: Rowman and Littlefield.

Souter, I. and Goodwin, T.M. (1998). Decision making in multifetal pregnancy reduction for triplets. *American Journal of Perinatology* **15**: 63.

Tribune News Services (1999). Two McGaughey septuplets being monitored for cerebral palsy. *Chicago Tribune*, 26 April, section 1: p. 13.

'Zoe' (1999). Personal communication to Feminist Approaches to Bioethics listserve: zoe@miht.net

Third trimester

Caesarean section: who chooses – the woman or her doctor?

Wendy Savage

Academic Department of Obstetrics and Gynaecology, St Bartholemew and Royal London Hospital School of Medicine, UK

Caesarean section (CS) is a major operation which may be life-saving for mother or child. Like any major operation it carries risks, needs adequate anaesthesia and requires the informed consent of the woman.

The procedure

The woman may receive a general anaesthetic which renders her unconscious after injection of a suitable agent. Anaesthesia is then maintained with volatile gases, passed into the lungs via a tube in the trachea. Care has to be taken when the woman has been in labour that stomach contents are not regurgitated and inhaled into the lungs, as emptying of the stomach is delayed during labour. Because of this risk and the unhappiness that many women feel at not being aware of their baby's birth, regional anaesthesia is the preferred method today.

These methods involve passing a needle in between the vertebrae in the spine and injecting local anaesthetic agents, which requires considerable skill. There is a risk of the blood pressure falling, so an intravenous infusion is set up beforehand. If the woman has already had a catheter introduced into the epidural space to administer drugs to relieve pain, this can be topped up to give a higher degree of pain relief. Alternatively a spinal anaesthetic can be given, where the needle is passed into the cerebro-spinal fluid surrounding the spinal cord. This usually lasts about an hour, whereas the epidural can be maintained to give post-operative pain relief, if there are sufficient staff to monitor the woman adequately in the postnatal ward.

One advantage of a regional technique is that the woman is conscious when the baby is born and can hold her whilst the abdomen is being closed. Once adequate anaesthesia has been induced, the bladder is catheterized, and most doctors today leave this in for 24 hours. The skin is cleaned with antiseptic solution and the abdomen covered with sterile drapes around the line of incision. Normally a horizontal cut 12 to 20 cm long is made above the pubic bone, through the skin, subcutaneous fat and rectus sheath. The rectus muscles are separated, the peritoneal cavity opened and the uterus comes into view. This is then opened in the lower part and the membranes ruptured and the baby delivered though the incision. The cord is cut and the baby passed to the paediatrician. As the baby has not experienced labour she may be slower to breathe and fluid may need to be sucked out of the mouth and nose. The baby is usually delivered within 10 minutes and then it takes from 20 to 60 minutes to close the abdomen, depending on whether this is a first or later CS.

Effects and complications of Caesarean section

As with any major operation, the wound is painful and analgesic agents are required, which may affect the breast-fed baby. Prophylactic antibiotics are usually given to prevent infection; thrombolytic agents may be needed to prevent blood clots forming in the veins and haemorrhage may occur during or after the operation. Despite the use of prophylactic antibiotics, studies have shown that 20–45 per cent of women have infection associated with the operation (Nice et al., 1996). Looking after a newborn baby with a scar in the abdomen and whilst recovering from surgery is not ideal. Blood transfusion is needed more often than following a normal birth. Pulmonary embolism is more common after CS; thus, as the rate of surgery continues to rise (even though the death rate per 1000 operations has declined over the last 20 years), the number of women dying following CS has remained much the same in the UK for the decade to 1993 – 80–90 per triennium (Confidential Inquiry, 1991–1993 by the Department of Health et al., published in 1997). The direct eath rate estimated by Marion Hall from the 1988–90 figures was 1.8 per 100 000 vaginal deliveries, 14.8/100 000 following elective CS and 25.2/100 000 following emergency CS (Hall, 1994: p. 191). In the last UK Confidential Inquiry (1994–1996, by the Department of Health et al., published in 1998) the chapter devoted to CS was omitted, ostensibly because of the poor quality of data about the CS rate. Better case ascertainment makes it difficult to compare with earlier inquiries; the overall maternal mortality figure rose from 9.9 in the previous two reports (Confidential Inquiry 1988–1990, 1991–1993 by the Department of Health et al., published in 1994 and 1997 respectively) to 12.2 per 100 000 maternities in 1994–96 (Department of Health et al., 1998). I estimate that the rate of death from pulmonary embolism, which is commoner after any surgical procedure, was nine times higher following CS than vaginal delivery (4.37 vs. 0.51 per 100 000 deliveries) assuming a 15 per cent CS rate during this period. If the CS rate was lower, the death rate would be at least 10 times higher following CS than a vaginal delivery.

Long-term problems are less well documented, but both voluntary and involuntary infertility is higher (Hemminki et al., 1985; Jolly et al., 1999).The risk of CS in a subsequent pregnancy is increased, as is the risk of placenta praevia (where the afterbirth is in the lower part of the uterus) and placenta accreta (where the afterbirth penetrates deep in the wall of the uterus). These are dangerous conditions which may cause massive haemorrhage or even death if hysterectomy (removal of the uterus) is not performed in time (Clark, Koonings and Phelan, 1985).

Epidemiology

Over 100 000 CS per year are performed in England, and over a million in the US. Caesarean section is now the most commonly performed major operation in the UK. Sixteen per cent of all UK women, and 19 per cent of women having their first baby in Scotland (which has accurate data), were delivered by CS in 1995 (Scottish Health Services, 1997). In England, where the data are less accurate, the overall rate in 1994–95 is also thought to be about 16 per cent, with some hospitals reaching rates of 25 per cent (Department of Health *Statistical Bulletin*, 1997). The English National Board midwifery audit for 1998 (based on replies from 87 per cent of maternal units in England) found that 68 per cent of units had a rate of 10.0–19.9 per cent, 25 per cent had 20.0–29.9 per cent, and 2 per cent had a rate of over 30 per cent (ENBNMHV, 1998).

The last decade has seen a continuing rise in the rate of CS in most countries in the world (McIlwaine *et al.*, 1985; Lomas and Enkin, 1989; Notzon, 1990; Savage, 1990). At the same time that public health physicians (and some obstetricians) in the western world fear that women are being subjected to unnecessary surgery, women who need CS are being denied it in the developing world. Thousands die every week in agony from obstructed labour or are left with fistulae that ruin their health and leave them socially isolated (de Costa, 1998). Even in the West, some women have complained that when they have asked for a CS, because they feel they are not going to deliver normally, it has been refused by the doctor, sometimes with disastrous consequences. Now in the UK, some obstetricians are saying that women are asking for CS (Jackson and Irvine, 1998; Mackenzie, 1999) although the information they have been given before making such a request is an unknown quantity (McIlwaine et al., 1998). In a later prospective study Graham et al. (1999) showed that in seven per cent of women having a CS, maternal preference was a direct factor in making the decision. In the US, the government set targets to reduce the rate (Department of Health and Human Services, 1991), which has fallen slightly from its peak of 24.7 per cent in 1989 to 22.8 per cent in 1994 (Clarke and Taffel, 1996).

In England in 1990, the government response to the House of Commons Select Committee report on maternity care (Select Committee Report, 1992; Department of Health, 1993) aimed to give women more choice and control over childbirth. These reports emphasized the need for better communication between professionals and with the woman, and for continuity of care by fewer people. One had hoped that if 30 per cent of women were looked after entirely by midwives (as in the Netherlands with a CS rate (CSR) under 10 per cent; Treffers et al., 1990), that this would reduce the CSR, but this has not happened. This is partly because this target 'indicator of success' set by the Changing Childbirth team has not been met (Rothwell, 1996) and partly because some obstetricians and midwives have interpreted this directive as 'allowing' or giving every woman the right to choose to have a CS (Paterson Browne and Fisk, 1999).

From the viewpoint of public health, i.e. the health of populations, there are also problems. The CSR is now 18 per cent; if it should be 10 per cent or less (World Health Organization, 1985) and if each one per cent rise in CSR costs the National Health Service £5 000 000 (Audit Commission, 1997), then unless it can be shown that there is health benefit from this high cost, there must be better ways to use £40 000 000.

The rising CSR is not just about medical or woman power, advances in medical technology or changing societal expectation, it is also about the organization of services and money. The highest rates are found in countries in which the medical system is dominated by private practice, as for example in the US and Australia (Sakala,1993). In South America the even higher rates are said to be due to social factors, while Chile, with a rate of 37 per cent nationally, is thought to have the highest rate in the world. The recent steep rise followed a change in the organization of payment for health care (Murray and Serani Pradenas, 1997).

A woman's right to choose a Caesarean section

As a professional, one has a duty to the individual patient, as well as a duty to society to use resources wisely (General Medical Council, 1995). At the individual level, one's advice should be based on good, unbiased, up-to-date evidence (if it exists), complemented by one's own experience. Decisions should be made in the best interests of the patient. The patient has the right to decline to take one's advice, but, in my view, does not have the right to ask the doctor to perform a procedure which the doctor considers unwarranted by the evidence and which is not in the patient's best interests. In contrast to induced abortion, where terminating a pregnancy up to 20 weeks is statistically safer than carrying a pregnancy to term, in the UK even elective CS carries a ninefold risk of death compared with vaginal delivery (Confidential

Inquiry, 1994–1996 by the Department of Health et al., published in 1998). So, whilst as a doctor I can support 'a woman's right to choose' an abortion, and as a feminist I also support it, I do not think that CS on demand is every woman's right. 'Physicians have the responsibility to inform and counsel women in this matter. At present, because hard evidence of net benefit does not exist, performing CS for non-medical reasons is ethically not justified' (FIGO, 1999).

Those who argue that CS is now so safe that women should be allowed to choose the mode of delivery quote the risk of damage to the pelvic floor and the risk of a baby dying during labour, but rarely discuss the disadvantages to the woman of having a major operation, whilst coping with breast-feeding, sleepless nights and the major life event of becoming a mother. Is death even mentioned? The overall risk of dying in association with pregnancy is about 1 in 10 000, about the same as one's risk of dying in a road accident. Following vaginal delivery it is about 1 in 50 000, and following elective CS it is about 1 in 7000 (Hall, 1994) The risk of a baby dying in labour at term is about 1 in 1000 (CESDI, 1998), and in about half of these cases, with different management the baby might have lived. I would prefer to improve the standard of care so that babies do not die needlessly. Midwifery care has been associated with good outcomes and low rates of CS – about 1.5 per cent (van Alten, Eskes and Treffers, 1989; Durand, 1992) – but obstetricians seem reluctant to look at this work.

The passage of a baby through the birth canal is an amazing process, and not unnaturally there are changes to the anatomy of the pelvic floor. Many women in middle age have some degree of prolapse of the uterus or vaginal walls, although with smaller families, and the abandonment of high forceps deliveries, the number is decreasing. Work done in the 1980s suggested that damage to the pudendal nerve during childbirth was related to urinary and faecal incontinence in later life (Snooks and Swash, 1984). Recently the use of ultrasound to demonstrate damage to the anal sphincter, a promising new research technique (Sultan et al., 1993), has been used to support the idea of elective CS to preserve the pelvic floor, but rejected in a *British Journal of Obstetricians and Gynaecologists* editorial (Sultan and Stanton, 1996). The high rates reported in this non-random sample do not necessarily fit with women's own perceptions or obstetricians' clinical observations.

Sleep et al. (1984) reported that two per cent of women (of 67 per cent followed up in their prospective randomized study of the use of episiotomy) had urinary stress incontinence three or more times a week, and half of these used a pad. Occasional stress incontinence was reported by at least a third. Faecal incontinence was reported occasionally by three per cent of women three months after delivery but not mentioned in their later follow-up study (Sleep and Grant, 1987). MacArthur et al. (1997) reported that four per cent of 916 (out of a total of 1667 women delivered consecutively) developed new faecal incontinence after childbirth, which persisted in 2.4 per cent at 10 months. A more recent study from Scandinavia (Zetterstrom et al., 1999) found lower rates. Forceps delivery, large babies, occipito-posterior positions (when the baby's back is towards the mother's back and a bigger diameter of the head passes through the pelvis) and previous constipation have been associated with higher rates. Third-degree tears, which vary in incidence from one in 1000 to one in 200 deliveries, are associated with continued faecal incontinence in up to 50 per cent of women (Tetzschner et al., 1996).

In my experience, women with severe problems with bowel and bladder control are rarely seen. Planned surgery when the woman is older and not caring for a newborn baby, for those who are shown to need it, seems a better use of resources. A review in 1998 concluded that studies on anal and faecal incontinence 'are weakened to various degrees by methodological error... There are no good longitudinal data to suggest whether anal incontinence is a persistent or remitting condition in large populations' (Bump and Norton, 1998: p. 746).

Why women ask for Caesarean section

Ryding (1993) studied 33 women requesting CS in a Swedish hospital in 1988–90, with a CSR of 8.2 per cent and a perinatal mortality rate of 4.8 per 1000. Half decided to have a vaginal delivery after consultation, giving a rate of CS on request of 2.7 per 1000, most of these following a difficult labour the first time round. Graham et al. (1999) reported the views of 166 women who had undergone CS; seven per cent of those women expressed a preference for this mode of delivery.

An editorial in the *British Journal of Obstetricians and Gynaecologists* in 1996 by a leading urogynaecologist and one of the researchers in the field concluded that it was difficult to pick out the women who would benefit from elective surgery. It would be premature to offer CS to all women, it was argued, and the morbidity of this approach would outweigh the benefits (Sultan and Stanton, 1996). If all women learned and practised pelvic floor exercises from the teenage years, it would probably provide greater benefit and protect against urinary problems in later life (J. Mantle, 1999, pers. comm.). The evidence about long-term problems following CS is lacking, as little research has been done in this field, so it is difficult to tell women how many will suffer from pain in the scar, secondary infertility or pelvic pain due to infection.

Forced Caesarean section: the law in England and Wales

Legal enforcement of the doctor's decision to perform a CS when the woman did not consent began in the US in 1973 and became an issue in the 1980s (Kolder et al., 1987). After 1990, following a successful posthumous appeal against a forced CS in the case of AC (*In re AC*, 1990) the climate has changed in the US. The first reported British case occurred in 1992 (*Re S*, 1992) and then in 1996 there followed a spate of five cases, two on the same day (Table 17.1).

The Royal College of Obstetricians and Gynaecologists (RCOG) Ethics Committee published its guidance in 1993 (RCOG, 1993) and stated un-equivocally that, 'It is inappropriate, and unlikely to be helpful or necessary, to invoke judicial intervention to overrule an informed or competent woman's refusal of a proposed medical treatment, even though her refusal might place her life and that of her fetus at risk'. Since then the Court of Appeal has clearly restated the legal situation in *Re MB* (February 1997) and *Re S* (1998; see *Re S*, 1996).

English law makes it quite clear that a competent adult has the right to refuse treatment and that surgery without consent is an assault on the person. As Wall J said in his judgment in the Tameside and Glossop case (1996):

- (i) It remains a criminal and tortious assault to perform physically invasive medical treatment without the patient's consent.
- (ii) A mentally competent patient has an absolute right to refuse medical treatment for any reason, rational or irrational, or for no reason at all, even where that decision will lead to his or her own death.
- (iii) Where it is impossible for the patient to communicate the decision through unconsciousness or lack of mental competence and the treatment is not contrary to a known competent previously expressed decision of the patient, it is lawful to provide treatment which is:
  (a) necessary to save the life or preserve or prevent deterioration of the physical and mental health of the patient;
  (b) in the patient's best interests.
- (iv) A patient lacks the relevant mental competence to make treatment decisions if he is incapable of:
  (a) comprehending and retaining treatment information;
  (b) believing such information;
  (c) weighing such information in the balance to make a choice.

The competence test relied on the judgment by Thorpe J in *Re C* (1994), who said 'I consider helpful Dr E's analysis of the decision-making process into three stages' – which are those given above. C was a paranoid schizophrenic in Broadmoor who did not want his leg amputated. Despite his long-standing mental illness, he was deemed to have the capacity to make an informed decision. In fact he recovered the use of his leg with only conservative surgery.

The question of competence to decide was modified in the MB case, where the Court of Appeal ruled that a person lacks capacity if some impairment or disturbance of mental functioning renders the person unable to make a decision whether to consent to or to refuse treatment. That inability to make a decision will occur when

(1) The patient is unable to comprehend and retain the information which is material to the decision, especially as to the likely consequence of having or not having the treatment in question.

(2) The patient is unable to use the information and weigh it in the balance as part of the process of arriving at the decision.

If, as Thorpe J observed in *Re C* (*supra*), a compulsive disorder or phobia from which the patient suffers stifles belief in the information presented to her, then the decision may not be a true one. Significantly, the question of belief was dropped, unless it was deemed part of a mental illness.

The Court of Appeal also dealt with the question of 'temporary factors' such as confusion, shock, fatigue, pain or drugs, which may erode a person's capacity, saying that those concerned must be satisfied that such factors are operating to such a degree that the ability to decide is absent. Another such influence may be panic induced by fear. Again, careful scrutiny of the evidence is necessary, because fear of an operation may be a rational reason for refusal to undergo it. Fear may also, however, paralyse the will and thus destroy the capacity to make a decision.

It is also clear that in English law the fetus is not a legal entity separate from its mother, it does not have legal rights. Balcombe LJ expressed this doctrine in a judgment in the Court of Appeal, *In re F (in utero)* (1988), where a local authority sought to make the fetus a Ward of Court and to detain a pregnant woman, who, despite a history of mental illness and a nomadic life-style, was not currently suffering from mental illness as defined by the Mental Health Act 1983. If the law is to be extended in this country, so as to impose control over the mother of an unborn child where such control may be necessary for the benefit of that child, then under our system of Parliamentary democracy it is for Parliament to decide whether such controls can be imposed, and if so, subject to what limitations or conditions.

The first English case where we know that a woman was forced to have a CS against her will occurred in April, 1992. Caroline Spear was booked for a home birth, but was transferred to hospital when the midwife found the presentation to be breech (when the bottom of the baby, not the head is entering the pelvis, as happens to about three per cent of women at term). Despite Ms Spear's objection that breech babies could be born vaginally, the doctor insisted on performing a CS. Ms Spear allegedly suffered from post-traumatic stress disorder following the birth, and then sued for assault. The action was settled out of court for £7000, although the North Middlesex Hospital did not admit liability. Ms Spear was unable to continue to fight the

Table 17.1. Cases of forced Caesarean section that have occurred in the UK (1992–97)

Court Case	Date	Ethnic origin	Medical outcome	Legal decision	In labour
Caroline Spear	17.4.92	English	CS for breech. Mother alleged PTSD	North Middlesex settled	Yes – transfer from home
Bloomsbury & Islington HA re S	12.10.92	Nigerian	Alleged assault. Baby A&W Mother alive after CS baby died ?SB	£7000 no liability admitted Judge 20 mins to decide	6 days
Tameside & Glossop Trust re CH	12.1.96		Mother schizophrenic detained IOL for IUGR may need CS	Lacked capacity to consent Rx for mental disorder	No
St Georges v Ms S	29.4.96	English	CS for 'PET'. Mother rejected baby initially. Baby well	Judge misled, case went to CA 1997, appeal allowed	No
Norfolk & Norwich v W	21.6.96	?	Forceps	Lacked capacity to balance risks	Yes – fully dilated all day
Rochdale v Choudhury	21.6.96	Bangladeshi	Previous 3 CS had been sterilized Agreed to CS whilst court in session	Denied was pregnant. Lacked capacity to consent	Yes
Re L Kirkwood J	5.12.96	?	Mother and baby well prev CS Mother and baby well Woman thanked doctors	Suing, gave consent before operation, under duress Lacked capacity to consent because of needle phobia	Yes
Re MB	18.2.97	?	Mother and baby well, elective CS for breech presentation	Lacked capacity to consent because of needle phobia	Yes

PTSD = Post traumatic stress disorder
A&W = Alive and well
CS = Caesarean Section

SB = Still birth
IOL = Induction of labour
IUGR = Intrauterine growth retardation

PET = Pre-eclamptic toxaemia
CA = Court of Appeal

case through the courts as she was not granted legal aid. However, childbirth activists felt that this was a victory, and despite Ms Spear's disappointment at not being able to take the case to court, she said she felt vindicated. Following her enforced CS, she had two babies born normally at home.

The second case, which was the first in the UK to involve a court order, was *Re S* (1992). This concerned a Nigerian woman with a transverse lie who refused a CS on religious grounds. The decision of the President of the Family Court, Sir Stephen Brown, was made in the interests of the fetus and has been criticized by many authorities, including the Court of Appeal in 1997. He relied upon a reference to the lower court's decision in the US Angela Carder case (*In re AC*, 1990), although that judgment, authorizing an enforced CS, had been reversed on appeal. Both Angela Carder and her baby died soon after the operation, and her estate sued the hospital, winning the appeal. The judgment stated that such interventions were 'virtually never' justified: 'Even a dying woman with a viable fetus has the final say' (Hewson, 1992). Surgery such as CS against the will of a competent patient was not justified, a view shared by the American Medical Association and the American College of Obstetricians and Gynecologists (ACOG, 1987). In the Court of Appeal judgment *Re MB* (1997) Butler Sloss LJ, Saville LJ and Ward LJ said of *Re S*:

The interest of the fetus prevailed. It is a decision the correctness of which we must now call in doubt. That is not to say that the ethical dilemma does not remain. Nonetheless, as has so often been said, this is not a court of morals...

(Re MB, 1997: p. 21.)

There was considerable debate within the medical and legal professions about this decision; in 1993 the Ethics Committee of the Royal College of Obstetricians and Gynaecologists (RCOG, 1993) published their guidance.

In January 1996, Tameside and Glossop health authority sought leave to perform a CS if necessary on a woman who was detained under the Mental Health Act (MHA). She was a schizophrenic, and in the opinion of the psychiatrist lacked the capacity to consent (although, as *Re C* demonstrates, people with mental illness do not necessarily lack capacity). The fetus was said to be growing poorly, and the obstetrician wished to induce her labour and, if the fetus became distressed, to carry out a CS. The order was granted, but because this was not an emergency there was time to discuss the issues. It was argued that if the baby were stillborn, the woman's mental health would suffer, and so the treatment was ordered under the MHA, a decision of dubious legal standing.

The next case in April of 1996 involved another Ms S who attended her new general practitioner (GP) for the first time at 36 weeks, having recently moved into the area. The GP diagnosed pre-eclampsia (raised blood pressure, protein in the urine and generalized swelling due to fluid retention, PET) and recommended admission to hospital. The woman said she believed in allowing nature to take its course. When it was explained that this was a dangerous condition that might lead to her having fits and the baby being stillborn, she apparently said that she did not care if she and her baby lived or died. The GP, alarmed by this attitude, rang her previous GP, who said she had been depressed, so the help of a social worker was invoked. The social worker, GP and the GP's partner arranged for Ms S to be admitted to Springfield Hospital for assessment under Section 2 of the 1983 MHA. Later that night she was transferred to St George's Hospital, as the staff in the psychiatric unit did not feel that they had the facilities to look after a pregnant woman with PET.

She was seen by the duty registrar and briefly by the senior registrar. The next day, despite a psychiatrist being called who said she was competent to make a decision about her treatment, the hospital obtained a court order from Hogg J, authorizing them to perform a CS, on the grounds that she was in labour and the PET was severe. The order required her to be delivered immediately. Ms S had instructed solicitors, but neither they nor she were informed that the hospital was going to court. When the order was obtained, Ms S did not struggle against the administration of the anaesthetic as she felt this would be undignified, but acquiesced. She refused to sign the consent form, and following the birth rejected the baby initially. After four days she was transferred back to Springfield Hospital where the psychiatrists did not find any mental illness. She then took her own discharge (*St. George's NHS Trust* v *S*, 1998). There was considerable disquiet about this case, which was widely reported in the media (Dyer, 1997; Gibb, 1997).

On 26th June 1996, two cases came before the High Court, one breaking off so that the second case could be heard urgently. The facts were presented within two minutes. A Bengali woman, Ms Choudhury, who had had a previous CS, said she would rather die than have another operation, but the consultant considered that the scar would rupture if she did not have a CS within the next hour. She was unrepresented by legal counsel. Despite the fact that there was no question of her lacking capacity to understand and believe information, the judge ordered her to have a CS. It was said that she lacked the third component of capacity, the ability to weigh up information (*Rochdale Healthcare NHS Trust* v *C*, 1997). Johnson J said:

I accepted the view of the consultant obstetrician in relation to the first two elements in the analysis of Wall J in Tameside as to the capacity of the patient in the sense of her ability to comprehend and retain information and to believe such information. However, I have concluded that the patient was not capable of weighing up the information she was given, the third element. The patient was in the throes of labour with all that is involved in terms of pain and emotional stress. I concluded that a patient who could, in these circumstances, speak in terms which seemed to accept the inevitability of her own death, was not a patient who was able properly to weigh up the considerations that arose so as to make any valid decision, about *anything of even the most trivial kind, surely less one which involved her own life.* [Emphasis added.]

(*Rochdale Healthcare NHS Trust* v *C*, 1997, p. 505.)

During the hearing Ms Choudhury agreed to sign the consent form, but is now suing as she said that this was done under duress. Following the Ms S appeal, it was held that if the woman was unrepresented, any court decision was unlawful.

The other case heard that day by Johnson J was *Norfolk and Norwich Healthcare (NHS) Trust* v *W* (1997). Here the woman had not realized that she was pregnant (she had previously been sterilized, having had three CS operations), and did not believe that she needed an assisted delivery by forceps. She had been diagnosed as being in the second stage for some hours. The Court authorized the obstetricians to perform an assisted delivery, if necessary proceeding to CS. The judge ruled that she lacked capacity because she could not balance the risks:

She was called upon to make the decision at a time of acute emotional stress and physical pain in the ordinary course of labour, made even more difficult for her because of her own particular mental history. I held that termination of this labour would be in the best interests of the patient. I was satisfied that unless the patient was delivered of the fetus she was carrying, whether by way of forceps delivery or by Caesarean section, then her own physical health would be put at risk. This risk would arise if the fetus died because of rupture of the old Caesarean scar or by suffocation in the birth canal. The death of the fetus would have immediate and increasing deleterious effects on the patient herself leading to serious damage and possible death. *Termination would end the stress and the pain of her labour, it would avoid the likelihood of damage to her physical health which might have potentially life-threatening consequences and, despite her present view about the fetus, would avoid her feeling any feeling of guilt in the future were she, by her refusal to consent, to cause the death of the fetus.*

Throughout the judgment I have referred to 'the fetus' because I wish to emphasise that the focus of my judicial attention was upon the interests of the patient herself and not upon the interests of the fetus which she bore. However, the reality was that the fetus was a fully formed child, capable of normal life if only it could be delivered from the mother.

[Emphasis added.]

The woman was safely delivered, but her reaction to the intervention is not known as she left the area.

On 5th December 1996, there was another application regarding a woman, Ms L, with alleged needle phobia. Kirkwood J heard this case over the telephone, speaking to her doctors and the Trust barrister but not to the woman.

In February 1996, Blackburn Hospital applied for an order, *Re MB*, for a woman with a footling breech presentation who had been advised to have a CS. She had agreed, but when the anaesthetic was about to be administered, she refused because she apparently had a needle phobia. The Court ordered the CS, ruling that she lacked capacity because of the panic induced by her fear of needles. The procedure was carried out the following day. Again the woman was not legally represented. She appealed, and in April 1997 the case was heard before three judges, who accepted that she had temporarily lacked the capacity to consent but strongly reiterated the right of a competent adult to refuse treatment. They said:

Every person is presumed to have the capacity to consent to or to refuse medical treatment unless and until that presumption is rebutted. A competent woman who has the capacity to decide may, for religious reasons, other reasons, for rational or irrational reasons or for no reason at all, choose not to have medical intervention, even though the consequence may be the death or serious handicap of the child she bears, or her own death. In that event, the courts do not have the jurisdiction to declare medical intervention lawful and the question of her own best interests, objectively considered, does not arise. (*Re MB*, 1997.)

The judges suggested some guidelines for hospitals faced with the situation where a woman might lack the capacity to consent to medical treatment because of mental illness or inability to comprehend the information.

In February 1998, Ms S appealed against the judgment in April 1996 which had forced her to undergo a CS whilst detained under the Mental Health Act. The Court of Appeal allowed the appeal and granted leave for judicial review (*St George's Healthcare NHS Trust* v *S*, 1998), saying:

Even when his or her own life depended on receiving medical treatment, an adult of sound mind was entitled to refuse it; ... although pregnancy increased the personal responsibilities of the woman, it did not diminish her entitlement to decide whether to undergo medical treatment. An unborn child was not a separate person from its mother and its need for medical assistance did not prevail over her right not to be forced to submit to an invasion of her body against her will, whether her own life or that of her unborn child depended on it, and that right was not reduced or diminished merely because her decision might appear morally repugnant.

Unless lawfully justified, the removal of the baby from within the applicant's body under physical compulsion constituted an infringement of her autonomy and amounted to a trespass, and the perceived needs of the foetus [sic] did not provide the necessary justification. Granting judicial review and ordering the appropriate declarations, the Court held that an individual was not suffering from mental disorder and could not be detained under the Mental Health Act 1983 against his will merely because his thinking process was unusual and contrary to the views of the overwhelming majority of the community at large. Unless an individual case fell within the prescribed conditions, the Mental Health Act of 1983 could not be used to justify detention for mental disorder, and a patient so detained could not be forced into medical procedures unconnected with his mental condition unless his capacity to consent to such treatment was diminished. The necessary care and treatment for the applicant's pregnancy was not treatment for which she could be admitted to hospital under the Act of 1983, nor could it be argued that the unborn child was a 'person' in need of protection.

The unlawfulness of the applicant's transfer and detention in the general hospital would have entitled her to make an application for habeas corpus which would have led to her immediate release; her transfer back to the mental hospital and subsequent detention before her final discharge ... were therefore unlawful.

There are several disturbing features about these cases, first the fact that five of the seven women in cases where orders were obtained were unrepresented by a solicitor or barrister, so that their side of the story was not heard. In the first case, *Re S* (1992), the Official Solicitor acted as the representative but had no discussion with the woman; in the *St George*'s case the hospital solicitors did not communicate with Ms S's solicitors, and the judge did not know she had instructed them.

A second disturbing element is the speed with which the cases were decided by the judges, often on inadequate or incorrect medical evidence. For example, the *St George*'s case (1998) was heard in the lunch break; the Court was told that the woman had been in labour for 24 hours and 'every minute counted', both statements being untrue.

Thirdly, some judges appeared to be acting to protect the fetus, as in the cases of *Re S* (1992) and Ms S of 1996, despite the fact that the fetus is not a person in English law. Is there a move to change the law, despite the forceful arguments that have been restated by Butler Sloss et al. in the *MB* and the *St George*'s cases? In 1988, Balcombe J turned down an application by social workers to admit a pregnant woman for the good of her fetus, stating:

Approaching the question as one of principle, in my judgement, there is no jurisdiction to make an unborn child a ward of court. Since an unborn child has, *ex hypothesi*, no existence independent of its mother, the only purpose of extending the jurisdiction to include a foetus [sic] is to enable the mother's actions to be controlled. Indeed that is the purpose of the present action.

Two cases where putative fathers aimed to prevent women from having a legal abortion, *Paton* v *British Pregnancy Advisory Service* (1979) and *C* v *S* (1987), both upheld the woman's right to have a legal abortion. Sir George Baker, president of the Family Court, said in the first case:

The first question is whether this plaintiff has a right at all. The foetus [sic] cannot, in English law, in my view have any right of its own at least until it is born and has a separate existence from its mother. That permeates the whole of the civil law of this country (I except the criminal law which is now irrelevant) and is, indeed the basis of the decisions in those countries where law is founded on the common law, that is today, in America, Canada, Australia and, I have no doubt, in others.

However, Lord Donaldson in *Re T* (1992), a case where a pregnant woman involved in a car accident required a blood transfusion, raised a question in his judgment:

An adult patient, who like Miss T, suffers from no mental incapacity, has an absolute right to choose one rather than another of the treatments being offered. The only possible qualification is a case in which the choice may lead to the death of a viable foetus [sic]. That is not this case and, if and when it arises, the courts will be faced with a novel problem of considerable legal and ethical complexity.

No one would have thought such a problem could be decided in 18 minutes, as occurred in the case of S in October of that year (Hewson, 1992).

American courts first forced pregnant women to have blood transfusions in 1974 (*Riley–Fitkin–Paul* v *Anderson*, 1964; *In re President of Georgetown College*, 1964) and later to undergo CS operations. From 1973, for the sake of the fetus, women in the US have been ordered to have treatment or given unusually heavy sentences for drug offences, but the climate has changed since 1990 after the Angela Carder appeal (see Chapter 7). More recently in 1997, in another such case involving glue-sniffing, the Canadian Supreme Court accepted a woman's autonomy by a 7–2 majority. McLachlin J said:

Judicial intervention ... ignores the basic components of women's fundamental human rights – the right to bodily integrity, and the right to equality, privacy and dignity... The common law does not clothe the courts with power to order the detention of a pregnant woman for the purpose of preventing her from harming her unborn child. Nor, given the magnitude of the changes and their potential ramifications, would it be appropriate for the courts to extend their power to make such an order. (*Winnipeg Child & Family Services*, 1997.)

In another early US case, the judge ordered a CS as the obstetrician said the woman could not deliver normally, because of a placenta praevia detected on ultrasound. The placenta lies in front of the baby in the lower part of the uterus, and bleeding may kill the woman if an operation is not done. The woman delivered normally before the operation could be performed (Kolder, Gallagher and Parsons, 1987).

In summary, women have been forced by the courts to undergo blood transfusions, operative deliveries and admission to hospital for treatment in the US and more recently in the UK. Judges have exhibited a paternalistic attitude, placing the non-existent legal rights of the fetus above the woman's autonomy. However, in the UK, the Court of Appeal judgments in 1997 and 1998 have stated clearly that a pregnant woman has the right to refuse medical treatment. There remains a possibility that some lawyers will try to use the European Court of Human Rights to attempt to change the law to give the fetus legal status.

Ethical issues

The debate about forced CS usually focuses on the conflict between maternal and fetal rights, but as Draper (1996) points out, the woman, as in the Angela Carder case, may consider that she knows best about her unborn child. Angela Carder considered the fetus was too immature to survive, and she was right. In another US case, a woman with nine children refused a CS advised by the doctors because the cord was round the baby's neck. She considered that her other children would suffer if she had a CS, which would also hurt her, whereas a dead baby she could accept. Judge Margaret Taylor in 1982 declined to order a CS. The baby was born normally and was healthy. Judge Taylor added that once women are denied the right to refuse treatment at delivery, there are logically no lengths to which doctors and courts cannot go to protect life (Hewson, 1992).

In the majority of cases it seems that there has been a breakdown in the doctor–patient relationship, either because of current or past mental illness, or because the doctor cannot accept the woman's right to make her own decisions. The ethical principles of autonomy, beneficence and non-maleficence may be difficult for a hard-pressed clinician to cope with, when faced with the dilemma of a woman refusing medical advice which may lead to her death or the death of her unborn child. The latter may benefit, but the woman may not. If her autonomy is to be overridden and she is forced to accept an invasion of her body for the sake of her child, the doctor or medical/midwifery team may be physically subduing her. Can this be ethical behaviour?

If women must accept such surgery for the sake of their children (and of course the vast majority do without any question) should not parents donate organs for the sake of their children? Naturally the majority would do so, but should they be compelled to make such a sacrifice? As Robert Francis QC said in a lecture to the Medico-Legal Society in 1995 (Francis, 1995):

The trouble with *Re S* is, if it is correct, that we have to face an expanding range of cases in which a patient is obliged to submit to surgery in the interests of a child. After all, if surgery is mandatory to save the life of a viable fetus, why should a parent not be compelled to donate bone marrow or a kidney to a child who will die without the benefit of such donation? If such cases are to be prevented on the grounds that the interests of the parents and child must coincide, how is that requirement squared with the established law where a person's objective best interests are to be subordinated to his express will?

In *McFall* v *Shimp* (1978), a US case, the cousin of a person who required a bone-marrow transplant as treatment for leukaemia, declined to donate. Flaherty J. ruled in his favour, saying:

Our society, contrary to many others, has as its first principle the respect for the individual, and that society and government exist to protect the individual from being invaded and hurt by another. Many societies accept a contrary view which has the individual existing to serve the society as a whole. In preserving such a society as we have it is bound to happen that great moral conflicts will arise and will appear harsh in a given instance ... Morally this decision rests with the defendant, and in the view of the court the refusal of the defendant is morally indefensible. For our law to compel the defendant to submit to an intrusion of his body would change every concept and principle upon which our society is founded. To do so would defeat the sanctity of the individual.

Medical issues

The quality of the medical care in these cases does not always seem to have been high; nor was there really a medical emergency, in some instances. For example, in the Caroline Spear case, there was no reason why she should not have been allowed a trial of vaginal breech delivery, and if the registrar was not competent to conduct this, the consultant could have come in to teach. Alternatively, as she was in early labour, she could have been transferred to another hospital where vaginal breech deliveries were done.

I have met with a refusal to have a CS only twice in 35 years of obstetric practice. The first, a woman in Nigeria, told me at about 5.00 a.m. that she did not want a CS, which I had recommended because she appeared to be in obstructed labour in her fifth pregnancy, as she always delivered when the sun rose. I told her that I thought this baby was bigger and she would not do so this time. When the sun rose at 6.45 a.m. and she was still not delivered, she agreed to a CS.

The second woman was only 16 years old, and did not speak English; her husband, who was a devout Muslim, would not agree to a CS. When it became apparent that she was not going to deliver after several hours of full dilatation, he agreed, but sadly the baby died. However, when she returned the next year, he accepted our advice and she went on to have six more children by CS because she had a small pelvis. At the age of 26 she had a premature baby at 28 weeks, born normally. If we had gone to court would he have tried to have his wife deliver at home the next time and perhaps die from a ruptured uterus? An unanswerable question.

George Annas writing in the *New England Journal of Medicine* in 1987, said:

It is not helpful to use the law to convert a woman's and society's moral responsibility to her fetus into the woman's legal responsibility alone. The best chance we have to protect fetuses is through enhancing the status of all women by fostering reasonable pay for the work they do, providing equal employment opportunities and adequate daycare, providing a reasonable social safety net, and ensuring all pregnant women access to high quality pre-natal services... By protecting the liberty of the pregnant woman and the integrity of the voluntary doctor–patient relationship, we not only promote autonomy, we also promote the well-being of the vast majority of fetuses.

If doctors lose the trust of women because they compel them to undergo surgery, they are flying in the face of patient autonomy and the shared decision-making that characterizes medicine today. But if we give up our professional training and merely act as a technician performing surgery at the behest of the woman, without questioning her reasons, we will lose our right to be considered a profession.

References

American College of Obstetricians and Gynecologists (ACOG) (1987). *Patients' Choice: Maternal/Fetal Conflict.* Washington, DC: ACOG Statement Committee on Ethics.

Annas, G. (1987). Protecting the liberty of pregnant patients. *New England Journal of Medicine* **316**: 1213–14.

Audit Commission (1997). *First-Class Delivery: Improving Maternity Services in England and Wales.* Abingdon: Audit Commission Publications.

Bump, H. and Norton, P. (1998). Epidemiology and natural history of pelvic floor dysfunction. *Clinics of North America Obstetrics and Gynecology* **25**: 723–46.

C v S [1987] All ER 1230.

Clark, S.L., Koonings, P.P. and Phelan, J.P. (1985). Placenta praevia/accreta and previous caesarean section. *Obstetrics and Gynaecology* **66**: 89–92.

Clarke, S.C. and Taffel, S.M. (1996). Rates of Cesarean and VBAC delivery, United States 1994. *Birth* **23**: 166–8.

Confidential Inquiry into Stillbirths and Deaths in Infancy (CESDI) (1998). *Fifth Annual Report.* Maternal and Child Health Research Consortium. London: Department of Health, HMSO.

de Costa, C. (1998). A sort of progress. *Lancet* **351**: 1202–3.

Department of Health (1993). *Changing Childbirth. Report of the Expert Maternity Group Chaired by Cumberledge J.* London: HMSO.

Department of Health (1997). *Statistical Bulletin: NHS Maternity Statistics 1989–90 to 1994–5.* London: HMSO.

Department of Health, Welsh Office, Scottish Office Home and Health Department, and Department of Health and Social Services, Northern Ireland (1994). *Report On Confidential Inquiries into Maternal Deaths in the United Kingdom 1988–90.* London: HMSO.

Department of Health, Welsh Office, Scottish Office Home and Health Department, and Department of Health and Social Services, Northern Ireland (1997). *Report On Confidential Inquiries into Maternal Deaths in the United Kingdom 1991–3.* London: HMSO.

Department of Health, Welsh Office, Scottish Office Home and Health Department, and Department of Health and Social Services, Northern Ireland (1998). *Why Mothers Die. Report On Confidential Inquiries into Maternal Deaths in the United Kingdom 1994–6.* London: HMSO.

Department of Health and Human Services (1991). *Healthy People 2000.* DHSS Pub. No. (PHS) 91–50212. Washington, DC: DHHS.

Draper, H. (1996). Women, forced Caesareans and antenatal responsibilities. *Journal of Medical Ethics* **22**: 327–33.

Durand, A.M. (1992). The safety of home birth: the farm study. *American Journal of Public Health* **82**: 450–2.

Dyer, C. (1997). Birth of a dilemma. *Guardian,* 3 March.

English National Board for Nursing, Midwifery and Health Visiting (ENBNMHV) (1998). *Report of the Audit of Midwifery Practice.* London: ENB.

FIGO Committee for the Ethical Aspects of Human Reproduction and Women's

Health (1999). *International Journal of Obstetrics and Gynecology* **64**: 317–22.

Francis, R. (1995). Lecture. *Medico-Legal Journal* **63**: 19.

General Medical Council (1995). *The Duties of a Doctor: Good Medical Practice.* London: GMC.

Gibb, F. (1997). Judge 'misled' into ordering a Caesarean section. *Times*, 15 March.

Graham, W.J., Hundley, V., McCheyne, A.L., Hall, M.H., Gurney, E. and Milne, J. (1999). An investigation of women's involvement in the decision to deliver by Caesarean section. *British Journal of Obstetrics and Gynaecology* **106**: 213–20.

Hall, M. (1994). 'Audit'. In *The Future of the Maternity Services,* ed. G. Chamberlain and N. Patel, pp. 190–4. London: RCOG Press.

Hemminki, E., Graubard, B.I., Hoffman, H.J., Mosher, W.D. and Fetterly, K. (1985). Cesarean section and subsequent fertility: results from the 1982 national survey of family growth, Birmingham, Alabama. *Fertility and Sterility* **43**: 520–8.

Hewson, B. (1992). When 'no' means 'yes'. *Law Society Gazette* **45**: 2.

In re AC [1990] 573 A 2d 1235 (D.C. App. 1990).

In re President of Georgetown College, Inc. [1964]. 331 F.2d 1000.

Jackson, N.V. and Irvine, L.M. (1998). The influence of maternal request on the elective Caesarean section rate. *Journal of Obstetrics and Gynaecology* **118**: 115–19.

Jolly, J., Walker, J. and Bhabra, K. (1999). Subsequent obstetric performance related to primary mode of delivery. *British Journal of Obstetrics and Gynaecology* **106**: 227–37.

Kolder, V.E., Gallagher, J. and Parsons, M.T. (1987). Court-ordered obstetrical interventions. *New England Journal of Medicine* **316**: 1192–6.

Lomas, J. and Enkin, M. (1989). Variations in operative delivery rates. In *Effective Care in Pregnancy and Childbirth,* ed. I. Chalmers, M. Enkin M and M. Kierse, pp. 1182–95. Oxford: Oxford University Press.

MacArthur, C., Bick, D.E. and Keighley, M.R.B. (1997). Faecal incontinence after childbirth. *British Journal of Obstetrics and Gynaecology* **104**: 46–50.

McFall v *Shimp* [1978]. 127 Pitts.L.J.14.

Mackenzie, I.Z. (1999). Should women who elect to have Caesarean sections pay for them? *British Medical Journal* **318**: 1070.

McIlwaine, G., Boulton-Jones, C., Cole, S. and Wilkinson, C. (1998). *Caesarean Section in Scotland 1994/5: A National Audit.* University of Edinburgh: Scottish Programme for Clinical Effectiveness in Reproductive Health.

McIlwaine, G., Cole, S. and Macnaughton, M. (1985). The rising Caesarean section rate – a matter for concern? *Health Bulletin* **43**: 301–5.

Murray, S.E. and Serani Pradenas, F. (1997). Caesarean birth trends in Chile, 1986 to 1994. *Birth* **24**: 258–63.

Nice, C., Feeney, A., Godwin, P. et al. (1996). A prospective audit of wound infection rates after Caesarean section in five West Yorkshire hospitals. *Journal of Hospital Infection* **33**: 55–61.

Norfolk and Norwich Healthcare (NHS) Trust v *W* [1997] 1 F.C.R 269.

Notzon, F.C. (1990). International differences in the use of obstetric interventions. *Journal of the American Medical Association* **263**: 3286–91.

Paterson Browne, S. and Fisk, N.M. (1999). Caesarean section: every woman's right to choose? *Current Opinion in Obstetrics and Gynaecology* **9**: 351–5.

Paton v *British Pregnancy Advisory Service* [1979] QB 276.

Re C (Refusal of Medical Treatment) [1994] 1 FLR 31.

Re F (in utero) [1988] 2 All ER 193.

Re MB (Adult: Medical treatment). [1997] 2 FCR 541. C.A.

Re S (Adult refusal of treatment) [1992] 4 All ER 671.

Re S (Hospital Patient: Court's Jurisdiction) [1996] Fam 123

Re T (An adult) (Consent to Medical Treatment) [1992] 4 All ER 649.

Riley-Fitkin-Paul Morgan Memorial Hospital v *Anderson* [1964] 42 NJ 421/201 A.2d 537.

Rochdale Healthcare (NHS) Trust v *C* [1997] 1 F.C.R 274, in *Hempson's Lawyer*, 1996.

Rothwell, H. (1996). Changing childbirth...changing nothing. *Midwives*, 109, **1306**: 291–4.

Royal College of Obstetricians and Gynaecologists Ethics Committee (RCOG) (1993). *A Consideration of the Law and Ethics in relation to Court-Authorised Obstetric Intervention*. London: RCOG Press.

Ryding, E.L. (1993). Investigation of 33 women who demanded CS for personal reasons. *Acta Obstetrica et Gynecologica Scandinavica* **72**: 280–5.

St George's Healthcare NHS Trust v *S* [1998] 3 W.L.R. 936 C.A.

Sakala, C. (1993). Medically unnecessary Cesarean section births: introduction to a symposium. *Social Science and Medicine* **37**: 1177–98.

Savage, W. (1990). The rising Caesarean section rate: anxiety, not science. In *Obstetrics for the 1990s: Current Controversies*, ed. T. Chard and M.P.M. Richards, pp. 177–91. London: MacKeith Press.

Scottish Health Services (1997). *Births in Scotland 1976–1995*. Edinburgh: Information and Statistics Division, Common Services Agency.

Select Committee Report (1992). *Maternity Services: Preconceptual Care, Antenatal Care and Delivery (The Winterton Report)*. House of Commons Health Committee, 1991–2 Session, vol. I-III, pp. xciv–xcv. London: HMSO.

Sleep, J., Grant, A., Garcia, J., et al. (1984). West Berkshire perineal management trial. *British Medical Journal* **289**: 587–91.

Sleep, J. and Grant, A. (1987). West Berkshire perineal management trial 3-year follow-up. *British Medical Journal* **295**: 49–51.

Snooks, S.J. and Swash, M. (1984). Abnormalities of innervation of the urethral striated sphincter musculature in incontinence. *British Journal of Urology* **56**: 401–5.

Sultan, A.H., Kamm, M.A., Hudson, C.H., et al. (1993). Anal-sphincter disruption during vaginal delivery. *New England Journal of Medicine* **329**: 1905–11.

Sultan, A. and Stanton, S. (1996). Preserving the pelvic floor and perineum-elective CS? *British Journal of Obstetrics and Gynaecology* **103**: 731–4.

Tameside and Glossop Acute Services NHS Trust v *C.H* [1996] 1 FCR. 753.

Tetzschner, T., Sorensen, M., Lose, G. and Christiansen, J. (1996). Anal and urinary incontinence in women with obstetric anal sphincter rupture. *British Journal of Obstetrics and Gynaecology* **103**: 1034–40.

Treffers, P.E., Eskes, M., Kleiverda, G. and van Alten, D. (1990). Home births and minimal medical intervention. *Journal of the American Medical Association* **17**: 2203–8.

van Alten, D., Eskes, M. and Treffers, P.E. (1989). Midwifery in the Netherlands: the Wormerveer study, selection, mode of delivery, perinatal mortality and infant morbidity. *British Journal of Obstetrics and. Gynaecology* **96**: 656–62.

Winnipeg Child and Family Services (North West Area) v G [1997] 3 B.H.R.C. 611.

World Health Organization (1985). Appropriate technology for birth. *Lancet* **2**: 436–7.

Zetterstrom, J.P., Lopez, A., Anzen, B., Dokk, A., Norman, M. and Mellgren, A. (1999). Anal incontinence after vaginal delivery: a prospective study in primiparous women. *British Journal of Obstetrics and Gynaecology* **106**: 324–30.

18

Judgements of non-compliance in pregnancy

Françoise Baylis[1] and Susan Sherwin[2]

Departments of Bioethics[1] and Philosophy[2], Dalhousie University, Halifax, Canada

Introduction

Medical knowledge regarding the ways in which women can actively pursue healthy pregnancies and the birth of healthy infants covers an increasingly broad spectrum of activities before, during and after the usual nine months of pregnancy. In fact, depending upon the clinical situation, the number and range of activities are such that, if a woman were to take all obstetrical advice seriously, she would be faced with a daunting list of instructions ranging from mere suggestions to strong professional recommendations. Few women could (or would want to) fully adapt their lives to the entire range of advice from physicians, midwives, nurses, nutritionists, physiotherapists and childbirth educators, and generally this is not a problem. In principle, professional advice is something that patients can choose to follow or not – this is the essence of informed choice (Faden and Beauchamp, 1986). In some instances, however, failure to follow professional recommendations elicits pejorative judgements of non-compliance, and while these judgements are provoked by a failure to comply with specific advice, typically they are applied to the patient as a whole. Moreover, even if the patient ultimately consents to the recommended course of action, she may continue to carry the label of non-compliant because of her initial efforts to resist medical authority, and this labelling frequently has repercussions for her subsequent interactions with health care professionals.

Some health care providers now use the terms adherence and non-adherence instead of compliance and non-compliance in an effort to promote more ethically sound interactions between themselves and their patients. We agree with Feinstein, however, that there is no 'preferred substitute for compliance. *Adherence* seems too sticky; *fidelity* has too many other connotations; and *maintenance* suggests a repair crew. Although *adherence* has its advocates, compliance continues to be the most popular term for lack of anything better' (Feinstein, 1990).

In this paper we explore the factors that go into judging a woman to be non-compliant in the context of pregnancy and consider the implications of such judgements. Though we recognize that these judgements can be made by one or more members of the health care team, we focus here on physician–

patient interactions. We are particularly interested in understanding what is problematic in the circumstances that elicit judgements of patient non-compliance from the perspectives of both the physician and the patient. Towards that end, we explore a number of scenarios in which these judgements may arise and try to understand the reasons for the patient's behaviour and for the physician's decision to apply that label. Further, we consider the implications for the patient–physician relationship of invoking a framework that evaluates patient behaviours and choices in terms of compliance and non-compliance. Finally, we suggest that a subset of the behaviours and choices that the language of non-compliance now captures are not inherently problematic. They ought not to be construed as non-compliance, but rather as informed or uninformed refusals. In our view, the only situations that are inherently problematic are those where the patient fails to comply with her own choices which may or may not be consistent with directions from her physician. A commitment to provide respectful health care requires that these situations be dealt with in a way that enhances, rather than undermines, autonomy-respecting, integrity-preserving patient–physician interactions.

The scope of compliance/non-compliance judgements

To situate the experience of women who are judged to be non-compliant with respect to obstetrical advice, we review the range of advice that women are likely to receive before, during and after pregnancy.

The advice

Medical advice about pregnancy and pregnancy-related behaviours begins before conception. There are medical opinions on who should become pregnant, when and under what circumstances. For example, women diagnosed with a serious medical condition that makes pregnancy extremely hazardous for themselves and/or their fetuses (e.g. cyanotic heart disease, brittle diabetes or AIDS) are among those who may be advised not to become pregnant. Frequently these women require medication to control their own illnesses, and in some cases their doctors worry that these medications may have an adverse effect on the developing fetus. Of equal concern are the health risks to the women should they decide to stop or alter their medications during pregnancy. Particularly troublesome in this regard are cases of mental illness such as schizophrenia or depression where women's ability to function in society is thought to be dependent upon continued use of the prescribed medication. In such circumstances, women who choose to become pregnant against medical advice are faced with the unpalatable choice of continuing their medication and risking the well-being of their future child, or abstaining from its use for the duration of the pregnancy and seriously risking their own health and independence.

For women who intend to become pregnant, there is also advice on the timing of conception. From a medical point of view, it is best to bear children in early adulthood (from late teens to early thirties). Pregnancy too late in a woman's life can increase the health risks to both the woman and the fetus. For example, women over 40 years of age face an increased rate of gestational diabetes and hypertension as well as an increased rate of fetal chromosomal anomalies. Further, in some cases there will be patient-specific advice regarding the timing of conception because of the woman's particular health status and needs. For example, a woman with severe cervical dysplasia could be advised to delay pregnancy until her treatment was complete. Sometimes advice about the timing of conception is followed, sometimes not; and sometimes this is intentional, sometimes not.

In addition to the above, there is medical advice about a range of pre-conception behaviours that may affect the medical outcome of pregnancy. For example, in the months before pregnancy it is important to eat a well-balanced diet and take folic acid supplements to reduce the risk of spina bifida and other neural tube defects. For this reason, family doctors and gynaecologists post notices in their offices directing women to consult them if they are 'thinking about becoming pregnant in the next few months.' Despite extensive efforts to educate fertile women about the benefits of pre-conceptual folic acid however, many remain unaware of these benefits. And among those who are aware of the benefits of folic acid supplementation there is still a high rate of incorrect usage (Metson et al., 1995; Roberts, 1996).

Further, before pregnancy is initiated women will be advised to overcome addictions to such dangerous substances as tobacco, crack cocaine, anabolic steroids and solvents. From a medical perspective this advice is hardly optional. From the woman's perspective this advice, though sound, may be impossible to follow; addictions are not simply about choice (Baylis, 1998). Unfortunately, some physicians seem to have little appreciation for the powers of addictions and become very angry with women who expose their fetuses to harm for the sake of a smoke or a high. (For further discussion see Chapter 8 by Susan Bewley.)

Once women do become pregnant, they are enjoined to become patients and the medical advice they receive typically becomes more direct and potentially overwhelming. Prenatal care usually includes advice on virtually all aspects of a woman's life, including:

- diet (eat plenty of green, leafy vegetables, consume lots of calcium, monitor weight gain);
- exercise (do this in moderation, with some activities curtailed);

- work, including unpaid housework (avoid exposure to dangerous chemicals, heavy lifting; reduce hours and stress; in certain circumstances, give up work altogether and remain confined to bed);
- prescription and over-the-counter drugs (avoid most, take care with others);
- tobacco (stop smoking and also avoid second-hand smoke)
- alcohol (avoid drinking)
- recreational drugs (stop);
- sex (continue as comfortable).

Further, women with pre-existing medical conditions that make pregnancy particularly hazardous, and those who develop serious conditions such as hypertension in the course of pregnancy, will receive much more urgent and case-specific instructions. With due diligence, but varying degrees of success, most women will try to follow these directives. Among those who fail, some will be labelled non-compliant.

Also, during pregnancy women are likely to be given advice regarding genetic counselling and testing, particularly if their pregnancy results from the use of reproductive technologies, or if they are considered at above average risk of giving birth to a child with a serious disease or disorder. This latter category includes women of 'advanced maternal age', women with a family history of genetic disease, and women who are members of an at-risk community (e.g. elevated risk of Tay–Sachs disease among Ashkenazi-derived communities). If a woman follows such advice and certain fetal anomalies are detected, or the woman is found to be carrying multiple embryos, more advice will likely be forthcoming (claims about non-directive counselling, notwithstanding). In some cases, the woman may be advised to terminate her pregnancy or undergo selective fetal reduction. In other cases, as when the fetus has a major congenital anomaly that could be corrected in utero, she may be encouraged to consent to fetal therapy or research (Caniano and Baylis, 1999). Not surprisingly, women's responses to such advice varies considerably.

Doctors also have firm opinions about the best ways of managing the potentially complicated and dangerous final stages of pregnancy – labour and delivery. The timing, mode and location of delivery are all subject to strong medical advice and are frequently the source of serious contests of will between patients and their doctors. For example, it is not uncommon for some women to question their doctors about the wisdom of initiating and continuing tocolysis for preterm labour or inducing labour for worsening gestational hypertension (Lettrie et al., 1993). There can also be serious disagreement regarding the need for Caesarean section, anaesthetic, episiotomy or forceps, as well as disagreement about the participants to be involved in the delivery including the roles of midwife, labour coach and children. A patient's resistance to medical preferences on such matters may be interpreted as non-compliance on the part of worried and exasperated physicians.

The location of delivery can also be a contentious issue. In North America, particularly, doctors tend to be wary of home births. Further, depending upon the circumstances of the pregnancy, physicians may want to insist that women travel to a tertiary care centre fully equipped with all necessary technology. For women in remote rural areas, these demands can be especially burdensome.

Finally, medical care does not end after women have given birth. The postpartum woman will be advised to return to her family physician for follow-up care to make sure that her uterus has involuted (returned to normal size), there are no infections or cervical abnormalities (pap smear), blood pressure has returned to normal, nutritional status is adequate, and so on. At this time, the woman will receive advice about the appropriate period of time to wait before becoming pregnant again and options for contraception. There will also be questions about, and advice relevant to, the mother–child relationship, nursing, coping and general fatigue. As well, the newborn(s) will be monitored to ensure adequate nutrition and appropriate growth. The general expectation is that 'good' mothers will comply with physician advice on how best to promote their own and their child's health and well-being.

Implications of the compliance and non-compliance framework

As the above clearly shows, there is an overwhelming amount of expert medical advice directed at women who are contemplating pregnancy or are currently pregnant. Moreover, this advice is layered on top of abundant general health advice (e.g. about good oral health, breast self-examinations, stress management and so on), as well as advice about proper care of existing children, households and partners. Few women will manage to follow all of this advice and most will diverge at least to some degree from the directions they are offered. Happily, most women none the less will emerge from pregnancy with their own health and that of their fetuses intact. Moreover, many will escape the label of non-compliant. It is worth observing, then, when physicians evaluate failure to act in accordance with medical advice in terms of the compliance and non-compliance framework, and when they do not.

It appears that judgements of compliance and non-compliance are reserved for circumstances in which there exists a physician–patient relationship or formal interaction. Since most healthy fertile women do not assume the role of obstetrical patient until they are pregnant and seeking routine prenatal care, it is unusual for these labels to be invoked (with respect to reproduction-related behaviours) prior to conception. Physicians may worry about women who conceive outside of the ideal time frame, eat inadequate diets, or consume dangerous substances – and some will make disapproving moral judgements regarding those who flagrantly ignore widely available medical knowledge – but most doctors are unlikely to label such women non-compliant. Failure to act in accordance with general directives for initiating a healthy pregnancy may be regretted, and may even be construed as evidence of poor judgement, but such failure is unlikely to be perceived as non-compliance. It is quite a different matter, however, when the women are in the specific role of patient 'under the care of' a physician (or clinic), where failure to comply involves the rejection of patient-specific medical advice.

None the less, not all divergence from physician opinion will evoke the label non-compliant. For example, the term is seldom used when the behaviour in question is within a morally contested realm such as prenatal genetic testing. In the face of public and professional debates about the appropriateness of the genetics agenda, refusal of genetic testing is generally tolerated. Also, the label non-compliant is seldom used when patients demonstrate excessive enthusiasm for medical interventions deemed unnecessary. For example, patients who request Caesarean deliveries that their doctors do not consider medically required may have their requests refused, but they are unlikely to be seen as non-compliant. (See Chapter 17.) The same is true with patients who request/demand an amniocentesis in the absence of professionally accepted risk factors. Thus, it appears that failure to act in accordance with patient-specific medical advice is a necessary but not a sufficient condition for being so labelled.

The label non-compliant is readily assigned, however, in cases where there is a perceived risk of serious harm for the fetus or the woman that is avoidable but for the woman's failure to comply with her physician's recommendations. The paradigm of non-compliance is women who continue to smoke or drink (or sniff solvents, use crack cocaine or other illegal drugs) during pregnancy, and women who do not defer to medical expertise during labour and delivery (Greenwall, 1990; Lescale et al., 1996).

Some clear patterns emerge regarding judgements of compliance and non-compliance. First, these judgements not only denote the existence of a doctor–patient (or health care professional–patient) relationship (or formal interaction), they also reflect certain assumptions about the nature of that relationship. Specifically, the framework of patient compliance and non-compliance expresses a commitment to an implicit hierarchical structure within medicine, in that these terms reflect an understanding of the doctor–patient relationship as inherently unequal. The labels compliant and non-compliant apply in cases where those with greater power have issued directives to those with less power, and these directives have either been followed or set aside. In marked contrast, those with lesser power can only make requests of those with greater authority. For example, patients who refuse to act in accordance with physicians' professional recommendations can be deemed non-compliant with medical advice. On the other hand, physicians who refuse to act in accordance with women's requests may be judged uncooperative, but not non-compliant. To be sure, it is possible for physicians to be labelled non-compliant, but in their case it is not for failure to respond to patients' demands, but rather for failure to comply with practice norms or professional guidelines, such as established protocols, prescription standards or research criteria. (See, for example, Cheon-Lee and Amstey, 1998; Helfgott et al., 1998.)

Furthermore, within the doctor–patient relationship the label non-compliant does not simply record the patient's divergence from prescribed behaviours, it also expresses/implies disapproval of, and disappointment in, the patient's behaviour. When the label is invoked, there is a presumption that something has gone seriously wrong in the relationship and that blame should be assigned. Physicians applying the label non-compliant generally intend to assign that blame to patients, particularly when patients refuse interventions that are standard care. From the physician's perspective such refusals not only represent needless risks with the future well-being of the patient and/or her offspring, but they also create potential problems of legal liability in the event of a 'bad outcome' and a later claim by the patient about inadequate care. Not surprisingly, physicians may seek to distance themselves from such responsibility.

Interestingly, however, much of the literature tracking this phenomenon suggests that blame for patient non-compliance should rest with physicians and not patients, since it is the responsibility of the former to inform properly and educate patients and, in so doing, to convey adequately the importance of conscientiously following medical advice (DiMatteo and DiNicola, 1982: esp. p. 251). Jonsen, for example, argues that '[t]o refer to the problem as compliance is to pose it as a problem of the behavior of patients and, consequently, to seek its causes in the patient. In so doing, the sins of the careless, irrational, authoritarian physician are visited on the heads of his patients' (Jonsen, 1979). Issues of blame and responsibility aside, there are good reasons to question the labelling of patients as non-compliant. Labelling particular patients in this way emphasizes the authoritarian nature of the physician–patient relationship without usually producing 'better' patient behaviour.

In addition, situating patient behaviours within a framework of compliance and non-compliance discourages development of the trust that is essential for a good doctor–patient relationship. In labelling a patient non-compliant, the physician is expressing his/her distrust in the patient's ability or motivation to make appropriate use of medical expertise. The term is pejorative and often functions as an expression of exasperation at the patient's 'irresponsible' behaviour. For her part, the patient may be sensitive to any moral judgements surrounding her behaviour. She may be wary of negative labels generally and, in particular, worried about being labelled non-compliant and abandoned by her physician if she is judged unworthy. Hence, she may feel anxious about being fully honest with her physician. Rather than bringing her questions and concerns to the forefront, she may tell the physician what she thinks he/she wants to hear and may also seek to minimize the time spent with her physician in order to hide her 'negative' behaviour and avoid disapproving lectures.

Finally, the decision to invoke the framework of compliance and non-compliance works against the goals of informed choice. It does not situate the woman's actions and choices in the context of her own life, but instead constructs and evaluates the patient's behaviour in response to her physician's expressed views regarding the means necessary to achieve a 'good outcome'. The woman's agency is reduced in that she is discouraged from determining her behaviour on the basis of her own perception of what constitutes a good outcome and how best to achieve it. She is expected to follow passively medical instructions or to find herself on the defensive, accounting for her failure to do so. This situation, where consent is *de rigueur,* is clearly at odds with the professed commitment to respect the autonomous choices (i.e. informed consents and informed refusals) of patients.

In sum, the framework of compliance and non-compliance trades on the unequal, hierarchical nature of the physician–patient relationship, potentially denigrates patients, undermines trust, reduces patient agency, and conflicts with the goals of informed choice. Given these problematic implications, it is curious that this framework is so prominent in obstetrics and other areas of medicine.

A closer look at judgements of non-compliance

While there is wide variation among physicians in the appropriate use of the term non-compliant, in general a physician will label a pregnant woman non-compliant when she fails to act in accordance with expressed medical advice that is believed to be of benefit to herself or her fetus. The physician worries that the woman's behaviour unnecessarily increases the risk of avoidable harm. In addition, other factors sometimes influence the physician's decision to apply the label non-compliant. For example, some physicians are personally affronted by their patients' unwillingness to follow their advice; they interpret such action as evidence that the patient lacks respect for their medical expertise. Further, some physicians worry that failure to follow their instructions may have serious economic consequences for the health care or social services system. As such, physicians may invoke the label non-compliant not only when they are concerned on behalf of their patient and her future child, but also when they have concerns about their own dignity and authority and/or about costs that will be borne by the state. And, as noted earlier, physicians sometimes seek to protect themselves from legal actions in anticipation of a preventable 'bad outcome.'

For their part, patients generally will not know that they have been labelled non-compliant, though they may experience the consequences of this labelling and not be able to make sense of their situation, especially if that label follows them through subsequent medical encounters. Some patients, however, will know that they have been labelled and will be angry about this, particularly if from their perspective the medical advice offered is insensitive to their circumstances and an unjust basis for the negative judgement that follows. Other patients will be more upset than angry, and may internalize the implicit negative moral judgement. That is, the labelling may engender guilt and undermine self-esteem. We note here that even though countless studies demonstrate that patients in all areas of medicine routinely diverge from medical directives and that judgements of non-compliance are common throughout medicine (Sackett and Snow, 1979; Cramer and Spilker, 1991), these judgements take on a particular urgency in obstetrics. This is because a non-compliant pregnant patient is thought to be risking not only her own health, but also the well-being of the future child she is expected to be nurturing. Social stereotypes that demand that women be self-sacrificing for the sake of their (future) children judge women especially harshly if they fail to make all reasonable efforts to protect the health of their developing fetuses. It is one thing to be bad at caring for oneself. It is generally considered a far greater flaw for women if they are bad at caring for their (future) children. These judgements are not entirely external. Women tend to internalize the social messages of good mothering and pregnant women may well feel guilt-laden if they suspect their own behaviour could harm their future children.

To understand better the problems that the compliance and non-compliance framework is meant to capture, and to help set the stage for an alternative approach, we review a fairly standard range of behaviours is which patients fail to follow the specific advice of their doctors. In identifying these behaviours, we are particularly interested in understanding whether patients and physicians agree about the nature of the problem. Our aim is to see if other responses might better address the perceived problem than the pejorative labelling represented by judgements of non-compliance and to determine whether the situations might be better described according to alternative frameworks.

Deliberate refusals: value conflict

As noted above, women sometimes make a deliberate decision to reject their physicians' advice because it runs contrary to their values. For example, a woman who has undergone infertility treatment and is carrying three or more fetuses may be advised to submit to selective termination in order to increase the chance of a healthy pregnancy, uncomplicated delivery and the birth of healthy infants. If she is adamantly opposed to abortion, however, she will reject the advice out of hand, as it is in direct conflict with her deep-seated values. As long as the values that the woman is following are clear and accepted within the culture, she is unlikely to be labelled non-compliant. None the less, she may experience less support from her physician as tensions mount because of potential harms associated with her choice. In the abstract, most physicians will formally acknowledge a patient's right to make her own deliberate value choices; in practice, though, some will find it extremely difficult to demonstrate full respect for what they perceive to be poor choices.

Deliberate refusals: epistemological conflict

In other cases, women may agree with the values that inform the physician's recommendation (e.g. promotion of their own health and that of their fetuses), but question the medical knowledge on which that advice is based. Medical knowledge is, after all, imperfect and continually subject to revision and re-interpretation. Consider, for example, how in the past 100 years medical advice regarding morning sickness has changed. In 1899, a pregnant woman might have been advised to take cocaine for nausea (ten minims of a three per cent solution), and to sip champagne to prevent vomiting (Merck, 1899). In the 1950s, tragically, thousands of women worldwide were advised to use thalidomide to control nausea in pregnancy until the disastrous effect on the fetuses' developing limbs became evident. Current wisdom is that soda crackers and a soft drink will frequently relieve nausea (Merck, 1999: pp. 2021–2). Similarly, in recent decades advice on weight gain during pregnancy has varied dramatically: first, women were told that all weight gain was good; subsequently, they were told that weight gain should not exceed the estimated total weight of the placenta and the baby; today, most women of average weight are advised to strive for a weight gain of between 25 and 35 pounds (c. 11 and 16 kg).

Not only are there inconsistencies over time with respect to the information on which medical advice is based, there are sometimes also significant inconsistencies among physicians at any one point in time. For example, there is significant variation in rates of Caesarean deliveries, use of fetal monitors, and numbers of ultrasounds performed in different geographical centres. Not surprisingly, such differences in professional practice patterns undermine patient confidence in expert medical opinion.

A second reason for some women to doubt medical knowledge is evidence of past mistakes. In the 1950s, for example, women considered at risk for miscarriage were advised to take DES (diethylstilboestrol) to reduce the likelihood of miscarriage, even though research failed to establish its effectiveness at this task. The tragic consequences of such marketing include an exceptionally high frequency of genital cancers among the young adults whose mothers took DES while they were pregnant. As this and other mistakes clearly demonstrate, medical opinion sometimes rests on incomplete and inaccurate data.

Finally, women may also doubt medical knowledge because they 'know' better, as when their lived experience (or that of a family member or close friend) contradicts medical dicta. A woman advised to exercise during pregnancy because this will help ease the labour may deny this claim based on personal knowledge – e.g. she may have experienced a long hard labour with her last pregnancy, despite having followed medical advice regarding exercise. Similarly, a woman informed of the need for a Caesarean delivery may remember having a successful vaginal delivery after having been told once before of the need for a Caesarean.

In addition to any doubts that women may have about the validity of particular medical knowledge, there may also be disagreement with the (problematic) epistemological assumption held by many physicians that medical knowledge is preferable to other forms of knowledge and should always be privileged. As feminist epistemologists have argued, there are multiple ways of knowing; scientific knowledge is one form among many. It is a particularly useful way of promoting some forms of understanding, but it cannot account for all types of important information. Experiential, and particularly, embodied ways of knowing provide other essential kinds of knowledge that cannot always be accessed through scientific methods. In the complex, embodied experience of pregnancy, women must depend upon both scientific and experiential forms of knowledge (Abel and Browner, 1998).

For many women an important test of whether their doctor values experiential knowledge is if the doctor is attentive to (and validates) the reports about their experiences through pregnancy. To care well for their obstetrical patients, physicians need to listen carefully to women's descriptions of their bodily experiences. If this is a repeat pregnancy, for example, they should be interested in learning what is different in this experience from that of earlier pregnancies. Often, it is women's own reports that give the first indication of complications or difficulties in a pregnancy. Physicians who disregard women's reports or concerns about their embodied experience in favour of abstract, scientific knowledge may find that their own advice is disregarded in turn because their patients do not believe it was based on all relevant information.

Deliberate refusals: distrust

Some women who intentionally reject medical advice do so not because of conflicting values, or problematic knowledge claims, but rather because of a deep-seated mistrust of physicians and the medical profession as a whole. There is some evidence, for example, that African-Americans who reject medical advice sometimes do so in part as 'a response to racially differentiated histories and sentiments concerning medical intervention and experimentation' (Rapp, 1998, p. 147). In some jurisdictions, women from ethnic-racial minorities are much more likely to be encouraged to accept sterilization as a form of contraception than are women who are part of the dominant social group (Lopez, 1998). So, too, are women with serious mental or physical disabilities. Poor women, especially those dependent on welfare, are subject to intense monitoring and regulation by the state in many aspects of their private life, and may assume that the physician is simply one more agent of the state, intent on extending the state's control ever further into their lives. Lesbian women may sense their doctor's disapproval of their plans to raise children in a non-standard family. And women with serious addictions, especially those with criminal records, may expect that the physician has only contempt for them and little concern for their welfare. Women from these various social groups have reason to see physicians as representing a culture that is hostile to them; hence, they may distrust the physician's commitment to their well-being and that of their children. Under such pervasive conditions of distrust, it is difficult to see why women would choose to follow medical advice unless the value to them of doing so is made very clear to them.

Failure of understanding

There are other cases, however, which differ markedly from the previous examples where patients deliberately decide against accepting medical advice. Specifically, there are many cases in which patients do not follow medical advice simply because they do not fully comprehend the recommendations or instructions they have been given or the reasons behind them. Consider, for example, patients who are taking prescribed medications at the wrong times or in the wrong ways (Lasagna and Hutt, 1991). Another classic example of this problem is missed appointments. A recent study of high-risk pregnant women who failed to keep appointments at an obstetric complications clinic documents a failure to understand the underlying medical condition, the possible impact of this condition on the health of the fetus and the benefits of attending the clinic (Blankson et al., 1994).

Failure of understanding also colours many decisions regarding prenatal testing where patients who are not scientifically literate may have difficulty deciphering the language. Consider, for example, the counter-intuitive use of the medical phrase 'positive test result' to denote a negative outcome. There are also patients who will have difficulty with statistical thinking and who may forgo or accept testing having misunderstood the risk of miscarriage or the risk of carrying a fetus with a chromosomal abnormality.

Inadvertent non-compliance

There are other, more complicated reasons for patients' failure to act according to medical directives, as well. It is not unusual for a patient and physician to agree on the goals of the medical advice, and the legitimacy of the knowledge base upon which it rests. As well, the patient believes in the good will of the physician, understands the advice given and agrees that it should be followed. Nevertheless, the patient does not act in accordance with the medical advice. One reason for this behaviour, as noted earlier, is that there is just too much advice directed at pregnant women and it is simply not practical for anyone to follow it all. It is not a deliberate rejection of the advice but just a reflection of other aims and commitments guiding her activities as well as medical interests.

Medical attention often focuses on specific behaviours without considering the full range of concerns and constraints that structure patients' lives. Consider for example, patients whose jobs depend on working long and unpredictable shifts. They may not eat properly, get adequate exercise or be able to keep their doctors' appointments. They may appear irresponsible to doctors who do not appreciate the lack of control these women have over their time. Similarly, pregnant women who work in unhealthy environments may not be able to change jobs and for financial reasons may not be able to quit working. They may be judged non-compliant if they have been advised that the workplace exposes the developing fetus to toxic substances. Another example of this problem is women who develop diabetes during pregnancy. They will need to learn to test their blood sugar levels frequently, to eat at regular intervals, to modify their diet significantly, and perhaps to administer insulin daily. They can agree with their physicians about the medical need for such adjustments, but still find that the stresses of daily life make adaptation to the recommended regimen very difficult. The demands of work, children, and possibly poverty may militate against their ability to meet some of these prescriptions. Further, their own conflicting emotions about having such a serious disease may foster ambivalent attitudes about fully acknowledging and addressing their state (Martins, 1999).

For other women, apprehension (possibly engendered by a failure of understanding) is another reason for diverging from recommended actions. For example, fear of amniocentesis, chorionic villus sampling and percutaneous umbilical cord sampling is often the reason for missed prenatal diagnosis appointments. In addition, some women will not have access to the support system necessary for them to comply with medical advice – for example, if they have serious addictions they may not be able to stop consuming the dangerous substance(s) on their own, and there are very few treatment programs willing to accept pregnant women.

In yet other cases, patients have difficulty explaining, even to themselves, the reasons for their failure to follow medical advice and feel very confused about their competence as future mothers. The underlying assumption with compliance and non-compliance judgements is that patients are purely rational beings who will follow medical advice if it is fully explained to them and they understand the likely consequences of their behaviour. Yet human beings are more complex than this simplistic picture suggests. Our actions reflect both conscious and unconscious motivations and our reasons for action are not always transparent to us. The biomedical model suggests that experiences should all be subject to rational evaluation and control, but daily life makes it evident that the experience of pregnancy cannot be reduced to this model without losing important dimensions. Emotional and physical experience – yes, even 'intuitions' – need to be acknowledged as part of a patient's motivational structure.

Judgments of non-compliance in review

In the ideal physician–patient relationship, responses to medical advice should be mutually satisfactory, based on mutual respect, mutual under- standing and mutual responsibility. There is no need to speak of non- compliance, since patient and physician come to an agreement on an accept- able and realistic plan. This ideal is not always attainable, however, and sometimes a consensual regimen cannot be negotiated, or, if it can be negotiated, it cannot always be precisely followed. Typically, this is when judgements of non-compliance are invoked.

From a physician perspective, the problem with each of the five categories of behaviour described above is the patient who ignores or rejects medical advice aimed at protecting and promoting her own and her fetus's health and well-being. Significantly, however, the nature of the problem varies with the perspective taken. From a patient perspective, a description of herself as the problem might only apply when failure to act in accordance with the advice received is inadvertent. When a pregnant woman wants and intends to follow her doctor's recommendation(s), but for one or more reasons is unable to do so, she (like her physician) may perceive herself as the problem. On the other hand, when there is a failure of understanding or a deliberate rejection of medical advice – because of a value-conflict, an epistemological conflict, or distrust – the patient may instead describe the problem in terms of physician limitations. For her, the problem is the physician who attempts to pressure her to comply with medical advice by reproaching her for her 'bad' behaviour, who unfairly judges her to be irresponsible, who treats her with suspicion in anticipation of further 'mistakes', or who appears to question her capacity for autonomous decision-making.

When patients choose not to conform to medical advice, physicians need to look for integrity-preserving ways of providing their patients with respectful health care. At the very least, this would involve 'no-fault' attitudes towards behaviour that diverges from what has been recommended (Fink, 1976). More specifically, when patients intentionally refuse medical advice, their behaviours and choices should be respected; to do otherwise is to misunderstand fundamentally where decision-making authority ultimately rests. Such cases should be clearly understood as patients choosing differently than their physicians might hope, not as instances of failures to comply with the instructions of a higher authority.

On the other hand, when patients do not conform to medical advice because they do not understand their situation and the available options before them, physicians should strive to help them make sense of the options before them, perhaps in a context of shared decision-making (Brock, 1991). Here, the aim is to help patients make responsible decisions by providing them with a full understanding of the relevant and available information, including the implications of their own behaviour.

Finally, when patients have understood their options and have chosen to follow medical advice but then fail to do so – for reasons they may or may not understand – they need to be engaged and empowered so that they can identify and effectively pursue their own short- and long-term goals. This is not about better educating or motivating patients or more effectively counselling or persuading them to pursue a particular course of action, but is rather about developing creative strategies for dealing with obstacles that may not be evident or acknowledged by either the patient or her physician.

In this schema, there is no place for the language of compliance and non-compliance – language that is imbued with the hierarchy of medicine and thus is fundamentally at odds with the commitment to promote agency and respect the autonomous choice of patients. Such language inappropriately obscures that which is important, namely, the context within which, and the reason(s) why, a patient does not conform with medical advice. To fashion an ethically acceptable response to situations where patients do not follow medical advice, it is necessary to understand the patient's motives and life setting, the legitimacy of goals other than the pursuit of health, and the limits of individual physicians and of medicine more generally. Seeking appropriate targets for blame inhibits rather than facilitates this task. Following the patient's sense of agency and control is more consistent with a commitment to respectful patient care, and, moreover, helps to support the patient's own desire for achieving a healthy pregnancy.

Acknowledgement

Thanks are owed to Drs Betty Flagler and Barbara Parish, both caring obstetricians, for helpful comments on an earlier draft of this paper.

References

Abel, E.K. and Browner, C.H. (1998). Selective compliance with biomedical authority and the uses of experiential knowledge. In *Pragmatic Women and Body Politics*, ed. M. Lock and P. Kaufert, pp. 310–26. Cambridge: Cambridge University Press.

Baylis, F. (1998). Dissenting with the dissent: Winnipeg Child and Family Services (Northwest Area) *v* G. (D.F.). *Alberta Law Review* **36**: 785–98.

Blankson, M.L., Goldenberg, R.L. and Keith, B. (1994). Noncompliance of high-risk pregnant women in keeping appointments at an obstetrics complications clinic. *Southern Medical Journal* **87**: 634–8.

Brock. D. (1991). The ideal of shared decision-making between physicians and patients. *Kennedy Institute of Ethics Journal* **1**: 28–47.

Caniano, D.A. and Baylis, F. (1999). Ethical considerations in prenatal surgical consultation. *Pediatric Surgery International* **15**: 303–9.

Cheon-Lee, E. and Amstey, M.S. (1998). Compliance with Centers for Disease Control and Prevention antenatal culture protocol for preventing group B strep-tococcal perinatal sepsis. *American Journal of Obstetrics and Gynecology* **179**: 77–9.

Cramer, J.A. and Spilker, B. (Eds) (1991). *Patient Compliance in Medical Practice and Clinical Trials*. New York: Raven Press.

DiMatteo, M.R. and DiNicola, D.D. (1982). *Achieving Patient Compliance: The Psychology of the Medical Practitioner's Role*. New York: Pergamon Press.

Faden, R. and Beauchamp, T.L. (1986). *A History and Theory of Informed Consent*. Oxford: Oxford University Press.

Feinstein, A.R. (1990). On white coat effects and the electronic monitoring of compliance. *Archives of Internal Medicine* **150**: 1377–8.

Fink, D.L. (1976). Tailoring the consensual regimen. In *Compliance with Therapeutic Regimens*, ed. D.L. Sackett and P.B. Haynes, pp. 110–18. Baltimore: Johns Hopkins University Press.

Greenwall, J.L. (1990). Treatment refusal, noncompliance and substance abuse in pregnancy: legal and ethical issues. *Birth* **17**: 152–6.

Helfgott, A.W., Taylor-Burton, J., Garcini, F.J., Ericksen, N.L. and Grimes, R. (1998). Compliance with universal precautions: knowledge and behavior of residents and students in a Department of Obstetrics and Gynecology. *Infectious Disease in Obstetrics and Gynecology* **6**: 123–8.

Jonsen, A.R. (1979). Ethical issues in compliance. In *Compliance in Health Care*, ed. B. Haynes, D.W. Taylor and D.L. Sackett, pp. 113–20. Baltimore: Johns Hopkins University Press.

Lasagna, L. and Hutt, P.B. (1991). Health care, research, and regulatory impact of noncompliance. In *Patient Compliance in Medical Practice and Clinical Trials*, ed.

J.A. Cramer and B. Spilker, pp. 393–403. New York: Raven Press.

Lescale, K.B., Inglis, S.R., Eddleman, K.A., et al. (1996). Conflicts between physicians and patients in non-elective cesarean delivery: incidence and the adequacy of informed consent. *American Journal of Pertinatalogy* **13**: 171–6.

Lettrie, G.S., Markenson, G.B. and Markenson, M.M. (1993). Discharge against medical advice in an obstetric unit. *Journal of Obstetric Medicine* **38**: 370–4.

Lopez, I. (1998). An ethnography of the medicalization of Puerto Rican women's reproduction. In *Pragmatic Women and Body Politics*, ed. M. Lock and P.A. Kaufert, pp. 240–59. Cambridge: Cambridge University Press.

Martins, D. (1999). Compliance as an exercise of agency? Or, the exercise of agency in the discourse of compliance. Paper presented at the conference on College Composition and Communication, Atlanta, 25 March. (Unpublished.)

Merck's 1899 Manual of the Materia Media. (1899). New York: Merck and Co. Reprinted in *The Merck Manual* (1999), 17th edn. New Jersey: Merck Research Laboratories.

The Merck Manual (1999), 17th edn. New Jersey: Merck Research Laboratories.

Metson, D., Kremner, M., Tobin, M. et al. (1995). Supplementation with folic acid. *British Medical Journal* **310**: 942.

Rapp, R. (1998). Refusing prenatal diagnosis: the uneven meanings of bioscience in a multicultural world. In *Cyborg Babies from Techno-Sex to Techno-Tots*, ed. R. Davis-Floyd and J. Dumit, pp. 143–67. New York: Routledge.

Roberts, L.J. (1996). Knowledge and use of periconceptual folic acid supplements by British Forces Germany personnel and dependents. *Journal of the Royal Army Medical Corps* **142**: 116–19.

Sackett, D.L. and Snow, J.C. (1979). The magnitude of compliance and noncompliance. In *Compliance in Health Care*, ed. B. Haynes, D.W. Taylor and D.L. Sackett, pp. 11–22. Baltimore: Johns Hopkins University Press.

Neonatal life

Do new reproductive technologies benefit or harm children?

Christine Overall

Department of Philosophy, Queen's University, Kingston, Canada

In the recent ethical and social scientific literature on new reproductive technologies (NRTs) and practices there is not much discussion about their impact on children (e.g. Birke, Himmelweit and Vines, 1990; Iglesias, 1990; Marrs, 1993; Robertson, 1994; Hartouni, 1997; Steinberg, 1997). As the final report of the Canadian Royal Commission on New Reproductive Technologies (Royal Commission on New Reproductive Technologies, 1993: p. 42) puts it,

> There is a dearth of information about, for instance, the direct outcomes of being conceived through assisted reproduction. Physical outcomes are important to monitor, but there may also be emotional and psychological outcomes to being born through the use of assisted methods of conception. For instance, we know very little about the effect on a child's sense of identity and belonging of being born through assisted insemination using donor sperm or following *in vitro* fertilisation using donated eggs.

Books and anthologies written from a feminist perspective mostly emphasize the effects of NRTs on women (e.g. Rowland, 1992; Spallone, 1989). None the less, there is a connection, in reproductive issues, between the status of women and the status of children. This connection is explicitly recognized within the United Nations Declaration of the Rights of the Child (United Nations, 1959), which calls for 'special care and protection' both for children and for their mothers, 'including adequate prenatal and postnatal care' (Principle 4). Hence, it can plausibly be argued that if NRTs either benefit or harm women, then their children may be comparably affected. For example, the criminalization of maternal substance abuse indirectly threatens the well-being of children, since the threat of criminal prosecution may deter pregnant women from seeking medical care (Blank and Merrick, 1995: p. 165).

In this chapter I evaluate, from a feminist perspective, a number of arguments about the direct benefits and harms of reproductive technologies and practices with respect to children. As a moral touchstone for their assessment, I use the United Nations Declaration of the Rights of the Child, which sets forth, in a reasonably clear and uncontroversial fashion, some basic and essential moral entitlements for children everywhere, entitlements that are widely acknowledged, even if they are not always acted upon.

I shall confine my discussion to the western world, since that is the context in which most of the arguments on both sides have been advanced. For the purposes of this chapter I define a 'child' as a human offspring, from the time of birth up until the end of adolescence. For reasons I shall not explore here, I do not regard a human embryo or fetus as an infant or child; hence I reject the approach taken, for example, by Jerome Lejeune, who claims, in the title of one of his papers, that 'Test Tube Babies are Babies' (Lejeune, 1992). None the less, what is done to embryos and fetuses obviously can affect the children they may become. For this reason, the treatment of embryos and fetuses can be highly relevant to – although it is not identical with – the issue of the treatment of children.

Alleged benefits of NRTs and practices

It is important to notice that NRTs and practices are rarely defended in terms of arguments about direct alleged benefits for children. The focus of argument is almost always on potential parents, both women and men, and what they will receive. However, there are a few recurrent claims about the benefits of NRTs to children that deserve attention. Three main benefits are repeatedly cited: existence itself; loving, motivated, prosperous parents; and the avoidance of disabilities.

Existence itself

One prominent argument is that technologies such as IVF (in vitro fertilization) are a benefit to offspring since without the technologies, some children wouldn't exist – even if their existence includes physical or psychological health problems and/or disabilities. Existence itself is a benefit conferred by NRTs upon some lucky children. Thus, John Robertson, a prominent defender of the use of NRTs, argues that however difficult the problems may be arising from a life created through reproductive technology, that life is unlikely ever to be so bad as to be not worth living (Robertson, 1994: p. 76). He states, 'Whatever psychological or social problems arise, they hardly rise to the level of severe handicap or disability that would make the child's very existence a net burden, and hence a wrongful life' (Robertson, 1994: p. 122).

How should we assess this argument? Thomas H. Murray points out that if it is accepted without analysis, then virtually no 'novel method of bringing children into the world' could be morally condemned (Murray, 1996: p. 37). The argument implies that criticizing a reproductive technology requires showing that the children thus created would have been better off never having been born. Of course it seems true that being alive is usually good; I have little doubt that most children created through NRTs and practices are glad to be alive. Still, this argument should not be allowed to trump all other evidence about possible harms generated by reproductive technologies.

For it would be a moral and conceptual mistake to assume that there are children who would have missed out on a benefit – life – if not for NRTs. It is not as if children exist in a limbo, waiting to be given the opportunity to live via NRTs. Never having existed would not make some hypothetical child worse off; there is no child to harm (Parfit, 1984: p. 487). So, even if coming into existence is a type of benefit, failing to come into existence is not a harm.

Having life is the precondition that makes all other benefits – and harms – possible. If a child suffers illness or disabilities because of the circumstances of his or her conception or prenatal existence, then we seem to have harmed him or her, in the process of benefiting him or her by causing his or her existence. It is arguable that every person has an interest in possessing a healthy, non-disabled body. If the damages incurred at conception are sufficiently great, there seems to be virtually no benefit to the child at all.

I conclude that, from a perspective before conception of a child, life is not a benefit, since there is no one to benefit; only from the perspective after conception has occurred is life arguably a benefit – and then, only if the life is not heavily damaged through the process of conception itself. Causing someone to exist is not a benefit, since there is no one to benefit; but once the person exists, she or he has life, which is usually a good thing.

Loving, motivated, prosperous parents

A second alleged benefit claimed for NRTs is based on the ostensible characteristics of the parents. Prospective parents who use NRTs are often prosperous, seem really to want children, are in some instances supposedly assessed for stability, and are ready to have children. More simply, the claim is that NRTs benefit (potential) parents, who want children (Snowden and Mitchell, 1983: p. 76; Macklin, 1994: p. 56) and are pleased to have them; hence they indirectly benefit the resulting child.

This argument usually takes its most explicit form in the context of debates about so-called surrogate motherhood, or what I prefer to call contract pregnancy, where the claim is made that the children resulting from the contract receive all the benefits of life within middle-class or wealthy families, who are equipped to provide the material, social and intellectual privileges seldom attained in working-class families. Thus, the American Fertility Society (1990: p. 312) claims,

Even if there are psychological risks, most infertile couples who go through with a reproduction arrangement that involves a third party do so as a last resort. In some cases, their willingness to make sacrifices to have a child may testify to their worthiness as loving parents. A child conceived through surrogate motherhood may be born into a much healthier climate than a child whose birth was unplanned.

However, this argument is not persuasive. Its classist bias is immediately obvious: the assumption is that life in a middle- or upper-class family is inevitably a greater benefit to a child than life in a working-class family. This assumption worked to the disadvantage of Mary Beth Whitehead, a working-class woman, when she sought custody of her biological daughter, so-called 'Baby M', whom she contracted to create for William Stern, a well-off professional.

More significantly, perhaps, the argument assumes that would-be parents who resort to NRTs and practices are especially motivated and beneficent toward their subsequent children. However, as I shall suggest later, there are also reasons to be concerned about the motives and goals of these people. And, at the very least, there is no empirical evidence that I know of to suggest that they make better parents than those who do not use technology in reproduction.

Avoidance of disabilities

The third main benefit claimed for some NRTs and practices is that they can help to reduce or eliminate disabilities in children (Tauer, 1990: p. 75). For example, Deborah Kaplan (1994: p. 50) lists several possible benefits to children of prenatal diagnosis (PND) and treatment. First:

Prevention or amelioration of the disability using methods such as treatment through dietary changes or supplements for the mother or infant; prenatal treatment of the fetus through pharmaceutical or surgical interventions; other forms of treatment or therapy for the infant that occur after prenatal diagnosis.

Second:

Prevention of family disruption through prenatal preparation by family members. This can entail obtaining information about the diagnosed condition and its consequences through reading or through talking to families who have children with similar disabilities or to adults who live with the disability themselves. It may also include such means as finding out about available public or private resources or forms of assistance, purchasing equipment, or making home modifications.

So, the suggestion is that the technologies of prenatal diagnosis benefit children directly through the prevention and amelioration of disabilities, and indirectly, by assisting parents. These claims seem justified.

However, it would be a mistake to accept the related claim, made by some, that NRTs produce better, or even perfect, babies (Spallone, 1989: pp. 113,

117; Snowden and Mitchell, 1983: p. 77); that, for example, babies generated by IVF or donor insemination (DI) using sperm from gifted fathers are smarter or prettier (Scutt, 1990: p. 285). There is no clear evidence to support these claims. And there are reasons to be cautious about them, since, as I shall later show, they betray a eugenicist agenda.

Possible harms of NRTs and practices

I turn now to those arguments that claim that NRTs and practices harm children. These claims arise from asking, what kind of future do NRTs give to children, specifically to those born as a result of them, but also to other children who may be affected by the attitudes that NRTs foster?

Some claims about harms to children of NRTs are not plausible. For example, I am unpersuaded of the necessity, insisted upon by some Roman Catholic critics of NRTs, of 'naturalness' in reproduction, and of marriage as the ideal or the only moral site for the raising of children (Iglesias, 1990: p. 159). For if naturalness is the criterion of moral acceptability, then many medical interventions are morally unjustified. If marriage is the criterion, it is hard to account for the growing number, and evident success, of common-law relationships in which children are being born and raised.

Among the problems of NRTs for children that I think are serious are five that deserve special examination: the emphasis on a genetic link with one's offspring and the possibility of eugenicist tendencies in the application of reproductive technologies; the sexism of sex preselection and the hetero-sexism and racism of selective access to NRTs; the possible dangers to children's health of some reproductive techniques; the selling of children through contract pregnancy arrangements; and the violation of the right of children who are created through sperm or egg 'donation' or contract motherhood to know the identity of their progenitors.

Genetic links and eugenicist tendencies

The motive behind many new reproductive technologies and related practices (e.g. contract pregnancy and IVF for male subfertility problems) is the goal of obtaining, particularly for the potential father, a genetic link with one's offspring. But this emphasis on a genetic link is thought by some commentators to reinforce a cultural notion of the child as possession, as a form of property. When producing (better) babies is treated as a business opportunity, infants are seen as commodities, as consumer goods marketed to the infertile (Rowland, 1992: pp. 3–4, 243).

Such a view of children is arguably incompatible with Principle 2 of the United Nations Declaration of the Rights of the Child (United Nations,

1959), which mandates 'opportunities and facilities' to enable children 'to develop physically, mentally, morally, spiritually, and socially in a healthy and normal manner and in conditions of freedom and dignity', and also with the recognition in Principle 6 that children need 'love and understanding' for 'the full and harmonious development' of their personalities.

The result of the longing for children, especially children of a certain kind, a longing which, to some extent, NRTs exacerbate, could be the generation of performance pressures on children to live up to parental expectations. Such pressures seem inconsistent with the spirit of Principle 7 of the United Nations Declaration of the Rights of the Child, which states that the 'best interests of the child shall be the guiding principle of those responsible for his education and guidance.'

A related concern, frequently expressed in the literature by feminist theorists, involves worries about eugenicist tendencies generated by the use of techniques of prenatal diagnosis (e.g. Birke et al., 1990: p. 184; Bopp, 1990: pp. 205–7). The concern is both for general effects on children (Blank and Merrick, 1995: p. 101), with the fear that the quest to improve the characteristics of infants may cause psychological hardship and exacerbate the commodification of children, and also, more specifically, for the negative impact of the existence and use of prenatal diagnosis on children with disabilities, who may be made to feel that they are mistakes who should never have existed (Kaplan, 1994; Murray, 1996: p. 132), and who may be made less welcome within this culture.

In response to the latter claim, however, the Canadian Royal Commission on New Reproductive Technologies argues that it 'does not seem likely' that 'funding for PND will affect the funds available for social support for people with disabilities' (Royal Commission on New Reproductive Technologies, 1993: p. 800). Their reason is that PND has little affect on the incidence of disabilities (Royal Commission, 1993: p. 799), and people who seek PND may already have a child with disabilities whom they love: '[E]vidence suggests that in countries where PND is practised, there is greater rather than less interest in the welfare of people with disabilities as a result of increased medical and social awareness of their needs and rights' (Royal Commission, 1993: p. 802).

My own view is that it is not inevitable or necessary that the use of PND for fetal impairment will lead to the devaluing of children with disabilities. Indeed, the informal evidence suggests that even while the use of PND is growing, attempts to integrate people with disabilities within 'mainstream' culture, while at the same time providing for and supporting their differences, are also growing. Although I am concerned about the potential commodification of children caused by the use of NRTs, I agree with Ruth Chadwick, who argues, 'If we say that it is better, all things considered, to produce a child who is not handicapped rather than one who is, this does not commit us to saying that handicapped children are less worthy of respect. It is just that, other things being equal, it is preferable for the individual, the family, and the society' (Chadwick, 1992: p. 112). The use of NRTs and practices to reduce or ameliorate disabilities seems acceptable, provided it can be separated from the expectation or use of NRTs to 'perfect' offspring or to set inappropriate standards for the health, achievements and acceptability of children (Murray, 1996: pp. 133–7).

Sexism, heterosexism, racism and NRTs

Another possible danger of NRTs and practices is connected to invidious forms of discrimination. For example, in the practices of sex selection and preselection, children are being sought or avoided on the basis of their sex. Some commentators have worried that the resulting children will be expected to conform to certain gender stereotypes; to be 'real girls' or 'real boys'. Gena Corea suggests that the social validation of the role of 'surrogate mother' also raises a general problem of sexism: 'Is it in the best interests of female children to be born into a world where there is a class of breeder women? How damaging might that be to the self-esteem of girl children?' (Corea, 1990a: p. 159).

Based on its own surveys, the Royal Commission claims that in Canada 'most prospective parents expressed a weak preference for an equal number of sons and daughters' (Royal Commission, 1993: p. 890). While the Commission takes this finding as evidence of the absence of sexism in offspring choice, I believe we should be uneasy. A truly gender-indifferent parent would probably not care about the balance of girls to boys. Certainly, a preference for equal numbers of boys and girls could lead to disappointment if, for example, only girls are born.

Moreover, within the practice of assisted reproduction, the pronounced tendency to favour heterosexual relationships, and in some jurisdictions, to explicitly deny DI or IVF to lesbians (Rowland, 1992: p. 251), socially sanctions a blatant form of discrimination which, in addition to its injustice to lesbians, may also harm children who are growing up with lesbian or gay parents.

In addition, the motive to preserve racial lines, avoid miscegenation, and protect the interests of white people over those of people of colour is another form of discriminatory behaviour revealed within some reproductive practices. For example, the solicitation of 'donor' ova often invokes racial criteria – only 'Caucasian' potential 'donors' need apply. Moreover, the principles and precedents governing the legal resolution of disputes about contract pregnancy show that racial bias is an active ingredient in determining who is considered to be the 'real' parent of a contractually produced child. In the dispute between Mark and Crispina Calvert, a white man and Filipina woman, and Anna Johnson, a black woman who gestated their embryo and then claimed to bond with the child she bore, the debate was framed to call into question the reality of any feeling a black woman might have for an unrelated putatively white child (Hartouni, 1997: pp. 94–6). Once again, the enactment of prejudice and stereotype – this time on the basis of race – is unlikely to have positive outcomes for children, especially those who are being raised within so-called 'mixed-race' families.

I suggest that discriminatory practices within the applications of reproductive technologies are incompatible with the spirit of Principle 10 of the United Nations Declaration of the Rights of the Child (United Nations, 1959), which mandates the protection of children from all forms of discrimination.

Possible dangers to children's health

Principle 4 of the United Nations Declaration of the Rights of Children (United Nations, 1959) says that children are entitled to 'grow and develop in health', and that children have a right to adequate medical services. But some commentators suggest that children's health is potentially jeopardized through certain reproductive technologies and practices. For example, in donor insemination, the existence of uneven standards and 'unsafe practices' with respect to sexually transmitted diseases and genetic diseases may compromise the health of the resulting children (Royal Commission, 1993: p. 471). Questions have also been raised about the potential for transmission to children of genetic diseases as a result of the use of intracytoplasmic sperm injection (ICSI) to treat male infertility (Tripp et al., 1997). In addition, it is argued that the experimental use of hormones in conjunction with NRTs may have long-term, unforeseen effects on the offspring (Rowland, 1992: pp. 50–2), much as the long-term effects of the hormone diethylstilboestrol (DES) were unforeseen.

Another significant potential danger of NRTs to children arises from being conceived as part of large multiples. The use of IVF, with the return of several embryos to the woman's uterus, increases the likelihood of multiple pregnancy (Templeton and Morris, 1998). But multiple pregnancy is not an optimal gestational condition. (See Chapter 16.) There is a greater risk of ectopic pregnancy, spontaneous abortion, pre-term delivery, low birth weight, Caesarean section, and stillbirth in IVF and GIFT (gamete intra-fallopian transfer) pregnancies (Baird, 1992; Rowland, 1992: pp. 46, 64–5). Low birth weight can result in breathing problems, and low birth weight infants are more likely than normal weight infants to have cerebral palsy, poor eyesight, short attention span, poor learning skills, hyperactivity, reading difficulties and poor co-ordination and motor skills in childhood (Royal Commission, 1993: p. 528).

Moreover, being born as part of a multiple may not result in optimal conditions for growing up, depending on the amount of practical help and financial assistance the parents receive (Raymond, 1992: p. 67; Royal Commission, 1993: p. 529): 'In one example, Hon Campbell in North London was virtually housebound for a year with her triplets. In 1989, one Perth woman had to relinquish three of her quads for adoption because of the strain associated with their unwanted arrival' (Raymond, 1992: p. 67). It is important to point out that all of these risks are, of course, undertaken without the consent of the children themselves, let alone their knowledge and understanding.

Contract pregnancy and the sale of children

One practice in which children are arguably harmed and their rights certainly violated is in contract pregnancy arrangements, in which children are bought and sold. The evidence for the claim that a purchase occurs lies in the fact that contracts stipulate that the full sum will not be paid if the child is stillborn; the complete fee is paid only on delivery of a living baby.

In earlier work (Overall, 1987, 1993) I have argued that the buying and selling of infants, no matter what the context, is a form of slavery, and hence morally inexcusable. It is in clear contravention of Principle 6 of the United Nations Declaration of the Rights of the Child, which states, 'a child of tender years shall not, save in exceptional circumstances, be separated from his mother.' It seems unlikely that the United Nations would be willing to regard a contract for selling the child as constituting a genuinely 'exceptional circumstance', for Principle 9 of the Declaration states clearly that the child 'shall not be subject of traffic, in any form'.

Defenders of so-called 'surrogacy' arrangements have argued that the practice is not baby-selling because:

the resulting child is never in a state of insecurity. From the moment of birth, he or she is under the care of the biological father and his wife, who cannot sell the child. ... Moreover, no matter how much money is paid through the surrogacy arrangement, the child, upon birth, cannot be treated like a commodity – a car or a television set. Laws against child abuse and neglect come into play. (Andrews, 1990: p. 176.)

True, the practice of contract pregnancy does not mean that the child is necessarily treated badly; 'Many material objects, after all, are treated with respect and kept for a long time; but they are objects nevertheless' (Capron and Radin, 1990: p. 63). But it does mean that in these arrangements, the child is treated as no more than a means to an end (Royal Commission, 1993: p. 677), the end being the purchasing father's acquisition of a child. Contrary to ordinary adoption practices, the ruling criteria in contract pregnancy are the interests of the adults involved, not the interests of the children (Annas,

1990: p. 45). The contracting parents are usually not screened; ability to pay is the only criterion for eligibility to buy a child (Royal Commission, 1993: p. 677).

> Moreover, even if a child once incorporated into a family is never again thought of as something acquired in an expensive transaction, the fact remains that during the *process* of transaction the child was a thing. People had a transferable ownership interest in it and bargained over it in a market in which other 'products' were also for sale and in which other potential buyers may also have been bidding.
>
> (Capron and Radin, 1990: p. 63, their emphasis.)

The fact that the child is '"bought at a price" could make the child feel like a commodity that can be bought and sold, and create pressure for him or her to live up to his or her "purchase price"' (Royal Commission, 1993: p. 677).

In addition, it is incorrect to say that the child produced through these arrangements is never in a state of insecurity. The child loses his or her connection with the gestational mother, and also misses out on the benefits of being breast-fed. If the contract arrangement runs into problems, the child is placed in an extreme state of insecurity, and may either become the target of custody battles between a purchasing father and a gestational mother no longer able to give up her child, or become unwanted by anyone, in situations where, for example, the child has a disability (Raymond, 1992: p. 191), as in the Stiver-Malahoff case.

Experience shows that difficulties can arise even when the child produced, while healthy, is just not what was ordered:

> When 'surrogate mother' Patty Nowakowski delivered twins – a girl and a boy – in 1988, one child was as intended and the other not. The Michigan man who hired Nowakowski to be inseminated with his sperm wanted a girl. So he took the girl child and left the boy behind... The boy was put into a foster home until Nowakowski, pained at his fate, claimed him as her own. (Corea, 1990b: pp. 171–2.)

Hence, contract pregnancy arrangements significantly contribute to insecurity for the children who are generated, and are harmful to them as a consequence.

A number of commentators have also expressed concern about the possible effects on the biological siblings of contract children of seeing their baby sibling sold – in some cases, against the wishes of their mother, who changes her mind (Rowland, 1992: pp. 189–91). Proponents of contract pregnancy have claimed that the so-called surrogate mother can anticipate the effects on her existing children of selling the baby, and can mitigate those effects through what she says to the children (Andrews 1990: p. 177). But there are reasons to doubt this:

> One woman reported that her daughter, now seventeen, who was eleven at the time of the surrogate birth, 'is still having problems with what I did, and as a result she is still

angry with me.' She explains: 'Nobody told me that a child could bond with a baby while you're still pregnant. I didn't realize then that all the times she listened to his heartbeat and felt his legs kick that she was becoming attached to him.'

A less sentimental explanation is possible. It seems likely that her daughter, seeing one child given away, was fearful that the same might be done to her. We can expect anxiety and resentment on the part of children whose mothers give away a brother or sister. The psychological harm to these children is clearly relevant to a determination of whether surrogacy is contrary to public policy. (Steinbock, 1990: pp. 134–5).

Moreover, there is reason to be concerned that the social ratification of arrangements for buying and selling individual children could lead to a more general attitude that children are commodities to be bought and sold (Royal Commission, 1993: p. 678). Contract pregnancy arrangements reinforce cultural beliefs about the ownership of children, beliefs that may affect perceptions of and relationships to children. I agree with Angela Holder (1990: p. 85), who says, 'Trying to convince voters that children are important is difficult at best. Trying to do so in a society that considers it "all right" to make contracts to buy children strikes me as impossible'.

Denial of the right of children to know the identity of their progenitors

Finally, some commentators have argued that 'The intentional separation of genetic, gestational, and social parenting ... may adversely affect the well-being of the children produced' (Tauer, 1990: p. 81). In my view, however, it is not the separation of different parenting roles that is, in itself, necessarily harmful to children, but rather the lack of knowledge about one's origins and identities that often accompanies that separation. For example, children are often deprived of knowledge about the identity of sperm vendors and egg donors, and of contract mothers and their biological siblings and grandparents (Robertson, 1990: p. 29; Scutt, 1990: pp. 285–6; Rowland, 1992: pp. 192–3; Robertson, 1993: p. 212). The Royal Commission has raised the question whether 'genealogical bewilderment', a term borrowed from adoption, may be appropriate to the situation of these children (Royal Commission, 1993: p. 42). The large degree of secrecy and the reinforcement of anonymity surrounding the use of donated or purchased gametes violate children's right to be provided with crucial information about their health and medical status. Some commentators have also worried that if no limits are made on sperm sales, and only inadequate records are kept, then individuals could unwittingly marry and even have children with a half-sibling. Although 'statistically unlikely', this possibility none the less worries many DI participants (Royal Commission, 1993: p. 470).

Although the United Nations Declaration of the Rights of the Child (United Nations, 1959) does not directly defend a right to know one's biological family, it does provide that 'The child shall be entitled from his birth to a name and a nationality' (Principle 3), and that children are entitled to education, an education which, among other goals, promotes the child's general culture and is guided by the best interests of the child (Principle 7). These provisions create, I believe, at least a presumption in favour of providing the opportunity for offspring to learn about their biological antecedents. In making this claim I am not suggesting that biological kinship is constitutive of individuals, that information about the identities of gamete providers can or should supersede what children already know about the persons who raised them, or that relationships with biological parents must be added to offspring's relationships with their rearing parents (Weir, 1998). Nor am I saying that information about their biological antecedents should be forced on offspring; I claim only that they ought to have the opportunity to acquire it.

Conclusion

Do NRTs and practices harm children? I would say that the answer is clearly yes in the case of contract pregnancy arrangements. Moreover, there are also real risks to children's health from some high-technology medical interventions in reproduction such as IVF and ICSI. Children also face potential harm when they are deliberately misled or deprived of any knowledge about their biological origins.

In other cases, the story is less clear. There are general tendencies of which we should be wary: for example, the tendencies to regard children as improvable products, to exert performance pressures on children, and to perpetuate sexist, heterosexist and racist arrangements. These tendencies are real, but because they operate on a general social level, and are compatible with the kind treatment of individual children, they are harder both to notice and to avoid.

Do NRTs and practices benefit children? There is reason to believe that they do so only in a limited way, partly insofar as existence itself can be a benefit, and possibly through reducing or ameliorating disabilities. However, we should be clear that NRTs are not an unmitigated benefit for children; in fact, if they benefit anyone, it is parents and potential parents. When NRT enthusiasts advocate the idea of protecting 'procreative choice', it is in order to give adults the chance to 'acquire the possibility of rearing a child of their own genes and gestation' (Robertson 1993: p. 201). The purpose and value of NRTs are **not** for children, but for people who want to be parents, or who want other benefits attached to having children.

Moreover, the alleged benefits of reproductive technologies and practices are closely tied to the harms they cause. In order to give the child existence, there is a risk of harming the child's health; the cost of securing possibly loving parents for the child may be the reinforcement of the spurious importance of the genetic link; and lowering the likelihood of the occurrence of disabilities possibly contributes to eugenicist tendencies within reproductive practice and policy.

Policy implications

This assessment implies not only that there is an urgent need for more research about the effects on children of NRTs and practices, but also that social policy must limit and in some cases prohibit certain technologies and practices, for the sake of children's rights and well-being. I shall briefly mention five of what I regard as necessary policy measures:

(1) All contract pregnancy arrangements should be made unenforceable, and there should be legal penalties both for individuals who attempt to buy children and for professionals who participate in such arrangements.

(2) IVF and related procedures such as ICSI and GIFT should be available, if at all, only under conditions that offer maximum information and protection to women, and safety for the resulting offspring.

(3) In order to preserve women's access to abortion it is not desirable to attempt to police the use of sex selection via abortion. However, there is no reason to provide public health funding for technologies of sex preselection.

(4) There should be no discrimination on the basis of sexual orientation, marital status, or race in access to or regulation of assisted reproductive technologies and practices.

(5) There should be adequate provisions for the offspring of sperm vendors and egg donors to know the identity and health status of their biological antecedents.

Without aware social policies such as these, we run the risk of allowing NRTs and practices, despite claims about their purported benefits, to continue to be liabilities for children.

References

American Fertility Society (1990). Surrogate mothers. In *Surrogate Motherhood: Politics and Privacy*, ed. L. Gostin, pp. 307–14. Bloomington: Indiana University.

Andrews, L.B. (1990). Surrogate motherhood: the challenge for feminists. In *Surrogate Motherhood: Politics and Privacy*, ed. L. Gostin, pp. 167–82. Bloomington: Indiana University.

Annas, G.J. (1990). Fairy tales surrogate mothers tell. In *Surrogate Motherhood: Politics and Privacy*, ed. L. Gostin, pp. 43–55. Bloomington: Indiana University.

Baird, P. (1992). Reproductive technology and child health. Speech delivered to 'Child Health 2000: A World Congress and Exposition on Child Health,' Vancouver, British Columbia, February 22.

Birke, L., Himmelweit, S. and Vines, G. (1990). *Tomorrow's Child: Reproductive Technologies in the 90s*. London: Virago.

Blank, R. and Merrick, J.C. (1995). *Human Reproduction, Emerging Technologies, and Conflicting Rights*. Washington, DC: Congressional Quarterly.

Bopp, J. Jr. (1990). Surrogate motherhood agreements: the risks to innocent human life. In *Beyond Baby M: Ethical Issues in New Reproductive Techniques*, ed. D.M. Bartels, R. Priester, D.E. Vawter and A.L. Caplan, pp. 201–20. Clifton, NJ: Humana.

Capron, A.M. and Radin, M.J. (1990). Choosing family law over contract law as a paradigm for surrogate motherhood. In *Surrogate Motherhood: Politics and Privacy*, ed. L. Gostin, pp. 59–76. Bloomington: Indiana University.

Chadwick, R.F. (1992). The perfect baby: introduction. In *Ethics, Reproduction and Genetic Control*, 2nd edn, ed. R.F. Chadwick, pp. 93–135. New York: Routledge.

Corea, G. (1990a). Industrial experimentation on 'surrogate' mothers. In *Reconstructing Babylon: Essays on Women and Technology*, ed. H. P. Hynes, pp. 155–9. London: Earthscan Publications.

Corea, G. (1990b). Junk liberty. In *Reconstructing Babylon: Essays on Women and Technology*, ed. H.P. Hynes, pp. 166–87. London: Earthscan Publications.

Hartouni, V. (1997). *Cultural Conceptions: On Reproductive Technologies and the Remaking of Life*. Minneapolis: University of Minnesota.

Holder, A. (1990). Surrogate motherhood and the best interests of children. In *Surrogate Motherhood: Politics and Privacy*, ed. L. Gostin, pp. 77–87. Bloomington: Indiana University.

Iglesias, T. (1990). *IVF and Justice: Moral, Social and Legal Issues Related to Human In Vitro Fertilisation*. London: The Linacre Centre.

Kaplan, D. (1994). Prenatal screening and diagnosis: the impact on persons with disabilities. In *Women and Prenatal Testing: Facing the Challenges of Genetic Technology*, ed. K.H. Rothenberg and E.J. Thomson, pp. 49–61. Columbus, Ohio: Ohio State University.

Lejeune, J. (1992). Test tube babies are babies. In *Ethics, Reproduction and Genetic Control*, 2nd edn, ed. R. F. Chadwick, pp. 44–52. New York: Routledge.

Macklin, R. (1994). *Surrogates and Other Mothers: The Debates Over Assisted Reproduction*. Philadelphia: Temple University.

Marrs, R.P. (Ed.) (1993). *Assisted Reproductive Technologies*. Oxford: Blackwell Scientific Publications.

Murray, T.H. (1996). *The Worth of a Child*. Berkeley: University of California.

Overall, C. (1987). *Ethics and Human Reproduction: A Feminist Analysis*. Boston: Allen & Unwin.

Overall, C. (1993). *Human Reproduction: Principles, Practices, Policies*. Toronto: Oxford University.

Parfit, D. (1984). *Reasons and Persons*. Oxford: Clarendon.

Robertson, J.A. (1990). Procreative liberty and the state's burden of proof in regulating noncoital reproduction. In *Surrogate Motherhood: Politics and Privacy*, ed. L. Gostin, pp. 24–42. Bloomington: Indiana University.

Robertson, J.A. (1993). Ethical and legal issues in assisted reproduction. In *Assisted*

Reproductive Technologies, ed. R. P. Marrs, pp. 200–17. Oxford: Blackwell Scientific Publications.

Robertson, J.A. (1994). *Children of Choice: Freedom and the New Reproductive Technologies*. Princeton, NJ: Princeton University.

Rowland, R. (1992). *Living Laboratories: Women and Reproductive Technologies*. Bloomington: Indiana University.

Royal Commission on New Reproductive Technologies (1993). *Proceed with Care: Final Report of the Royal Commission on New Reproductive Technologies*, vols. 1 and 2. Ottawa: Canada Communications Group.

Scutt, J.A. (1990). Epilogue. In *The Baby Machine: Reproductive Technology and the Commercialisation of Motherhood*, ed. J.A. Scutt, pp. 274–320. London: Merlin.

Snowden, R. and Mitchell, G.D. (1983). *The Artificial Family: A Consideration of Artificial Insemination by Donor*. London: Unwin Paperbacks.

Spallone, P. (1989). *Beyond Conception: The New Politics of Reproduction*. Granby, MA: Bergin and Garvey Publishers.

Steinberg, D.L. (1997). *Bodies in Glass: Genetics, Eugenics, Embryo Ethics*. Manchester: Manchester University.

Steinbock, B. (1990). Surrogate motherhood as prenatal adoption. In *Surrogate Motherhood: Politics and Privacy*, ed. L. Gostin, pp. 123–35. Bloomington: Indiana University.

Tauer, C. (1990). Essential considerations for public policy on assisted reproduction. In *Beyond Baby M: Ethical Issues in New Reproductive Techniques*, ed. D. M. Bartels, R. Priester, D.E. Vawter and A.L. Caplan, pp. 65–86. Clifton, NJ: Humana.

Templeton, A. and Morris, J.K. (1998). Reducing the risk of multiple births by transfer of two embryos after in vitro fertilization. *New England Journal of Medicine* **339**: 573–7.

Tripp, B.M., Kolon, K.F., Bishop, C., Lipshultz, L.I. and Lamb, D.J. (1997). Letter. *Journal of the American Medical Association* **277**: 963–4.

United Nations (1959). Declaration of the Rights of the Child. General Assembly Resolution 1386 (XIV).

Weir, L. (1998). Commentary on 'Children, Oppression and New Reproductive Technologies and Practices'. Annual Meeting of the Canadian Sociology and Anthropology Association, Ottawa.

20

Are there lives not worth living? When is it morally wrong to reproduce?

Rebecca Bennett and John Harris

Centre for Social Ethics and Policy, University of Manchester, Manchester, UK

The idea that it might be a moral crime to have a baby, that it might be wrong to bring a new human individual into the world is to many people simply bizarre. Having a baby is a wonderful thing to do, it is usually regarded as the unproblematic choice from the moral if not from the 'social' or medical point of view. It is only having an abortion and perhaps also refraining from having children that is regarded as requiring justification ... [T]he idea that one might be harmed or wronged by being brought into existence in less than a satisfactory state is very important indeed, for, as we have seen, it challenges many of our moral presumptions about having children. Moreover, if the alleged wrong can give rise to legal actions for compensation, and perhaps also to criminal liability then a number of further problems arise.

(Harris, 1998: pp. 99 and 101.)

In this chapter we attempt to investigate the possible wrongs and harms for which people might be responsible in having or attempting to have children. We start 'together', so to speak, but as the argument develops points of difference arise. In charting both the points of agreement and those of difference we hope to throw light on and diffuse heat from a debate that is so often characterized by little of the former and a swelter of the latter.

Beginning together

The alleged wrong involved in bringing to birth a disabled child has been at the centre of so-called 'wrongful life' law suits. In wrongful life suits those brought to birth in a 'disabled' state seek compensation from allegedly negligent physicians for this disability through the courts. The claim in a wrongful life suit is not that the negligence of the health professional involved caused the 'disability' but that the negligence involved was that of failing to inform the patients adequately and thus being responsible for the birth of a child in a less than satisfactory condition who would otherwise not have been born. In such cases the physician is not held responsible for causing the impairment in the child but of causing the impaired child to be born, implying that the child would have been 'better off' if he or she had never been born. Thus in wrongful life suits we are not considering the difference

between being born impaired rather than unimpaired but rather the difference between being born and not being born – existing and not existing.

We will not go into detail here of such law suits; we are interested in the
philosophical issue at the heart of such cases, that is, is it morally wrong to
bring to birth a disabled child?

Worthwhile lives?

There is a strong obligation not to harm the future person or seriously
damage his or her welfare or other significant needs or interests. There is
obviously a strong obligation not to damage a fetus in utero, for example by
taking drugs that would damage its hearing or stunt its growth. However, this
is not the issue in wrongful life suits. The individual is not suing for
negligence of the harm inflicted but for the wrong of being brought to birth
in a damaged state. The claim is, it seems that the wrong they are suffering is
the wrong of being brought to birth.

The answer given to the question 'Would I, or anyone, wrong this child by
bringing it into being, in this condition?' will depend greatly on the value
which is placed on life itself. If it is thought that being brought to birth and
thus enabled to have the experience of being alive is usually a valuable and
positive experience, then it would seem that the only plausible answer to this
question is this – unless the child's condition is predicted to be so bad that it
would not have a worthwhile life, a life worth living, then it will always *be in
that child's interests* to be brought into being. It is in the interests of any child
whose life will be likely worth living overall, that he or she is brought to birth.
It is, after all, that child's only chance of existing at all. Unless the child is
likely to be born with a condition so severe that it is likely to cause suffering
so great as to outweigh the good of life then it is in the interests of the
individual to exist despite the possibility of a life compromised by disability
(Harris, 2000b).

It may be considered that this argument comparing existence to non-
existence is logically problematic. Bonnie Steinbock (1992: p. 117) explains
this difficulty:

> This argument maintains that it is impossible for a person to be better off never having
> been born. For if I had never been born, then I never was; if I never was, then I cannot
> be said to have been better off. The problem can be put another way. To be harmed is
> to be made worse off; but no individual is made worse off by coming to exist, for that
> suggests that we can compare the person before he existed with the person after he
> existed, which is absurd. Therefore, it is logically impossible that anyone is harmed by
> coming to exist and wrongful life suits are both illogical and unfair in that they require
> the defendant to compensate someone he has not harmed.

Even if it is deemed impossible to compare existence with non-existence in any meaningful way, it does seem reasonable to argue that as long as an individual does not have a life so blighted by suffering that it outweighs any pleasure gained by living, that individual has not been wronged by being brought to birth. It may well be that it does not make sense to talk of someone being made better or worse off by being brought into existence, but it does appear to make sense to talk about lives that are worth living and those that are so blighted by suffering that they may be considered 'unworthwhile'.

Where it is rational to judge that an individual would not only not have a worthwhile life, but would have a life so bad that it would be a cruelty rather than a kindness to bring it into existence, then we have not only powerful reasons not to make such choices ourselves, but also powerful moral reasons to object to those choices when made by others. Whether or not those objections should extend to attempts to prevent others from doing so if we can, by legislation or regulation if necessary, is a further and separate question. Certainly in such cases there must be a presumption that it would be morally right to prevent such cruelty if we can, but there are of course independent reasons why attempts to implement preventive measures by whatever means may themselves be problematic – for example, because they involve invasions of privacy, violations of bodily integrity or interferences with civil liberties which might be as or more morally problematic than the cruelty they are designed to prevent.

However, where we judge the circumstances of a future person to be less than ideal, but not so bad as to deprive that individual of a worthwhile existence, then we certainly lack the moral justification to impose our ideals on others (Harris, 1998: ch. 4).

Morally wrong worthwhile lives?

If it is morally wrong to bring to birth a child who will have a life blighted by suffering, it is morally wrong because we have created an individual to have an overwhelmingly negative experience which will not improve. It has been suggested (Feinberg, 1984; Harris, 1992: ch. 4) that not only is it morally wrong to bring such extreme cases to birth, but that it is also morally wrong to bring to birth children who, while expected to have 'worthwhile' lives, will be born with some kind of physical or mental impairment. As bringing to birth impaired children with worthwhile lives cannot be considered morally wrong based on the reasoning that their experience will be overwhelmingly negative, what if anything is morally wrong about bringing into existence an impaired but worthwhile life?

Beginning to diverge

We will present two different ways of thinking about what, if anything, is morally wrong about bringing into existence an impaired but worthwhile life. The chapter will proceed in the form of a commentary by Bennett on Harris and rejoinders by Harris. We end with a summary designed to point ways forward in the light of disagreement.

Harris argues that 'to deliberately make a reproductive choice knowing that the resulting child will be significantly disabled is morally problematic and often morally wrong' (Harris, 2000a: p. 96). For Harris the mother has not wronged her *child* by bringing it to birth. Far from it, he argues (Harris, 1998: p. 117) that:

It [the resulting child] has a life worth living because of her choice. The idea that she might have an obligation to compensate her child for benefiting him is nonsense. In such circumstances wrongful life cases are simply misconceived. Not because the life in question has not been impaired, not because the individuals are not suffering, not because they have not been harmed; it has, they are, and they have: rather because it is not plausible to regard them as being wronged.

But if the child has not been wronged by his mother's choice to bring him to birth, what sense can be made of the claim that the mother's choice to do so is morally questionable or even wrong?

Harris considers the example of a congenitally deaf couple who, after undergoing IVF (in vitro fertilization), are faced with a choice of embryos to implant. We are asked to suppose that pre-implantation screening has shown that among the embryos available for implantation are two congenitally 'deaf' embryos. Harris claims that to choose to implant the 'deaf' embryos rather than the 'healthy' embryos would be morally wrong. He argues (Harris, 2000a: p. 97) that:

In a case like this the parents have wronged no one, but have harmed some children unnecessarily, but those who were harmed had no complaint because for them the alternative was non-existence.

Harris argues that if it is possible for a parent to have a child who is not disabled, and that parent chooses to bring to birth a disabled child, the parent is choosing to bring disability into the world. He argues that it is morally wrong in such a situation to choose to bring a disabled child to birth. This wrong might be classified as 'the wrong of bringing avoidable suffering into the world' (Harris, 1998: p. 111). The wrong done by those who 'choose', in this sense, to bring a disabled child to birth is not the wrong of creating a life of overall negative experience but of creating lives that are likely to have more suffering than other possible lives.

What counts as suffering?

Harris argues that it may be morally wrong to 'choose' to bring to birth an individual with any impairment, however slight, if a healthy individual could be brought to birth instead. He argues (Harris, 1998: p. 109) that the impaired child has been harmed:

[T]o be harmed is to be put in a condition that is harmful. A condition that is harmful, ... is one in which the individual is disabled or suffering in some way or in which his interests or rights are frustrated. The disability or suffering may be slight, just as harms may be trivial ... I would want to claim that a harmed condition obtains whenever someone is in a disabling or hurtful condition, even though that condition is only marginally disabling and even though it is not possible for that particular individual to avoid the condition in question.

Thus, for Harris, to be born with any impairment that one could have a rational preference to be born without, even something as slight as being born without a little finger, is to be born in a harmed state. Bringing to birth a child in a 'harmed state', in Harris's sense, rather than in an 'unharmed' state, is to make the world a worse place than it need have been and is thus morally wrong proportionately to the degree of gratuitous harm created. If the disabling condition is relatively trivial, e.g. the loss of a finger, the moral wrong done is relatively trivial.

Who suffers?

For Harris the choice to bring to birth a 'disabled' child is partly wrongful because it causes a child to be born in a 'harmed' condition and partly wrongful because it creates a world which needlessly contains more suffering, hardship or disability than would have been created by an alternative choice. There is clearly a strong moral obligation to avoid harming others and to attempt to minimize suffering. Is it plausible to suppose that bringing to birth children who, while 'disabled' have worthwhile lives, can be considered as harming these children, and in what sense does a choice to give birth to a disabled child create more suffering in the world?

Harris claims that to choose to have a deaf child is analogous to not curing curable deafness in a child. Just as the deaf child denied the cure is harmed by this decision, so the child with incurable deafness is harmed by the choice to bring him to birth. Harris (2000a: p. 97) argues:

[A] cure for this congenital deafness is discovered, it is risk-free and there are no side effects. Would the parents, in this case, be right to withhold this cure for deafness from their child? Would the child have any legitimate complaint if they did not remove the deafness? Could this child say to its parents: 'I could have enjoyed Mozart and Beethoven and dance music and the sound of the wind in the trees and the waves on the shore, I could have heard the beauty of the spoken word and in my turn spoken fluently but for your deliberate denial.'

If deaf parents decided to deny their deaf child such an effective cure, this would seem morally wrong. Even if the parents felt that it would be more 'convenient' for them to have a child with similar disabilities to themselves, this does not seem to justify them in denying their child the valuable experience of hearing where that experience is possible. However, while it would be morally wrong to deprive a child of hearing by denying him a cure for deafness, these cases are not clearly analogous with the case of 'choosing' to have a child who will be deaf. In making the analogy Harris (2000a: p. 97) argues:

I do not believe there is a difference between choosing a preimplantation deaf embryo and refusing a cure to a newborn. Nor do I see an important difference between refusing a cure and deliberately deafening a child.

A possible response to this line of reasoning is as follows. There is no moral difference between refusing a cure and deliberately deafening a child; however, choosing to implant a 'deaf' embryo rather than a 'hearing' embryo is not deliberately deafening a child. (But of course it does involve deliberately creating a 'deaf' child rather than the equally viable alternative of a 'hearing' child.) For the analogy to be sound, the 'deaf' embryo would have to have the option of hearing or being deaf. However the 'deaf' embryo does not have these options – it can either exist deaf or not exist at all. Harris talks of 'depriving it [the deaf child] of one of its senses' (Harris, 2000a: p. 99). The 'deaf' embryo is not *denied* anything by not being able to hear; it can only be denied something that it could possibly have. Thus, it would be wrong to deny a deaf child the possibility of hearing by denying him an effective cure, but it is not wrong to give birth to a child who has incurable deafness as *that child* has not been denied anything – he has not been harmed. A child who is deafened or denied hearing by being denied a cure is harmed by this lack of hearing. However, a child born with congenital incurable deafness has not been harmed and has not been denied anything he could have ever possibly had.

Harris (1998: p. 110) explains responsibility for harming thus:

Where B is in a condition that is harmed and A and/or C is responsible for B's being in that condition then A and/or C have harmed B.

He claims (Harris, 1998: p. 110) that:

In the case of wrongful birth, A and/or C have not only caused B to be in a condition which is harmful but are also morally responsible for B's being in that condition, therefore A and/or C have harmed B. A thus harms B whenever A puts B in a harmful condition. Where A is morally responsible for putting B in such a condition, then A is morally responsible for B's condition.

While it seems uncontroversial that those who choose to bring a disabled child to birth are responsible for that decision, it is not clear that that child is harmed. The mother of such a child has not put the child 'in such a condition', unless by this it is meant that she is responsible for putting the child in the position of existing. If the mother had disabled her 'healthy' child by her deliberate actions, then she would be responsible for the harm incurred. However, in the case of a congenital malformation, neither has the child been harmed, nor is the mother morally responsible for that harm by bringing the child to birth. The child has not been denied anything by being born – he has gained a chance to live in the only state it is possible for him to live in. The child has not been harmed, as this child could not be born in any other way than he is born. The child does not suffer having his interests or rights frustrated. This child may be denied opportunities that other children are not denied, but he is not 'harmed' by this as these opportunities were never available to him. As a female, Bennett would argue, I am not denied the opportunity to experience life as a male; I am not harmed by my inability to do so.

However, here Harris would respond to Bennett that this is because being a female rather than a male is in no sense a 'worse' condition. However, if a person's gender had been chosen for them by someone else, their parents perhaps, it would be the case that others had determined, not that *you* would never experience being a male, but that the child to which they gave birth would never experience being a male.

Who is harmed/wronged by disability?

Harris argues that a child denied an effective cure for his deafness is both harmed and wronged. He also argues that a child with incurable deafness is harmed by being brought into existence but not wronged. He is brought into existence in a 'harmed' state but has not been wronged as this is the only state he could exist in. In both cases Harris claims that the child has been 'harmed', but that this harm constitutes a wrong to the child only in the case of the child denied treatment.

Bennett, on the other hand, would argue that it makes no sense to talk about harming or wronging a disabled child brought to birth, unless he has a life that would be considered not worth living. She argues that comparing a child's life with or without disability, when to be without disability is not an option, suffers from the same logical problems as the argument that attempts to compare non-existence with existence. It makes no sense to talk of the disabled child as being denied something he could never have or being harmed by coming into existence in the only state in which he could have existed. It does make sense to say bringing to birth individuals with very severe disabilities that overwhelm any positive aspects of life would not be something that we should strive to do, but this is a very different case than the one we have been discussing here.

Even if we concede that we are comparing not a child's life with or without disability but rather the lives of different possible children, the argument still suffers from trying to make an impossible and puzzling comparison. We will consider this argument in more detail below.

Two separate questions

According to Bennett, Harris, is answering two very different and separate questions in his analysis of the moral responsibility for bringing to birth disabled children. These questions are: 'What counts as a worthwhile life?'; and 'What sort of people should there be?'.

The question 'What counts as a worthwhile life?' has to do with the particular child who will or will not be born and whether it will have a life worth living despite possible impairments or disabilities. On this Harris's position is clear, that what counts as a worthwhile life is one which is not overwhelmed by suffering, one which we would rationally consider as valuable.

On the other hand, the question 'What sort of people should there be?' does not lead us to consider the possible welfare of any individual child but rather what sorts of children it might be better to bring into existence. This is a more general question about possible future worlds rather than the welfare of individuals. The question here is not which individuals have worthwhile lives but which of two possible worlds would be better: a world where disabled individuals are brought to birth and a world where non-disabled individuals are brought to birth. In this discussion it is not appropriate to talk of the disabled individuals as being harmed unless they have lives that are not worth living – what is the issue here is that a world which contains disabled individuals *instead* of 'healthy' individuals is a world of more net suffering and thus a less desirable world.

It is in this sense that Harris believes it is morally wrong to bring a disabled child to birth. The resultant child is not wronged by its existence; rather, it is the case that individuals have been harmed unnecessarily, since individuals have been created with worse lives than possible alternative individuals. Thus a worse society has been created than need have been.

Bennett's position

Bennett holds that Harris's argument regarding the question 'what sort of people should there be?' is a difficult argument in a number of ways. Typically arguments regarding moral obligations and pregnancy deal with the tension between respecting the procreative autonomy of parents and the interests of their future children. The impetus for most procreation is the wishes of the parents; parents choose to have children for reasons that concern their lives, rather than the welfare of the children who will be born as a result of those choices. When dealing with this argument about future possible worlds we are asked to consider neither the wishes of parents nor the welfare of the children – no parents or children suffer in the 'worse world' where disabled children are born. (In the 'worse world' it is only morally wrong to have a child whose life is not worth living or to frustrate the procreative autonomy of those who wish to have children who will lead worthwhile lives.) What we are asked to consider is the very abstract idea of net happiness and suffering of a population as a whole. As a concept it is difficult to see why this should be important or at least *more* important than an attempt to maximize the number of lives that are considered valuable and worthwhile.

In its detail this argument is also problematic. It seems that the world with disabled rather than 'healthy' children being born can only be a 'worse' world in terms of net suffering if a disabled child's life is held to have less value than that of a 'healthy' child (a view which Harris would not support). Moreover, Harris's assumption that the life of a disabled individual will contain more suffering than that of a non-disabled individual is far from self-evident. Arguments attempting to compare the lives of different possible children are both impossible and puzzling. Firstly, how can we estimate that to create a 'deaf' child rather than a 'healthy' child will involve the introduction of unnecessary suffering in the world? Predicting with any accuracy the expected quality of life of individuals before their birth would seem to be an impossible task. It may be that some predictable disadvantages can be determined before birth, such as congenital physical or mental impairments, but what of other factors important to an individual's quality of life? For instance, whether a child is likely to be an optimist or a pessimist, or whether he or she will suffer from depression or schizophrenia, cannot be predicted at this early stage in development. Secondly, even if we were able to make a meaningful estimate of the likely quality of life of two alternative persons, what sense does it make to ask whether one life is a 'better' life than the other? Surely, while both lives are worthwhile and valued by those who live them, they have equal value although they may have different qualities.

Harris's position

Again the Harris view is somewhat different. It is clear that it cannot be said that no one necessarily suffers if children are knowingly produced with disabilities. If I am born with a condition that for me was unavoidable because congenital, say, and I suffer from that condition, then someone suffers and it is me. Of course I am not worse off than I would have been because without the condition I would not exist.

Bennett has two main objections: 'Firstly, how can we estimate that to create a "deaf" child rather than a "healthy" child will involve the introduction of unnecessary suffering in the world? Predicting with any accuracy the expected quality of life of individuals before their birth would seem to be an impossible task.' In so far as this is true it gives us no reason to cure deafness in a newborn, for if we really have no reason to suppose a life with the ability to hear would be in some sense a better life, we have no reason to interfere.

Bennett's second point is that 'even if we were able to make a meaningful estimate of the likely quality of life of two alternative persons, what sense does it make to ask whether one life is a "better" life than the other? Surely, while both lives are worthwhile and valued by those who live them, they have equal value although they may have different qualities.' Here Bennett is equivocating over two different senses of the term 'value' or 'valuable' when applied to lives. All existing people have lives that are equally 'valuable' in the existential sense that they are equally morally important and that the individuals whose lives they are have equal rights and entitlements to equal consideration of interests. It does not follow that the lives of any two equals in this existential sense are equally valuable in terms of the quality of the lives lived as subjectively experienced.

The point about interpersonal comparisons of quality of life may be put in the following way. It makes sense to say that my life would be better if I were healthier, happier and more successful. I do not deny that it might make sense to say that Bennett's life is healthier, happier and more successful than mine (if it is). It does not follow from such judgements either that my life is more worth saving if its quality improves than it was before, or that Bennett's life is more worth saving than mine if she is healthier, happier and more successful than me. On this we agree. It is false, however, to deny that we cannot make interpersonal judgements between lives with respect to their quality or 'value' in this second sense, the sense in which I concede that Bennett's life is objectively a better life than mine.

Suppose John and Becky are each affected by a condition which makes a particular diet imperative if they are to stay alive. John's diet, unhappily for him, consists solely of bread and water; Becky can survive only on pre-phylloxera claret and plovers' eggs. It does not follow from the fact that John would be happier with Becky's condition that there is a greater moral imperative to feed Becky, if resources can only purchase food for one, but not both, of them. In conceding that claret and plovers' eggs is a pleasanter diet than bread and water, John is not conceding that Becky's life is more valuable than his, nor that Becky has a greater interest in living. (This point was also missed by Peter Singer in his exchange with Per Sundstrom – Singer, 1995; Sundstrom, 1995.) A life on the bread line is not less worth saving than a life on the egg line.

This does not of course show that some lives are not more valuable than others. It shows only that it does not follow from the fact that some lives are more desirable in virtue of their objective features than others, that those with more desirable lives have more valuable lives. Each person has a powerful interest in living their own life – the life available to them. Each person has a powerful interest in making that life as good as it can be. In striving to make my life more like Becky's, I am not conceding that Becky's is more valuable in what I have called the existential sense, more worth living, more worthy to be lived. These are different senses of terms like 'worth' and 'value' (Harris, 1996).

So, while we can make meaningful interpersonal comparisons between existing lives from the perspective of their quality or value, these judgements do not support conclusions about the respective moral importance or the respective existential value of the lives compared. However, when we are talking about *possible* lives rather than actual people things are different. Here there is no life that has value in the existential sense because there is no existence, only the *hypothesis* of existence. Here the interpersonal judgements about the respective value of different possible lives can be made without wronging (or insulting) anyone whose existential value might thereby be discounted, counted for nothing.

Conclusions

Both Bennett and Harris agree that as long as a life is worth living, or worthwhile, it should count equally with any other life, whatever the quality that life has. If the person whose life it is values it, then it is worth the same as any other valued life, both to that person and, for example, in any general utilitarian calculus which may compare alternative worlds. This will be true of all actual lives, that is to say all lives in being. Bennett would extend this principle to cover possible lives. In such a case she would argue that the only kind of life that has a different value is one of overwhelming suffering, and that hence that it is a matter of moral indifference to choose to bring into being a child with disabilities or impairments so long as that child will benefit overall from existence.

We wish to emphasize that both authors accept the importance of reproductive autonomy. This is the idea that there is a powerful interest or 'right' in the freedom to make reproductive choices, even where these choices may be thought unwise, frivolous or contrary to the public interest. The American philosopher and legal theorist Ronald Dworkin has outlined arguments for such a right, which he defines as 'a right to control their own role in procreation unless the state has a compelling reason for denying them that control' (Dworkin, 1993: p. 148; see also Robertson, 1994: esp. ch. 2). The principle of reproductive autonomy defends liberty and privacy in matters of reproduction unless especially powerful moral reasons can be demonstrated as to the wrong of a particular exercise of that liberty. If reproductive autonomy is accepted, then those who would object to a particular exercise of that autonomy must show more than the fact that such exercise would result in disutilities to either the parents of the child or the wider society. Moreover they must show more than that the exercise in question is foolish or ill-judged or offensive to others. Reproductive liberty may only be interfered with either if substantial and serious harm may be shown to be the likely result or if serious moral wrong is involved (Harris, 1999).

We also agree that where someone can only have a disabled child, where for them the choice is between having a child with disabilities or no children at all, parents are not wrong to choose to have a child with disabilities so long as the child will, none the less, have a worthwhile life (so far as this can be judged). It is quite clear to us that most disabilities fall far short of the high standard of awfulness required to judge a life to be not worth living. This is why Harris, for example, has consistently distinguished the moral reasons for avoiding producing new disabled individuals from reasons that would support enforcement, regulation or prevention of such activities. This is why he has repeatedly said that for those who can only have disabled children, having such children may be morally better than having no children at all (Harris, 1992: p. 72). On this we both agree.

The main point on which we see things differently is as to whether would-be parents have moral reasons to avoid bringing children with disabilities into existence where they do have the alternative of having children who will not be affected by disabilities, or at least of trying with some prospect of success. In this case Harris believes doing so is to risk, unnecessarily, bringing people with disabilities into existence. For Harris this is needlessly making a worse world than might have been made. For Harris it is not a matter of moral indifference to choose between pre-implantation embryos, some of which will be disabled and some not. In such a case we have moral reasons to choose the embryos without disabilities when we cannot choose all. The same would be true when choosing sequentially between embryos, as is more usually the case with prenatal testing for example.

If we use deafness as an example of disability the differences are clear. For Harris, if it is conceded that it would be wrong not to restore hearing to a 'deaf' child if such was possible, it is conceded that it would be better for any child not to be 'deaf'. From this it follows that it would be better to create a child that is not 'deaf', if one can choose between the creation of two possible children, for to choose the embryo that will become a deaf child is to choose to bring unnecessary harm into being. While this is morally wrong, it should not be prevented if that is what parents choose. Considerations of reproductive autonomy here trump the moral reasons for choosing not to increase the level of disbility in the world (Harris, 1999). What does not follow is that there is any sense in which, when comparing two existing children, the hearing child is better or more valuable in any existential sense than the 'deaf' child.

Bennett, on the other hand, believes such choices are genuinely morally indifferent. She would say while there may be reasons for preferring a 'non-disabled' child, these are not moral reasons but reasons arising from preferences we have about what sort of children we would like to have. Choosing to implant embryos with disabilities is not a morally wrong or a morally worthy decision but a morally neutral one. In choosing to bring to birth a disabled child (providing he or she is likely to have a worthwhile life) no one is harmed by that decision – the resultant disabled child gains existence and a worthwhile life, and parents are not condemned by their choice. The only sense in which this can be considered a morally questionable choice is a highly problematic and puzzling sense to do with the creation of a 'worse world' where 'suffering' is unnecessarily introduced to the world.

Harris is arguing that a world where 'hearing' children rather than 'deaf' children are brought to birth is a morally preferable world; but why? It is clear that it would be wrong not to restore the hearing of a 'deaf' child. It is also clear that it would be better for any particular child not to be 'deaf'. For a child to be 'deaf' when it could hear is for that child to be denied something it could value. We should not harm persons when this harm is avoidable, and to prevent a particular child from hearing when hearing is an option is to harm that child. However, to choose to implant a 'deaf' embryo rather than a 'hearing' one is not to deny that 'deaf' child anything he or she could have had. He or she is not harmed by this choice. It may be that most of us would prefer to implant the 'hearing' embryo rather than the 'deaf' embryo but this does not make it morally wrong to make a different choice. We choose the 'hearing' embryo because we prefer to have a child who hears rather than a 'deaf' child. If we choose the 'hearing' embryo no one is harmed by the choice and a worthwhile life is created. If we choose the 'deaf' embryo no one is harmed by the choice and a worthwhile life is created. The choice between the two embryos is a morally indifferent choice, in Bennett's view. While lives are worthwhile they are of equal value; it seems puzzling to describe as 'worse' the possible world in which disabled individuals with worthwhile lives exist, instead of non-disabled individuals with equally worthwhile lives.

References

Dworkin, R. (1993). *Life's Dominion*. London: Harper Collins.

Feinberg, J. (1984). *Harm to Others*. New York: Oxford University Press.

Harris, J. (1992). *Wonderwoman and Superman: The Ethics of Human Biotechnology*. Oxford: Oxford University Press.

Harris, J. (1996). Debate: Would Aristotle have played Russian roulette? *Journal of Medical Ethics* **22**: 209–15.

Harris, J. (1998). *Clones, Genes and Immortality*. Oxford: Oxford University Press.

Harris, J. (1999). Genes, clones and human rights. In *The Genetic Revolution and Human Rights: The Amnesty Lectures 1998*, ed. J.C. Burley, pp. 61–95. Oxford: Oxford University Press.

Harris, J. (2000a). Is there a coherent social conception of disability? *Journal of Medical Ethics* **26**: 95–100.

Harris, J. (2000b). The welfare of the child. (2000). *Health Care Analysis* **8**: 27–34.

Robertson, J.A. (1994). *Children of Choice*. Princeton: Princeton University Press.

Singer, P. (1995). Debate: Straw men with broken legs: a response to Per Sundstrom. *Journal of Medical Ethics* **21**: 89–90.

Steinbock, B. (1992). *Life Before Birth: The Moral and Legal Status of Embryos and Fetuses*. New York: Oxford University Press.

Sundstrom, P. (1995). Debate: Peter Singer and 'lives not worth living' – comments on a flawed argument from analogy. *Journal of Medical Ethics* **21**: 35–8.

21

Ethical issues in withdrawing life-sustaining treatment from handicapped neonates

Neil McIntosh

Department of Child Life and Health, University of Edinburgh, Edinburgh, UK

Introduction

Life-sustaining treatment is often classed as medical care, with palliative treatment being regarded as nursing care. However, optimal care of each type requires the full involvement of both medical and nursing staff in addition to the close commitment of the wider family. Life-sustaining treatment implies that treatment is being given in order to maintain or create the best possible outcome for the child's future life. This future might be abnormal but it would be assumed to be compatible with the self-respect of the family and later of the infant and child. Such management should be in the best interests of the child concerned. If life-sustaining treatment is not felt to be in the best interest of the child by the parents and the medical team, then UK law accepts that life-sustaining treatment (aimed at alleviating or curing the illness) may be inappropriately burdensome and may be reasonably withdrawn (*Re J*, 1981; *Re C*, 1989; *Re J*, 1992).

When the clinical team (in conjunction with the parents) makes a decision of this nature, the same medical and nursing staff then have a duty to offer the best possible palliative care. Palliative care should not only consider the patient's physical requirements, such as the relief of discomfort, pain or agitation and other symptoms, but should also address the emotional, social and spiritual needs. When life-sustaining care is withheld or withdrawn from an infant, the emotional, social and spiritual needs pertain more to the parents, but infants are human beings in their own right and it is important to respect their dignity, however small, sick or apparently damaged they may be. Even though the decision to withdraw life-saving treatment may be perceived as a failure of medical care, palliative treatment must be applied with no less enthusiasm. It is important that all in the clinical team in addition to the parents see this simply as an important reorientation of care for the better management of the infant. The infant should be kept clean and in a pleasant environment with appropriate attention and should not be forgotten for more pressing ward problems. The ethical provision of nutrition is a difficult concept area and will be mentioned further below. It is usually appropriate to offer food or fluid on a regular basis, but feeding by nasogastric tube or gastrostomy may not be for the best.

Background

Considerations about withholding or withdrawing life-saving medical treatment from a handicapped newborn may arise at two different times. At the moment of birth abnormalities may be so gross as to be obviously incompatible with any length or quality of life to even the most junior medical or non-medical person present. Such problems would include anencephaly (now rare in many countries due to antenatal screening programmes) or the baby with cyclops and a proboscis. In these instances cerebral function will be severely compromised even if survival is possible. Multiple and gross abnormalities such as sirenomyelia (the mermaid) will also be evident at birth, where, even though the head may look normal indicating possible cerebral potential, there are the gross deformities of lower limbs. Closer observation will reveal abnormalities of the genitalia and anal region, and, in this example, there would be severe gastrointestinal abnormalities and renal agenesis making death inevitable from renal failure within a very few days.

Consideration of withholding or withdrawing life-saving medical treatment may also arise later in the neonatal period. This may be because less obvious but equally compromising abnormalities have come to light, e.g. the grosser forms of hypoplastic left heart syndrome, or because a marked lack of cerebral potential following birth injury or birth asphyxia becomes obvious. Decisions at this time can take no account of the wishes or feelings of the child him- or herself; parents have the duty of decision-making in conjunction with the clinical team. There are three broad areas where such decisions may arise.

- Firstly, the extremely preterm infant (born, for example, at 23 weeks' gestation), where although life may be possible, it may depend on many months of highly invasive treatment, during which the chances of death are significant and morbidity more than likely. At this gestation the recent UK National EPICURE study has indicated only a six per cent survival of liveborn infants and in the survivors a 60 per cent incidence of disability (Wood and Marlow, 1999). Although medical management of the extremely immature infant with intensive care may improve the outcome, as the boundaries of gestation are pushed back, the anxieties about these outcomes are also moved back. It seems unlikely that this issue will disappear.
- The second area is that of multiple congenital abnormality – often evident right from the moment of birth (see above). These infants are becoming fewer in number with the introduction of antenatal physical abnormality scans and blood tests. When such diagnoses are picked up in early pregnancy, counselling followed by termination is often now a logical and legitimate choice for the parents.
- The third area in which these issues arise are the term babies who are

severely asphyxiated around the time of birth. Even with the best obstetric management, occasional infants are delivered in a severely neurologically depressed condition. Such infants in the past have been labelled as having suffered birth asphyxia. This reflex diagnosis is not helpful and in only a minority of cases is it likely to be accurate. In the majority of cases the attachment of this phraseology leads to a finger-pointing medico-legal exercise which can be expensive both in cash terms and in terms of emotional stress on both the parents and the involved staff. Epidemiological data and careful examination of the individual case more usually fail to reveal any mismanagement, and it is now believed that many of these cases may represent babies damaged antenatally, who then have difficulty sustaining the stress of a normal labour and delivery (Michaelis et al., 1980; Coorssen et al., 1991). This problem may be reduced by better obstetric monitoring, but how to do this is not established – indeed, it is one of the Holy Grails of obstetric care. Although 'birth asphyxia' has become far less common in the last 50 years, we have now reached a plateau for the last 10–15 years. Unless a more sophisticated monitoring technique is developed, these problems, and hence the ethical questions they raise about withdrawal of therapy around them, will continue.

The outlook for these three groups should be considered on the basis of their intellectual and physical future. Since Duff and Campbell wrote their seminal paper in 1973 when they described (or revealed) that 14 per cent of infants at the Yale University Neonatal Service who died did so because of the withdrawal of life-saving medical treatment, the number of such cases has risen (Duff and Campbell, 1973). Whitelaw in 1986 monitored a 30 per cent active withdrawal in such situations (Whitelaw, 1986). Hazeborek et al. (1993) and Caniano et al. (1995), writing in the late 1980s, suggested a prevalence of approximately 50 per cent; more recently, Wall and Partridge recorded 75 per cent (Wall and Partridge, 1997). In the western world at least, this practice is established, and it is likely to occur elsewhere.

Rights and duties of parents and doctors in the newborn period

The newborn infant is unable to make choices, so it is generally assumed that the parent will give or refuse consent on his or her behalf. This is perhaps logical, as the parents can generally be expected to have significant interests in their children and can be expected to safeguard these interests. Parental rights are not absolute, however, and infants are now recognized to have the same rights to life, liberty and autonomy as others. Although paternalism is justified, the choice is on the child's behalf and must represent the child's best interest at the time and for the future. Even if the parents have strongly held religious beliefs or other views, they are not at liberty to imperil their children by their decisions. The Children Act 1989 lays more overt stress on parental responsibility than on parental rights; the United Nations Convention on the Rights of the Child (1989) also enshrines principles of respect for children (particularly in Article 12) and has been ratified by the British government.

Doctors and nurses also have a duty of care that compels them to protect their patient's life and health. If the doctor fails in this duty, she or he may be guilty of negligence, although a negligence action is not to be expected in every case that turns out badly. The standard of competence expected of a doctor is that he or she should act in accordance with practice accepted by a responsible body of medical people skilled in that particular branch of medicine, the 'Bolam' test for England and Wales (*Bolam* v *Friern HMC*, 1957) and the 'Hunter and Hanley' test for Scotland (*Hunter* v *Hanley*, 1955). In other words, the specialist must practice with the ordinary skill of his or her specialty. The acknowledgement that this is a special skill, and in the UK a skill that follows considerable training, gives doctors alone the right to decide whether a treatment is medically appropriate. Parents do not have the right to *demand* treatments that a doctor may deem to be outside of the child's best interest, although they may *refuse* treatment which they view as not in the child's best interest. Doctors have no legal authority to institute treatments in the absence of a valid consent from someone with parental responsibility, but emergency treatment deemed to be in the infant's best interest can be given. Withdrawal of treatment that is life-saving would only in very rare circumstances be done without parental acceptance and consent. Thus communication, consisting of regular and frequent discussion by the clinical team with the parents, is crucial to all decisions in the neonatal unit. Information at all stages must be given in an understandable form to allow reason, deliberation and comfortable decision-making. Decisions on withholding or withdrawing life-sustaining treatment are unlikely to go well in the absence of previous communication. This is not to say that responsibility for such decisions should be left to the parents alone, but that it must be obvious that the parents are in agreement before such decisions are enacted.

The issues

The principles of modern medical ethics, often taken to consist of autonomy, beneficence, non-maleficence and justice (Gillon, 1986; Beauchamp and Childress, 1994) are as important for the newborn, and the handicapped newborn in particular, as for other age groups. The infant's own autonomy is largely replaced by 'autonomy within the family'. The parents take on the consenting role on behalf of their child for both therapy and research;

whereas the assent of the competent older child may be important (*Re W*, 1992), this is not an issue in infancy. Beneficence and non-maleficence relate to a therapy being in the infant's best interest, with a balance of benefit compared to harm – this is the crux of this chapter. Justice requires that the infant is not prejudiced in any way by his or her state as an individual – a treatment, if effective and necessary, should not be dependent on race, social background or ability to pay. Justice also demands that the standards of decision-making are as rigorous for the infant, and the handicapped infant especially, as for a sentient adult.

The Royal College of Paediatrics and Child Health have delimited three areas where the withholding or withdrawing of life-sustaining treatment might reasonably be considered in the newborn period (Royal College of Paediatrics and Child Health, 1997).

(1) In the no hope or no chance situation, life-sustaining treatment is simply delaying death without improving life quality or potential. If suffering is not to any significant extent alleviated, medical treatment would be deemed inappropriate. There is no legal obligation for the doctor to provide medical treatment in this situation which cannot be in the best interest of the patient. Indeed if this is done knowingly, it is futile treatment.

(2) The no purpose situation describes the case where the child's potential of having an extremely significant degree of impairment is inevitable, and it would not be reasonable to expect him or her to bear it. Such an impossibly poor quality of life may relate to the future, in which case treatment might reasonably not be initiated (e.g. ventilation for congenital myotonic dystrophy) or to the present, with the likelihood of it continuing with no foreseeable improvement, in which case the treatment might reasonably be withdrawn. This might apply to the severely asphyxiated infant where microcephaly, profound developmental delay, blindness and quadraplegia are believed to be inevitable. This could also reflect conditions where brain damage is not necessarily the worrying outcome. For instance, in severe myotonic dystrophy or for the ventilator-dependent infant with broncho-pulmonary dysplasia in *cor pulmonale*, compromise of potential cerebral function may not be a concern, but the likelihood of getting the child off the ventilator to any form of independent existence may be negligible.

(3) The third case is the unbearable situation, where a family may feel that further treatment is more than can be borne. They wish to have treatment withdrawn or wish to refuse further treatment irrespective of medical opinion. Parents may be able to recognize that it is reasonable to put up with short-term suffering for a good later outcome. There is a limit, however, to this tolerance – if there are likely to be repeated and severe problems and invasive therapy, parents may feel that treatment

withholding or withdrawal is the most appropriate option. An example might be the newborn infant with hypoplastic left heart syndrome, where successful survival is likely only to be possible with multiple and severe cardiac bypass operations.

These criteria illustrate the relationship between beneficence and non-maleficence – harm must always be exceeded by benefit.

The legal framework

In the UK, euthanasia is illegal, a prohibition supported by the Royal College of Paediatrics and Child Health working group that provided the above framework for the consideration and practice of withholding and withdrawal of care (Royal College of Paediatrics and Child Health, 1997). Giving medication that shortens life is not in itself illegal. Both English and Scottish law allow for the principle of double effect, whereby giving a medicine with the primary intent to hasten death is illicit but giving a medicine to relieve suffering, which may have the side effect of hastening death, is allowed (as was demonstrated for England by the 1997 High Court case of Annie Lindsell). Such prescription (usually of opiates) is viewed as being for the benefit of the patient during life, not as intended to cause or hasten death (Finnis, 1995).

Early UK case law around the subject of withdrawing or withholding medical treatment was based on knowledge or presumption of severe brain damage (Re J, 1981; Re C, 1989; Re J, 1992). If very severe brain damage leading to a very poor quality of life is anticipated (the no purpose situation) withholding or withdrawing treatment may be sanctioned (Re J, 1990). If the child will die soon irrespective of treatment and in the presence of normal cerebral function (the no hope situation) withholding or withdrawing of treatment has also been sanctioned (Re C, 1989). In the majority of cases, the issue of not providing or withdrawing medical treatment arises because of anxieties about the future function of the brain. However, treatment was held to be required for a baby with Down's syndrome and atresia of the gut (Re B, 1981), on the grounds that in this child the outcome was not so demonstrably awful. Lord Donaldson (Re J, 1981) said that decisions of awfulness must be based from the infant's viewpoint. Overall, however, the implications are that if the burden of suffering and the quality of survival outweigh the benefits, even without brain injury, then withdrawal may be appropriate.

Knowledge, evidence and certainty

Before the issue of withholding or withdrawing life-sustaining treatment can be considered, the present condition of the infant must be assessed in the

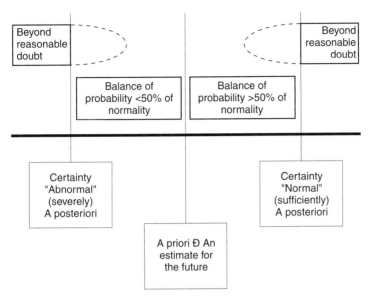

Figure 21.1. Ethical issues in withdrawing life-sustaining treatment from handicapped neonates – in the presence of uncertainty.

light of the best scientific knowledge available. The future for the infant must be estimated at least from the perspective of currently available therapies, and possibly also from the perspective of what therapies may eventually be available (e.g. small-intestine transplants or heart/lung transplants). For the newborn infant it is probably realistic and objective to assess the prognosis from the point of the currently available therapies and the future quality of life they can create. The dilemma generated by poor or inadequate evidence for the condition in question does not absolve the clinical team from seeking it, and if there is genuinely no such evidence to be found, then a second opinion may be appropriate from an experienced perinatologist, geneticist or neurologist.

For many medical conditions, the outlook may be uncertain because there are degrees of severity to be assessed within the condition. For a few cases, the severely abnormal outcome will be quite certain, and for a few others, sufficiently certain. In the presence of uncertainty, the issues may be seen in Figure 21.1. Either side of an equipoise of uncertainty, there is a balance of probability – to one side, that there will be a poor outcome, and to the other, that there will be a good outcome. As certainty becomes more secure because of further evidence about the diagnosis, or about the severity of the diagnosis, one moves to the theoretical area of complete certainty (that the outcome will be either bad or normal). One rarely becomes absolutely certain of the outcome, except in retrospect. At what stage 'the balance of probability' becomes 'beyond reasonable doubt' will depend on the condition and its severity in the patient, and also on the views of the medical team and the parents. Most neonatologists would wish the certainty of outcome to be in the 'beyond reasonable doubt' area before any discussion arose with the parents about withholding or withdrawing life-sustaining treatment.

Parental and societal pressures and second opinions

It is abhorrent for practising neonatologists to believe that economic or eugenic pressures would influence their clinical decisions. The realist, though, has to take account of the amount of parental and societal help that will be available for the child when considering their best interests. Parents who are able and prepared to put in huge amounts of time and love will create a better quality of life for a severely damaged infant than parents who lack the necessary financial or emotional resources, no matter how much help is available from the state. Clinicians' value judgements about the degree of support available to and from parents will impact pragmatically on any consideration of withholding or withdrawal of life-sustaining care in the situation of severe handicap, where the assumption is that there is no purpose in continuing treatment because of an extremely poor quality of life. However, when considering the best interests of the child, we must be clear that it is the child's best interest that is being considered and not that of the parents or wider family (Children Act 1989, s.1).

The gradation from balance of probability to beyond reasonable doubt and on to near-certainty about a condition or its prognosis ensures that rules and protocols are seldom, if ever, appropriate when these issues are considered. The organization of a second opinion is easy for the diagnostic or therapeutic elements in a difficult case, but the ethical and moral pressures that arise are usually not clear-cut. In the US and in some UK hospitals (including St Mary's and Great Ormond Street in London), multidisciplinary institutional ethics committees have been set up to review cases where these issues seem apparent (American Academy of Pediatrics, 1994). There are practical difficulties – the committees may need to be convened at short notice, and it may be difficult for the members to become aware of the nuances relating to the particular case. Such committees also remove the sole responsibility for making a decision from the clinical team, although typically the committee's function is advisory. In the majority of UK hospitals, where there is no clinical ethics committee, the consultant in charge of the infant bears the final responsibility for the decision-making, although this is done in the context of advice from the clinical team, and in partnership with the parents. If there is dissent from any of the clinical team, the consultant can accept or override it. In a situation where one or both parents disagree with such a decision, it is usually further time that is required for the parent to become convinced. If this disagreement persists, then the consultant would be prudent to get the advice of the court. In all cases the consultant, if wise, will take advice and opinion from experienced colleagues who have been working in the same field for a period of years.

Conclusion

The practicalities of withholding or withdrawing life-sustaining treatments from handicapped neonates revolve around good discussion within the clinical team and with the parents. All should have equal involvement in the discussion, although the final decision will be the consultant's alone (within the limits of the law and professional bodies' guidelines on good practice). Discussions on withholding or withdrawing are intimately bound up with palliative care. The use of opiates and other sedatives and symptomatic treatment is well accepted to provide comfort for the terminally ill child, even when this is likely to shorten the infant's life. In handicapped neonates, the ethical issues may also include the appropriateness or otherwise of artificial and natural feeding. Tube feeding is not completely innocuous. Many older children and adults find the positioning of a nasogastric tube worse than a venepuncture, and the restlessness of the handicapped child may be partly related to the discomfort of the tube. Nevertheless, there is at least a mental association between the withdrawal of tube feeding and starvation. However, some hospital guidelines regard it as undesirable to prolong an inevitable death through maintaining hydration but withdrawing nutrition (St Mary's Hospital Trust Clinical Ethics Committee, 2000). The clinical team, and in particular the nursing staff who will be carrying through the management plan, must be in agreement with the alternative of regularly offering food by bottle or spoon at appropriate intervals, recognizing that in this situation little food or fluid will be taken. These decisions are never easy, and all involved must be comfortable with the implementation of the decisions. In neonatal units, when life-sustaining treatment is withheld or withdrawn, it is almost inevitable that the baby dies, though this is not an inevitability in older children (Levetown et al., 1994).

Although there may have been a clear diagnosis in life, representation should always be made for a post-mortem examination. In many cases extra information will become available at an autopsy which was not known during life, and it is not infrequent for this additional information to aid counselling and decisions about future pregnancies. If autopsy is sanctioned, the results should be given to the parents as soon as they are available, not waiting for the subtleties or the microscopy or the fixation of the brain; these results should be communicated subsequently. Frank discussion about the results of the autopsy and how this relates to the decisions made in almost all cases consolidates the appropriateness of the decision that the staff and parents have made. From the parents' perspective, the realism provided by the results of the autopsy ease any remaining guilt feelings that they may have.

References

American Academy of Pediatrics, Committee on Bioethics (1994). Guidelines on forgoing life-sustaining medical treatment. *Pediatrics* **93**: 532–6.
Beauchamp, T.L. and Childress, J.F. (1994). *Principles of Biomedical Ethics*, 4th edn. Oxford: Oxford University Press.
Bolam v *Friern Hospital Management Committee* [1957] 2 All ER 118.
Caniano, D.A., Hazebroek, F.W.J., DenBesten, K.E. et al. (1995). End-of-life decisions for surgical neonates: experience in the Netherlands and United States. *Journal of Pediatric Surgery* **30**: 1420–4.
Children Act 1989 (1991). London: HMSO.
Children (Scotland) Act 1995. London: HMSO.
Coorssen, E.A., Msall, M.E. and Duffy, L.C. (1991) Multiple minor malformations as a marker for prenatal etiology of cerebral palsy. *Developmental Medicine and Child Neurology* **33**: 730–6.
Duff, R.S. and Campbell, A.G.M. (1973). Moral and ethical dilemmas in the special care nursery. *New England Journal of Medicine* **289**: 890–4.
Finnis, J. (1995). A philosophical case against euthanasia. In *Euthanasia Examined*, ed. J. Keown, pp. 23–35. Cambridge: Cambridge University Press.
Gillon, R. (1986). *Philosophical Medical Ethics*. Chichester: John Wiley.
Hazebroek, F.W.J., Tibboel, D., Mourik, M. et al. (1993) Withholding and withdrawal of life support from surgical neonates with life-threatening congenital anomalies. *Journal of Pediatric Surgery* **28**: 1093–7.
Hunter v *Hanley* [1955] Session Cases 200.
Levetown, M., Pollack, M.M., Cuerdon, T.T. et al. (1994). Limitations and withdrawals of medical interventions in pediatric critical care. *Journal of the American Medical Association* **272**: 1271–5.
Michaelis, R., Rooschuz, B. and Dopper, R. (1980). Prenatal origin of congenital spastic hemiparesis. *Early Human Development* **4**: 243–55.
Re B (a minor) [1981] 1 WLR 1421.
Re C (a minor) [1989] 2 All ER 782.
Re J (a minor) [1981] Fam 33?
Re J (a minor) [1990] 3 All ER 930.
Re J (a minor) [1992] 4 All ER 614.
Re W [1992] 4 All ER 627.
Royal College of Paediatrics and Child Health, Ethics Advisory Committee (1997). *Withholding and Withdrawal of Life-saving Treatment in Children: A Framework for Practice.* London: Royal College of Paediatrics and Child Health.
St Mary's NHS Trust Clinical Ethics Committee (2000). *Guidelines on Withdrawing*

and Withholding Treatment. London: St Mary's NHS Trust.

United Nations Convention on the Rights of the Child (1989), Article 12.

Wall, S.N. and Partridge, J.C. (1997). Death in the intensive care nursery: physician practice of withdrawing and withholding life support. *Pediatrics* **99**: 64–70.

Whitelaw, A. (1986). Death as an option in neonatal intensive care. *Lancet* **2**: 328–31.

Wood, N.S. and Marlow, N. (1999). Neurological and developmental morbidity in children less than 26 weeks gestation at 2.5 years of age. *Pediatric Research* **45**: 259A.

Index